# 50% OFF Nurse Executive Test Prep Course!

By Mometrix

Dear Customer,

We consider it an honor and a privilege that you chose our Nurse Executive Study Guide. As a way of showing our appreciation and to help us better serve you, we are offering **50% off our online Nurse Executive Prep Course.** Many Nurse Executive courses are needlessly expensive and don't deliver enough value. With our course, you get access to the best Nurse Executive prep material, and **you only pay half price.**

**We have structured our online course to perfectly complement your printed study guide.** The Nurse Executive Test Prep Course contains **in-depth lessons** that cover all the most important topics, over **700+ practice questions** to ensure you feel prepared, and more than **350 flashcards** for studying on the go.

## *Online Nurse Executive Prep Course*

**Topics Covered**:

- Human Resource Management
    - Communication
    - Staffing Fundamentals
    - Organizational Structure and Culture
- Quality and Safety
    - Change Management Frameworks
    - Continuous Process Improvement
    - Clinical Practice Innovation and Advocating for Research
- Business Management
    - Financial Management and Budgeting
    - Leadership
    - Strategic Planning
- Health Care Delivery
    - Ethics
    - Regulatory Standards
    - Care Delivery Evaluation
- And More!

**Course Features**:

- Nurse Executive Study Guide
    - Get access to content from the best reviewed study guide available.
- Track Your Progress
    - Our customized course allows you to check off content you have studied or feel confident with.
- 5 Full-Length Practice Tests
    - With 700+ practice questions and lesson reviews, you can test yourself again and again to build confidence.
- Nurse Executive Flashcards
    - Our course includes a flashcard mode consisting of over 350 content cards to help you study.

To receive this discount, visit us at mometrix.com/university/nurseexec or simply scan this QR code with your smartphone. At the checkout page, enter the discount code: **NURSEEXEC50OFF**

If you have any questions or concerns, please contact us at support@mometrix.com.

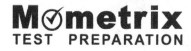

SCAN HERE

# FREE Study Skills Videos/DVD Offer

Dear Customer,

Thank you for your purchase from Mometrix! We consider it an honor and a privilege that you have purchased our product and we want to ensure your satisfaction.

As part of our ongoing effort to meet the needs of test takers, we have developed a set of Study Skills Videos that we would like to give you for FREE. These videos cover our *best practices* for getting ready for your exam, from how to use our study materials to how to best prepare for the day of the test.

All that we ask is that you email us with feedback that would describe your experience so far with our product. Good, bad, or indifferent, we want to know what you think!

To get your FREE Study Skills Videos, you can use the **QR code** below, or send us an **email** at studyvideos@mometrix.com with *FREE VIDEOS* in the subject line and the following information in the body of the email:

- The name of the product you purchased.
- Your product rating on a scale of 1-5, with 5 being the highest rating.
- Your feedback. It can be long, short, or anything in between. We just want to know your impressions and experience so far with our product. (Good feedback might include how our study material met your needs and ways we might be able to make it even better. You could highlight features that you found helpful or features that you think we should add.)

If you have any questions or concerns, please don't hesitate to contact me directly.

Thanks again!

Sincerely,

Jay Willis
Vice President
jay.willis@mometrix.com
1-800-673-8175

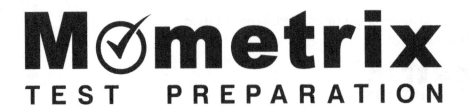

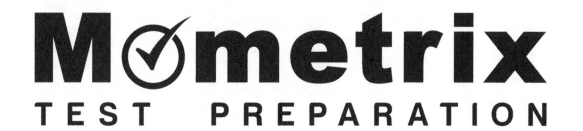

# Nurse Executive

## Study Guide 2024-2025

**3** Full-Length Practice Tests

Exam Secrets Review Book for the ANCC Certification

5th Edition

Written and edited by Mometrix Test Preparation

Printed in the United States of America

This paper meets the requirements of ANSI/NISO Z39.48-1992 (Permanence of Paper).

Mometrix offers volume discount pricing to institutions. For more information or a price quote, please contact our sales department at sales@mometrix.com or 888-248-1219.

Mometrix Media LLC is not affiliated with or endorsed by any official testing organization. All organizational and test names are trademarks of their respective owners.

Paperback
ISBN 13: 978-1-5167-2358-4

# DEAR FUTURE EXAM SUCCESS STORY

First of all, **THANK YOU** for purchasing Mometrix study materials!

Second, congratulations! You are one of the few determined test-takers who are committed to doing whatever it takes to excel on your exam. **You have come to the right place.** We developed these study materials with one goal in mind: to deliver you the information you need in a format that's concise and easy to use.

In addition to optimizing your guide for the content of the test, we've outlined our recommended steps for breaking down the preparation process into small, attainable goals so you can make sure you stay on track.

We've also analyzed the entire test-taking process, identifying the most common pitfalls and showing how you can overcome them and be ready for any curveball the test throws you.

Standardized testing is one of the biggest obstacles on your road to success, which only increases the importance of doing well in the high-pressure, high-stakes environment of test day. Your results on this test could have a significant impact on your future, and this guide provides the information and practical advice to help you achieve your full potential on test day.

### Your success is our success

**We would love to hear from you!** If you would like to share the story of your exam success or if you have any questions or comments in regard to our products, please contact us at **800-673-8175** or **support@mometrix.com**.

Thanks again for your business and we wish you continued success!

Sincerely,
The Mometrix Test Preparation Team

> **Need more help? Check out our flashcards at:**
> **http://mometrixflashcards.com/NursingAdmin**

# TABLE OF CONTENTS

INTRODUCTION _____ 1

SECRET KEY #1 – PLAN BIG, STUDY SMALL _____ 2

SECRET KEY #2 – MAKE YOUR STUDYING COUNT _____ 3

SECRET KEY #3 – PRACTICE THE RIGHT WAY _____ 4

SECRET KEY #4 – PACE YOURSELF _____ 6

SECRET KEY #5 – HAVE A PLAN FOR GUESSING _____ 7

TEST-TAKING STRATEGIES _____ 10

HUMAN RESOURCE MANAGEMENT _____ 15
    FEDERAL EMPLOYMENT LAWS _____ 15
    COMMUNICATION _____ 20
    STAFFING FUNDAMENTALS _____ 30
    EMPLOYEE PERFORMANCE MANAGEMENT _____ 35
    EMPLOYEE ENGAGEMENT STRATEGIES _____ 41
    TEAM PERFORMANCE MANAGEMENT _____ 43
    CHAPTER QUIZ _____ 58

QUALITY AND SAFETY _____ 59
    CHANGE MANAGEMENT FRAMEWORKS _____ 59
    CULTURE OF SAFETY _____ 66
    CONTINUOUS PROCESS IMPROVEMENT _____ 72
    RESEARCH AND EVIDENCE BASED PRACTICE _____ 81
    CHAPTER QUIZ _____ 95

BUSINESS MANAGEMENT _____ 96
    REIMBURSEMENT METHODS _____ 96
    FINANCIAL MANAGEMENT AND BUDGETING _____ 97
    LEADERSHIP _____ 104
    STRATEGIC PLANNING _____ 107
    PROGRAM DEVELOPMENT _____ 110
    CHAPTER QUIZ _____ 114

HEALTH CARE DELIVERY _____ 115
    ETHICS _____ 115
    SCOPE AND STANDARDS OF PRACTICE _____ 117
    REGULATORY STANDARDS _____ 119
    LEGAL ISSUES _____ 123
    COMMUNITY AND CONSUMER NEEDS _____ 126
    COMPLIANCE POLICY DEVELOPMENT _____ 127
    HEALTHCARE DELIVERY MODELS _____ 129
    WORKFLOWS _____ 133
    EMERGENCY PREPAREDNESS _____ 136
    FACILITATION OF PATIENT EXPERIENCE _____ 137
    CARE DELIVERY EVALUATION _____ 140

ADVOCATING FOR THE NURSING PROFESSION _____ 143

CHAPTER QUIZ _____ 144

## NURSE EXECUTIVE PRACTICE TEST #1 _____ 145

## ANSWER KEY AND EXPLANATIONS FOR TEST #1 _____ 169

## NURSE EXECUTIVE PRACTICE TEST #2 _____ 193

## ANSWER KEY AND EXPLANATIONS FOR TEST #2 _____ 216

## NURSE EXECUTIVE PRACTICE TEST #3 _____ 239

## HOW TO OVERCOME TEST ANXIETY _____ 240

## ADDITIONAL BONUS MATERIAL _____ 246

# Introduction

**Thank you for purchasing this resource!** You have made the choice to prepare yourself for a test that could have a huge impact on your future, and this guide is designed to help you be fully ready for test day. Obviously, it's important to have a solid understanding of the test material, but you also need to be prepared for the unique environment and stressors of the test, so that you can perform to the best of your abilities.

For this purpose, the first section that appears in this guide is the **Secret Keys**. We've devoted countless hours to meticulously researching what works and what doesn't, and we've boiled down our findings to the five most impactful steps you can take to improve your performance on the test. We start at the beginning with study planning and move through the preparation process, all the way to the testing strategies that will help you get the most out of what you know when you're finally sitting in front of the test.

We recommend that you start preparing for your test as far in advance as possible. However, if you've bought this guide as a last-minute study resource and only have a few days before your test, we recommend that you skip over the first two Secret Keys since they address a long-term study plan.

If you struggle with **test anxiety**, we strongly encourage you to check out our recommendations for how you can overcome it. Test anxiety is a formidable foe, but it can be beaten, and we want to make sure you have the tools you need to defeat it.

1

# Secret Key #1 – Plan Big, Study Small

There's a lot riding on your performance. If you want to ace this test, you're going to need to keep your skills sharp and the material fresh in your mind. You need a plan that lets you review everything you need to know while still fitting in your schedule. We'll break this strategy down into three categories.

## Information Organization

Start with the information you already have: the official test outline. From this, you can make a complete list of all the concepts you need to cover before the test. Organize these concepts into groups that can be studied together, and create a list of any related vocabulary you need to learn so you can brush up on any difficult terms. You'll want to keep this vocabulary list handy once you actually start studying since you may need to add to it along the way.

## Time Management

Once you have your set of study concepts, decide how to spread them out over the time you have left before the test. Break your study plan into small, clear goals so you have a manageable task for each day and know exactly what you're doing. Then just focus on one small step at a time. When you manage your time this way, you don't need to spend hours at a time studying. Studying a small block of content for a short period each day helps you retain information better and avoid stressing over how much you have left to do. You can relax knowing that you have a plan to cover everything in time. In order for this strategy to be effective though, you have to start studying early and stick to your schedule. Avoid the exhaustion and futility that comes from last-minute cramming!

## Study Environment

The environment you study in has a big impact on your learning. Studying in a coffee shop, while probably more enjoyable, is not likely to be as fruitful as studying in a quiet room. It's important to keep distractions to a minimum. You're only planning to study for a short block of time, so make the most of it. Don't pause to check your phone or get up to find a snack. It's also important to **avoid multitasking**. Research has consistently shown that multitasking will make your studying dramatically less effective. Your study area should also be comfortable and well-lit so you don't have the distraction of straining your eyes or sitting on an uncomfortable chair.

 The time of day you study is also important. You want to be rested and alert. Don't wait until just before bedtime. Study when you'll be most likely to comprehend and remember. Even better, if you know what time of day your test will be, set that time aside for study. That way your brain will be used to working on that subject at that specific time and you'll have a better chance of recalling information.

Finally, it can be helpful to team up with others who are studying for the same test. Your actual studying should be done in as isolated an environment as possible, but the work of organizing the information and setting up the study plan can be divided up. In between study sessions, you can discuss with your teammates the concepts that you're all studying and quiz each other on the details. Just be sure that your teammates are as serious about the test as you are. If you find that your study time is being replaced with social time, you might need to find a new team.

2

# Secret Key #2 – Make Your Studying Count

You're devoting a lot of time and effort to preparing for this test, so you want to be absolutely certain it will pay off. This means doing more than just reading the content and hoping you can remember it on test day. It's important to make every minute of study count. There are two main areas you can focus on to make your studying count.

## Retention

It doesn't matter how much time you study if you can't remember the material. You need to make sure you are retaining the concepts. To check your retention of the information you're learning, try recalling it at later times with minimal prompting. Try carrying around flashcards and glance at one or two from time to time or ask a friend who's also studying for the test to quiz you.

To enhance your retention, look for ways to put the information into practice so that you can apply it rather than simply recalling it. If you're using the information in practical ways, it will be much easier to remember. Similarly, it helps to solidify a concept in your mind if you're not only reading it to yourself but also explaining it to someone else. Ask a friend to let you teach them about a concept you're a little shaky on (or speak aloud to an imaginary audience if necessary). As you try to summarize, define, give examples, and answer your friend's questions, you'll understand the concepts better and they will stay with you longer. Finally, step back for a big picture view and ask yourself how each piece of information fits with the whole subject. When you link the different concepts together and see them working together as a whole, it's easier to remember the individual components.

Finally, practice showing your work on any multi-step problems, even if you're just studying. Writing out each step you take to solve a problem will help solidify the process in your mind, and you'll be more likely to remember it during the test.

## Modality

*Modality* simply refers to the means or method by which you study. Choosing a study modality that fits your own individual learning style is crucial. No two people learn best in exactly the same way, so it's important to know your strengths and use them to your advantage.

For example, if you learn best by visualization, focus on visualizing a concept in your mind and draw an image or a diagram. Try color-coding your notes, illustrating them, or creating symbols that will trigger your mind to recall a learned concept. If you learn best by hearing or discussing information, find a study partner who learns the same way or read aloud to yourself. Think about how to put the information in your own words. Imagine that you are giving a lecture on the topic and record yourself so you can listen to it later.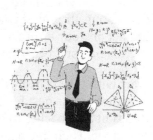

For any learning style, flashcards can be helpful. Organize the information so you can take advantage of spare moments to review. Underline key words or phrases. Use different colors for different categories. Mnemonic devices (such as creating a short list in which every item starts with the same letter) can also help with retention. Find what works best for you and use it to store the information in your mind most effectively and easily.

3

# Secret Key #3 – Practice the Right Way

Your success on test day depends not only on how many hours you put into preparing, but also on whether you prepared the right way. It's good to check along the way to see if your studying is paying off. One of the most effective ways to do this is by taking practice tests to evaluate your progress. Practice tests are useful because they show exactly where you need to improve. Every time you take a practice test, pay special attention to these three groups of questions:

- The questions you got wrong
- The questions you had to guess on, even if you guessed right
- The questions you found difficult or slow to work through

This will show you exactly what your weak areas are, and where you need to devote more study time. Ask yourself why each of these questions gave you trouble. Was it because you didn't understand the material? Was it because you didn't remember the vocabulary? Do you need more repetitions on this type of question to build speed and confidence? Dig into those questions and figure out how you can strengthen your weak areas as you go back to review the material.

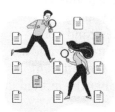 Additionally, many practice tests have a section explaining the answer choices. It can be tempting to read the explanation and think that you now have a good understanding of the concept. However, an explanation likely only covers part of the question's broader context. Even if the explanation makes perfect sense, **go back and investigate** every concept related to the question until you're positive you have a thorough understanding.

As you go along, keep in mind that the practice test is just that: practice. Memorizing these questions and answers will not be very helpful on the actual test because it is unlikely to have any of the same exact questions. If you only know the right answers to the sample questions, you won't be prepared for the real thing. **Study the concepts** until you understand them fully, and then you'll be able to answer any question that shows up on the test.

It's important to wait on the practice tests until you're ready. If you take a test on your first day of study, you may be overwhelmed by the amount of material covered and how much you need to learn. Work up to it gradually.

On test day, you'll need to be prepared for answering questions, managing your time, and using the test-taking strategies you've learned. It's a lot to balance, like a mental marathon that will have a big impact on your future. Like training for a marathon, you'll need to start slowly and work your way up. When test day arrives, you'll be ready.

Start with the strategies you've read in the first two Secret Keys—plan your course and study in the way that works best for you. If you have time, consider using multiple study resources to get different approaches to the same concepts. It can be helpful to see difficult concepts from more than one angle. Then find a good source for practice tests. Many times, the test website will suggest potential study resources or provide sample tests.

# Practice Test Strategy

If you're able to find at least three practice tests, we recommend this strategy:

## UNTIMED AND OPEN-BOOK PRACTICE

Take the first test with no time constraints and with your notes and study guide handy. Take your time and focus on applying the strategies you've learned.

## TIMED AND OPEN-BOOK PRACTICE

Take the second practice test open-book as well, but set a timer and practice pacing yourself to finish in time.

## TIMED AND CLOSED-BOOK PRACTICE

Take any other practice tests as if it were test day. Set a timer and put away your study materials. Sit at a table or desk in a quiet room, imagine yourself at the testing center, and answer questions as quickly and accurately as possible.

Keep repeating timed and closed-book tests on a regular basis until you run out of practice tests or it's time for the actual test. Your mind will be ready for the schedule and stress of test day, and you'll be able to focus on recalling the material you've learned.

# Secret Key #4 – Pace Yourself

Once you're fully prepared for the material on the test, your biggest challenge on test day will be managing your time. Just knowing that the clock is ticking can make you panic even if you have plenty of time left. Work on pacing yourself so you can build confidence against the time constraints of the exam. Pacing is a difficult skill to master, especially in a high-pressure environment, so **practice is vital**.

Set time expectations for your pace based on how much time is available. For example, if a section has 60 questions and the time limit is 30 minutes, you know you have to average 30 seconds or less per question in order to answer them all. Although 30 seconds is the hard limit, set 25 seconds per question as your goal, so you reserve extra time to spend on harder questions. When you budget extra time for the harder questions, you no longer have any reason to stress when those questions take longer to answer.

Don't let this time expectation distract you from working through the test at a calm, steady pace, but keep it in mind so you don't spend too much time on any one question. Recognize that taking extra time on one question you don't understand may keep you from answering two that you do understand later in the test. If your time limit for a question is up and you're still not sure of the answer, mark it and move on, and come back to it later if the time and the test format allow. If the testing format doesn't allow you to return to earlier questions, just make an educated guess; then put it out of your mind and move on.

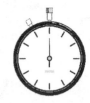

On the easier questions, be careful not to rush. It may seem wise to hurry through them so you have more time for the challenging ones, but it's not worth missing one if you know the concept and just didn't take the time to read the question fully. Work efficiently but make sure you understand the question and have looked at all of the answer choices, since more than one may seem right at first.

Even if you're paying attention to the time, you may find yourself a little behind at some point. You should speed up to get back on track, but do so wisely. Don't panic; just take a few seconds less on each question until you're caught up. Don't guess without thinking, but do look through the answer choices and eliminate any you know are wrong. If you can get down to two choices, it is often worthwhile to guess from those. Once you've chosen an answer, move on and don't dwell on any that you skipped or had to hurry through. If a question was taking too long, chances are it was one of the harder ones, so you weren't as likely to get it right anyway.

On the other hand, if you find yourself getting ahead of schedule, it may be beneficial to slow down a little. The more quickly you work, the more likely you are to make a careless mistake that will affect your score. You've budgeted time for each question, so don't be afraid to spend that time. Practice an efficient but careful pace to get the most out of the time you have.

# Secret Key #5 – Have a Plan for Guessing

When you're taking the test, you may find yourself stuck on a question. Some of the answer choices seem better than others, but you don't see the one answer choice that is obviously correct. What do you do?

The scenario described above is very common, yet most test takers have not effectively prepared for it. Developing and practicing a plan for guessing may be one of the single most effective uses of your time as you get ready for the exam.

In developing your plan for guessing, there are three questions to address:

- When should you start the guessing process?
- How should you narrow down the choices?
- Which answer should you choose?

## When to Start the Guessing Process

Unless your plan for guessing is to select C every time (which, despite its merits, is not what we recommend), you need to leave yourself enough time to apply your answer elimination strategies. Since you have a limited amount of time for each question, that means that if you're going to give yourself the best shot at guessing correctly, you have to decide quickly whether or not you will guess.

Of course, the best-case scenario is that you don't have to guess at all, so first, see if you can answer the question based on your knowledge of the subject and basic reasoning skills. Focus on the key words in the question and try to jog your memory of related topics. Give yourself a chance to bring the knowledge to mind, but once you realize that you don't have (or you can't access) the knowledge you need to answer the question, it's time to start the guessing process.

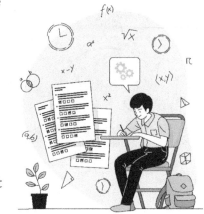

It's almost always better to start the guessing process too early than too late. It only takes a few seconds to remember something and answer the question from knowledge. Carefully eliminating wrong answer choices takes longer. Plus, going through the process of eliminating answer choices can actually help jog your memory.

**Summary**: Start the guessing process as soon as you decide that you can't answer the question based on your knowledge.

7

# How to Narrow Down the Choices

The next chapter in this book (**Test-Taking Strategies**) includes a wide range of strategies for how to approach questions and how to look for answer choices to eliminate. You will definitely want to read those carefully, practice them, and figure out which ones work best for you. Here though, we're going to address a mindset rather than a particular strategy.

Your odds of guessing an answer correctly depend on how many options you are choosing from.

| Number of options left | 5 | 4 | 3 | 2 | 1 |
|---|---|---|---|---|---|
| Odds of guessing correctly | 20% | 25% | 33% | 50% | 100% |

You can see from this chart just how valuable it is to be able to eliminate incorrect answers and make an educated guess, but there are two things that many test takers do that cause them to miss out on the benefits of guessing:

- Accidentally eliminating the correct answer
- Selecting an answer based on an impression

We'll look at the first one here, and the second one in the next section.

To avoid accidentally eliminating the correct answer, we recommend a thought exercise called **the $5 challenge**. In this challenge, you only eliminate an answer choice from contention if you are willing to bet $5 on it being wrong. Why $5? Five dollars is a small but not insignificant amount of money. It's an amount you could afford to lose but wouldn't want to throw away. And while losing

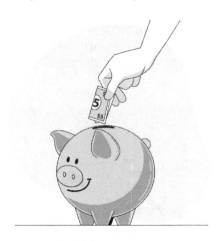

$5 once might not hurt too much, doing it twenty times will set you back $100. In the same way, each small decision you make—eliminating a choice here, guessing on a question there—won't by itself impact your score very much, but when you put them all together, they can make a big difference. By holding each answer choice elimination decision to a higher standard, you can reduce the risk of accidentally eliminating the correct answer.

The $5 challenge can also be applied in a positive sense: If you are willing to bet $5 that an answer choice *is* correct, go ahead and mark it as correct.

**Summary**: Only eliminate an answer choice if you are willing to bet $5 that it is wrong.

8

# Which Answer to Choose

You're taking the test. You've run into a hard question and decided you'll have to guess. You've eliminated all the answer choices you're willing to bet $5 on. Now you have to pick an answer. Why do we even need to talk about this? Why can't you just pick whichever one you feel like when the time comes?

The answer to these questions is that if you don't come into the test with a plan, you'll rely on your impression to select an answer choice, and if you do that, you risk falling into a trap. The test writers know that everyone who takes their test will be guessing on some of the questions, so they intentionally write wrong answer choices to seem plausible. You still have to pick an answer though, and if the wrong answer choices are designed to look right, how can you ever be sure that you're not falling for their trap? The best solution we've found to this dilemma is to take the decision out of your hands entirely. Here is the process we recommend:

**Once you've eliminated any choices that you are confident (willing to bet $5) are wrong, select the first remaining choice as your answer.**

Whether you choose to select the first remaining choice, the second, or the last, the important thing is that you use some preselected standard. Using this approach guarantees that you will not be enticed into selecting an answer choice that looks right, because you are not basing your decision on how the answer choices look.

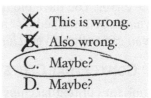

This is not meant to make you question your knowledge. Instead, it is to help you recognize the difference between your knowledge and your impressions. There's a huge difference between thinking an answer is right because of what you know, and thinking an answer is right because it looks or sounds like it should be right.

**Summary**: To ensure that your selection is appropriately random, make a predetermined selection from among all answer choices you have not eliminated.

# Test-Taking Strategies

This section contains a list of test-taking strategies that you may find helpful as you work through the test. By taking what you know and applying logical thought, you can maximize your chances of answering any question correctly!

It is very important to realize that every question is different and every person is different: no single strategy will work on every question, and no single strategy will work for every person. That's why we've included all of them here, so you can try them out and determine which ones work best for different types of questions and which ones work best for you.

## Question Strategies

### ⊘ READ CAREFULLY

Read the question and the answer choices carefully. Don't miss the question because you misread the terms. You have plenty of time to read each question thoroughly and make sure you understand what is being asked. Yet a happy medium must be attained, so don't waste too much time. You must read carefully and efficiently.

### ⊘ CONTEXTUAL CLUES

Look for contextual clues. If the question includes a word you are not familiar with, look at the immediate context for some indication of what the word might mean. Contextual clues can often give you all the information you need to decipher the meaning of an unfamiliar word. Even if you can't determine the meaning, you may be able to narrow down the possibilities enough to make a solid guess at the answer to the question.

### ⊘ PREFIXES

If you're having trouble with a word in the question or answer choices, try dissecting it. Take advantage of every clue that the word might include. Prefixes can be a huge help. Usually, they allow you to determine a basic meaning. *Pre-* means before, *post-* means after, *pro-* is positive, *de-* is negative. From prefixes, you can get an idea of the general meaning of the word and try to put it into context.

### ⊘ HEDGE WORDS

Watch out for critical hedge words, such as *likely, may, can, sometimes, often, almost, mostly, usually, generally, rarely,* and *sometimes.* Question writers insert these hedge phrases to cover every possibility. Often an answer choice will be wrong simply because it leaves no room for exception. Be on guard for answer choices that have definitive words such as *exactly* and *always.*

### ⊘ SWITCHBACK WORDS

Stay alert for *switchbacks.* These are the words and phrases frequently used to alert you to shifts in thought. The most common switchback words are *but, although,* and *however.* Others include *nevertheless, on the other hand, even though, while, in spite of, despite,* and *regardless of.* Switchback words are important to catch because they can change the direction of the question or an answer choice.

## ⊘ Face Value

When in doubt, use common sense. Accept the situation in the problem at face value. Don't read too much into it. These problems will not require you to make wild assumptions. If you have to go beyond creativity and warp time or space in order to have an answer choice fit the question, then you should move on and consider the other answer choices. These are normal problems rooted in reality. The applicable relationship or explanation may not be readily apparent, but it is there for you to figure out. Use your common sense to interpret anything that isn't clear.

# Answer Choice Strategies

## ⊘ Answer Selection

The most thorough way to pick an answer choice is to identify and eliminate wrong answers until only one is left, then confirm it is the correct answer. Sometimes an answer choice may immediately seem right, but be careful. The test writers will usually put more than one reasonable answer choice on each question, so take a second to read all of them and make sure that the other choices are not equally obvious. As long as you have time left, it is better to read every answer choice than to pick the first one that looks right without checking the others.

## ⊘ Answer Choice Families

An answer choice family consists of two (in rare cases, three) answer choices that are very similar in construction and cannot all be true at the same time. If you see two answer choices that are direct opposites or parallels, one of them is usually the correct answer. For instance, if one answer choice says that quantity $x$ increases and another either says that quantity $x$ decreases (opposite) or says that quantity $y$ increases (parallel), then those answer choices would fall into the same family. An answer choice that doesn't match the construction of the answer choice family is more likely to be incorrect. Most questions will not have answer choice families, but when they do appear, you should be prepared to recognize them.

## ⊘ Eliminate Answers

Eliminate answer choices as soon as you realize they are wrong, but make sure you consider all possibilities. If you are eliminating answer choices and realize that the last one you are left with is also wrong, don't panic. Start over and consider each choice again. There may be something you missed the first time that you will realize on the second pass.

## ⊘ Avoid Fact Traps

Don't be distracted by an answer choice that is factually true but doesn't answer the question. You are looking for the choice that answers the question. Stay focused on what the question is asking for so you don't accidentally pick an answer that is true but incorrect. Always go back to the question and make sure the answer choice you've selected actually answers the question and is not merely a true statement.

## ⊘ Extreme Statements

In general, you should avoid answers that put forth extreme actions as standard practice or proclaim controversial ideas as established fact. An answer choice that states the "process should be used in certain situations, if..." is much more likely to be correct than one that states the "process should be discontinued completely." The first is a calm rational statement and doesn't even make a definitive, uncompromising stance, using a hedge word *if* to provide wiggle room, whereas the second choice is far more extreme.

### ⊘ BENCHMARK

As you read through the answer choices and you come across one that seems to answer the question well, mentally select that answer choice. This is not your final answer, but it's the one that will help you evaluate the other answer choices. The one that you selected is your benchmark or standard for judging each of the other answer choices. Every other answer choice must be compared to your benchmark. That choice is correct until proven otherwise by another answer choice beating it. If you find a better answer, then that one becomes your new benchmark. Once you've decided that no other choice answers the question as well as your benchmark, you have your final answer.

### ⊘ PREDICT THE ANSWER

Before you even start looking at the answer choices, it is often best to try to predict the answer. When you come up with the answer on your own, it is easier to avoid distractions and traps because you will know exactly what to look for. The right answer choice is unlikely to be word-for-word what you came up with, but it should be a close match. Even if you are confident that you have the right answer, you should still take the time to read each option before moving on.

## General Strategies

### ⊘ TOUGH QUESTIONS

If you are stumped on a problem or it appears too hard or too difficult, don't waste time. Move on! Remember though, if you can quickly check for obviously incorrect answer choices, your chances of guessing correctly are greatly improved. Before you completely give up, at least try to knock out a couple of possible answers. Eliminate what you can and then guess at the remaining answer choices before moving on.

### ⊘ CHECK YOUR WORK

Since you will probably not know every term listed and the answer to every question, it is important that you get credit for the ones that you do know. Don't miss any questions through careless mistakes. If at all possible, try to take a second to look back over your answer selection and make sure you've selected the correct answer choice and haven't made a costly careless mistake (such as marking an answer choice that you didn't mean to mark). This quick double check should more than pay for itself in caught mistakes for the time it costs.

### ⊘ PACE YOURSELF

It's easy to be overwhelmed when you're looking at a page full of questions; your mind is confused and full of random thoughts, and the clock is ticking down faster than you would like. Calm down and maintain the pace that you have set for yourself. Especially as you get down to the last few minutes of the test, don't let the small numbers on the clock make you panic. As long as you are on track by monitoring your pace, you are guaranteed to have time for each question.

### ⊘ DON'T RUSH

It is very easy to make errors when you are in a hurry. Maintaining a fast pace in answering questions is pointless if it makes you miss questions that you would have gotten right otherwise. Test writers like to include distracting information and wrong answers that seem right. Taking a little extra time to avoid careless mistakes can make all the difference in your test score. Find a pace that allows you to be confident in the answers that you select.

## ⊘ KEEP MOVING

Panicking will not help you pass the test, so do your best to stay calm and keep moving. Taking deep breaths and going through the answer elimination steps you practiced can help to break through a stress barrier and keep your pace.

# Final Notes

The combination of a solid foundation of content knowledge and the confidence that comes from practicing your plan for applying that knowledge is the key to maximizing your performance on test day. As your foundation of content knowledge is built up and strengthened, you'll find that the strategies included in this chapter become more and more effective in helping you quickly sift through the distractions and traps of the test to isolate the correct answer.

Now that you're preparing to move forward into the test content chapters of this book, be sure to keep your goal in mind. As you read, think about how you will be able to apply this information on the test. If you've already seen sample questions for the test and you have an idea of the question format and style, try to come up with questions of your own that you can answer based on what you're reading. This will give you valuable practice applying your knowledge in the same ways you can expect to on test day.

**Good luck and good studying!**

# Human Resource Management

Transform passive reading into active learning! After immersing yourself in this chapter, put your comprehension to the test by taking a quiz. The insights you gained will stay with you longer this way. Scan the QR code to go directly to the chapter quiz interface for this study guide. If you're using a computer, simply visit the bonus page at **mometrix.com/bonus948/nurseexec** and click the Chapter Quizzes link.

## Federal Employment Laws

### FAMILY AND MEDICAL LEAVE ACT (FMLA)

The Family and Medical Leave Act (FMLA) (1993) is a federal law that requires employers with 50 or more employees to provide unpaid leave and job-protected time off up to 12 weeks during any 12-month period for medical and family reasons to fulltime and part-time employees who have worked more than 1,250 hours within the previous year. During leave time, the employer must continue the same benefits and insurance coverage and must maintain the position or provide another that is approximately equal in salary, benefits, and area of responsibility. Leave may be used to care for a newborn, adopted, or fostered child, sick spouse, child, or parent, and for adverse health conditions that prevent the employee from carrying out work functions. FMLA allows extended leave of up to 26 workweeks in a 12-month period to care for a service member's spouse, parent, or children.

### AMERICANS WITH DISABILITIES ACT (ADA)

The 1992 Americans with Disabilities Act is civil rights legislation that provides the disabled, including those with mental impairment, access to employment and the community. Under this act, employers must make reasonable accommodations for the disabled. The ADA covers not only obvious disabilities but also disorders such as arthritis, seizure disorders, and cardiovascular and respiratory disorders. Communities must provide transportation services for the disabled, including accommodation for wheelchairs. Public facilities (schools, museums, physician's offices, post offices, restaurants) must be accessible with ramps and elevators as needed. Telecommunications must also be accessible through devices or accommodations for the deaf and blind. Full compliance is not yet complete because older buildings are required to provide access that is possible without "undue hardship," but newer construction of public facilities must meet ADA regulations.

### FAIR LABOR STANDARDS ACT

The Fair Labor Standards Act establishes standards for minimum wage, record keeping, overtime pay, and standards for child labor. These standards apply to all workers of covered enterprises, although there are exemptions. As of July 24, 2009, the federal minimum wage was $7.25 per hour. States have the right to dictate their own minimum wage, but the worker has the right to the higher wage, if different than the federal wage. Workers must receive overtime pay at the rate of at least 1.5 times usual rates for work in excess of 40 hours/week. People employed in businesses where they earn more than $30 per month in tips must be paid directly at a rate of at least $2.13 per hour. The FLSA also outlines which workers may be paid at a rate lower than the minimum wage. These include student learners and impaired/disabled workers whose disability interferes with productivity. Hospitals and residential care facilities may have a partial exemption from overtime pay in that they may have a 14-day work period instead of 7 but must pay overtime for hours worked over 8 in one day or 80 hours in 14 days.

## WAGE AND HOUR LAWS

Wage and hour laws include:

- **Davis-Bacon Act**: Requires contractors and sub-contractors in public works projects to be paid prevailing wages.
- **Walsh-Healy Public Contracts Act**: Establishes overtime wages and minimum wage for government contracts worth more than $15,000 for manufacturing or supplying goods or equipment.
- **Contract Work Hours and Safety Standards Act**: Requires contractors and subcontractors on federal projects worth over $100,000 to pay overtime of 1.5 times hourly wages for hours over 40/week and prohibits unsanitary or unsafe working conditions.
- **McNamara-O'Hara Service Contract Act**: Requires contractors and subcontractors on prime contracts over $2500 to pay workers prevailing wages and benefits and minimum wage or better on contracts of less than $2500.
- **Federal Wage Garnishment Law**: Sets limits on the amount of a worker's wages that can be garnished and protects workers from being fired for having wages garnished.

## EQUAL EMPLOYMENT OPPORTUNITY COMMISSION

The Equal Employment Opportunity Commission enforces federal laws against discrimination in employment for employers with at least 15 employees or at least 20 employees in age-discrimination cases. The EEOC investigates, provides guidance, and enforces a number of laws:

- **Civil Rights Act (1964), Title VII, including Pregnancy Discrimination Act**: Employers cannot discriminate based on race, color, gender, pregnancy, religion, and national origin.
- **Civil Rights Act (1991), Sections 102 and 103**: Amends previous laws to allow jury trials and punitive and compensatory damages.
- **Equal Pay Act (1963)**: Males and females must receive equal pay for equal work.
- **Age Discrimination in Employment Act (ADEA) (1967)**: Law provides protection against age discrimination for those 40 or older.
- **Rehabilitation Act (1973), Sections 501 and 505**: Law is similar to ADA but applies to discrimination against those with disabilities in the federal government.
- **Genetic Information Nondiscrimination Act (GINA) (2008)**: Employers cannot discriminate based on genetic information.

## OCCUPATIONAL SAFETY AND HEALTH ADMINISTRATION (OSHA)

The Occupational Safety and Health Administration (OSHA) requires that safeguards to prevent occupational exposure and incidents be a part of infection control policies. Additionally, the FDA has requirements related to the safety of medical devices. Some states have regulations that are more restrictive than those of OSHA. Important elements include:

- An **exposure control plan** that outlines methods to reduce staff injury/ exposure.
- Use of universal **precautions** at all times with all individuals.
- Planning **work practices** to minimize danger and using newer and safer technologies as they become available, such as needles engineered to prevent injury.
- **Sharps disposal methods** that prohibit bending, recapping, shearing, breaking, or handling contaminated needles or other sharps. Scooping with one hand may be used if recapping is essential.

- Workers must be **trained** in the use of universal precautions and methods to decrease exposure.
- Procedures for **post-exposure evaluation and treatment** must be part of the exposure control plan.
- Immunization with **Hepatitis B vaccine** must be available to healthcare workers.

> **Review Video: Intro to OSHA**
> Visit mometrix.com/academy and enter code: 913559

## WORKERS' COMPENSATION

The primary focus of Workers' Compensation, a type of insurance, is to return people to work as quickly and safely as possible. Workers' Compensation is intended for those who are injured on the job or whose health is impaired because of their jobs. Workers' Compensation provides three different types of benefits: cash to replace lost wages, reimbursement for medical costs associated with the injury, and death benefits to survivors. Workers' Compensation laws may vary somewhat from one state to another. Workers' Compensation data are not available on a national basis, and criteria for data collection may vary from state to state along with state regulations, but even limited (statewide) data may provide an estimate of the frequency and severity of particular occupational injuries as well as associated costs. The data may help guide the institution of work safety measures and the development of safety training. The employer is, with few exceptions, immune from further liability because accepting benefits generally incudes waiving the right to sue.

> **Review Video: US Employment Compensation Laws**
> Visit mometrix.com/academy and enter code: 613448

## NURSING HOME REFORM AMENDMENTS

The **Omnibus Budget Reconciliation Act (OBRA)** of 1987 contains the **Nursing Home Reform Amendments (NHRA)**. These amendments establish guidelines for nursing facilities (such as long-term care facilities). Provisions include:

- A complete physical and mental **assessment** of each patient is required on admission, annually, and with change of condition.
- Requirement for **24-hour nursing** with RNs on duty for at least one shift.
- **Nurse aide training** is mandated as well as regular in-service and state registry of trained/qualified aides.
- Rehabilitative services must be available.
- A physician/physician's assistant/nurse practitioner must **visit** every 30 days for the first 3 months and then every 90 days.
- Outlawing/Discouraging **Medicaid discrimination**.
- Requirement for **independent monitoring** of psychopharmacologic drugs.
- Recognition of **patients' rights**.
- **Survey protocols** to assess patient care and patient outcomes.
- **State sanctions** to enforce nursing home regulations.

## OLDER AMERICANS ACT (OAA)

The Older Americans Act (OAA) (Title III) of 1965 (reauthorized in 2020 through 2024) provides improved access to services for older adults and Native Americans, including community services (meals, transportation, home health care, adult day care, legal assistance, and home repair). The OAA provides funding to local Area Agencies on Aging (AAA) or state or tribal agencies, which

17

administer funding. These local agencies can assess community needs and contract for services. One of the programs that is commonly supported with funds from the OAA is meals-on-wheels. Low-cost adult day care is also offered in some communities. The OAA includes the National Family Caregivers Support Act, which provides services for caregivers of older adults. The OAA also provides grants for programs that combat violence against older adults and others to provide computer training for older adults. Additionally, the OAA mandates that each state have an ombudsman program. Ombudsmen provide services to residents of nursing homes and other facilities to ensure that care meets state standards.

## EMERGENCY MEDICAL TREATMENT AND ACTIVE LABOR ACT (EMTALA)

The Emergency Medical Treatment and Active Labor Act (EMTALA) is designed to prevent patient "dumping" from emergency departments (ED) and is an issue of concern for risk management, requiring staff training for compliance.

- **Transfers** from the ED may be intrahospital or to another facility.
- Stabilization of the patient with emergency conditions or active labor must be done in the ED **prior to transfer**, and initial screening must be given prior to inquiring about insurance or ability to pay.
- Stabilization requires **treatment** for emergency conditions and reasonable belief that, although the emergency condition may not be completely resolved, the patient's condition will not deteriorate during transfer.
- (Not applicable to older adults) Women in the ED in **active labor** should deliver both the child and placenta before transfer.
- The receiving department or facility should be capable of **treating** the patient and dealing with **complications** that might occur.
- Transfer to another facility is indicated if the patient requires **specialized services** not available intrahospital, such as to burn centers.

## LABOR RELATIONS

### COLLECTIVE BARGAINING

Collective bargaining is a process involving negotiations, usually about salary and working conditions, between the administration of an organization and representatives of a group of employees, often those represented by a labor union (such as the United American Nurses). The negotiated terms of the agreement reached are outlined in a collective bargaining agreement. Both federal and state laws govern collective bargaining. In collective bargaining, each side usually has a team of 5 to 7 members that meet around a bargaining table. The existing contract is generally used as a starting point. **Types** of bargaining include:

- **Distributive**: A competitive process in which one side wins and the other loses (zero-sum, win-lose). May lead to compromise or stalemate.
- **Integrative**: A collaborative process (win-win). The parties involved bargain jointly, trying to solve problems. Integrative bargaining is most successful if the parties have developed trust.
- **Mixed**: Combines some aspects of distributive and integrative.

## CONTRACT NEGOTIATIONS

Contract negotiations usually entail two teams (administrative and personnel) meeting to reach an agreement. Preparation for contract negotiations includes:

- **Reviewing notes and reports** from the previous contract negotiations, including tactics used, key issues, and key stakeholders
- Developing a contract bargaining unit/team
- **Gathering data**, including key labor costs, average work hours, income vs expenses, and paid leave costs
- **Comparing** current data with data from previous negotiation
- Developing a bargaining strategy
- **Prioritizing** issues for negotiation, anticipating options, and determining bottom-line expectation
- Making a **plan**
- Creating a **schedule** for meetings

During negotiations, it's important to control the meeting as much as possible and to deal with **facts** and avoid expressing feelings or emotions. Negotiations often start with statements from both sides, indicating what they hope to accomplish though negotiations. Team members generally avoid giving the best offer first, leaving room to negotiate.

## GRIEVANCES AND ARBITRATIONS

Grievances, also known as contract disputes, are disputes about the terms of employment (administration, violation, understanding) that may occur between administration and personnel who are in a collective bargaining relationship. Grievance processes may vary depending on the collective bargaining contract; however, grievances are usually submitted in writing to an immediate supervisor. If the grievance is not resolved, it is taken to the next level in the chain of command. If again there is no resolution, then the issue is referred for **grievance arbitration**, which is a formal procedure in which an impartial third-party arbitrator holds a hearing to consider both sides of the dispute. The decision that the arbitrator makes based on evidence is binding to both parties of the dispute. The arbitrator is selected from a list of arbitrators and paid in accordance to contract stipulations, with both parties usually sharing costs.

## NATIONAL LABOR RELATIONS BOARD (NLRB)

The National Labor Relations Board **(NLRB)**, an independent federal agency, protects workers' right to organize and have labor unions in the private sector as their bargaining representatives and prevents unfair labor practices. The NLRB has statutory jurisdiction over almost all private sector jobs, whether unionized or not, including non-profits and interstate commerce. The NLRB has 32 regional offices. Functions include:

- Providing framework for organizing and conducting **elections** to certify or decertify labor unions.
- Investigating charges of **unfair labor practices** after a complaint is filed at a regional office.
- Facilitating **settlements** between disputing parties.
- Adjudicating **cases** (30 administrative judges and a board).
- Enforcing **compliance** through the US Court of Appeals.

Employers are prohibited from discouraging workers from **unionizing** or interfering with the process. Additionally, employers must post a notice of **employee rights**. Employees have the right to choose union representation or to reject union representation.

19

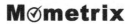

# Communication

## PRINCIPLES OF COMMUNICATION

### ACTIVE LISTENING

Active listening implies more than passively listening to another individual. Active listening includes observing the other individual carefully for nonverbal behaviors, such as posture, eye contact, and facial expression, as well as understanding and reflecting on what the person is saying. The listener should observe carefully for inconsistencies in what the individual is saying or comments that require clarification. Feedback is critical to active listening because it shows the speaker that one is paying attention and showing interest and respect. Feedback may be as simple as nodding the head in agreement but should also include asking questions or making comments to show full engagement. Listening with empathy is especially important because it helps to build a connection with the speaker. The listener should communicate empathy with words: "You feel (emotion) because (experience)," because the speaker may not be sensitive to what the listener is comprehending.

### REFLECTIVE COMMUNICATION

Reflective communication utilizes techniques to assist individuals to understand their personal thoughts and feelings by directing actions, feelings, and thoughts back to the individual. For example, if a person asks, "Do you think I should...," a reflective comment is "Do you think you should...." However, this type of reflective comment should be used sparingly. A better choice is often to reflect on what is implied. For example, if a person complains that his boss is unfair and shows favoritism, a reflective comment would be: "This makes you feel angry and upset." Reflection helps speakers to recognize their feelings, as they may not realize the impact that their feelings are having on their attitude and behavior. Reflection also helps individuals accept their feelings and find ways to work through them.

### SENDER-RECEIVER FEEDBACK LOOP

The communication process, which includes the **sender-receiver feedback loop,** is based on Claude Shannon's information theory (1948) in which he describes three necessary steps:

1.  **Encoding** the message
2.  **Transmitting** the message through a channel
3.  **Decoding** the message

The resultant communication process begins with the sender, who serves as the encoder and determines the content of the message. The medium is the form the message takes (digital, written, audiovisual), and the channel is the method of delivery (mail, radio, TV, phone). The recipient (receiver) who acts as the decoder determines the meaning from the message. Feedback helps to determine whether or not the communication is successful and the message understood as intended. This process is referred to as the send-receiver feedback loop. Context is the environment (physical and psychological) in which the communication occurs, and interference is any factor that impacts the communication process. Interference may be external (such as environmental noise) or internal (such as emotional distress or anxiety).

### TWO-WAY COMMUNICATION

Two-way communication is a process of interpersonal communication in which both parties participate and provide information. Examples of two-way communication include telephone conversations, amateur radio, in-person conversations, instant messaging, and chat rooms. Two-way communication incorporates the sender-receiver feedback loop because feedback is a critical component of communication, assuring the sender that the message was received as intended. In business communication, two-way communication occurs when a message receives a response (feedback). This is the most common type of business communication. Two-way communication tends to be more accurate than one-way communication but is more time-consuming and less orderly; however, two-way communication allows for corrections and modifications and results in greater understanding. Two-way communication may be horizontal (such as between two nurses) or vertical (such as between the nurse executive and subordinates).

## SELECTING COMMUNICATION METHODS

Selecting appropriate communication methods requires a number of steps:

1. Consider the **purpose** of the communication.
2. Identify the person or persons who will be the **recipients** and obtain or consider information about them, what influences them, and how best to reach them.
3. Consider the **message** to be conveyed and the best way to communicate so that the message is received as intended.
4. Determine whether the communication is intended as **one-way** or requires **feedback**. Choose an interactive channel if feedback is desired.
5. Determine the **cost or effort** involved in communicating through the chosen channel.
6. Develop the correct **format** for the communication (letter, FAX, email, phone call, face to face), using or developing a template as is appropriate.
7. Complete the message and **carry out** the communication using the channel selected.
8. **Monitor feedback** if appropriate.
9. **Respond to feedback** if indicated by comments.

## COMMUNICATION STYLES

### PERSUASIVE COMMUNICATION

The purpose of persuasive communication is to convince people to do or believe something, a crucial skill in the healthcare environment. The essential steps to persuasive communication include:

- **Understanding the audience**: The message should be directed at the needs of the listeners and should be presented in a language that is appropriate to their levels of education and experience, avoiding excess data and statistics.
- **Getting attention**: The speaker should begin with an anecdote or interesting information to get people's attention rather than immediately launching into the direct purpose of the communication.
- **Establishing credibility**: The speaker should outline authority or expertise.
- **Outlining benefits**: The listener's biggest concern is often how something will affect them personally, so explaining how they will benefit from the content communicated is crucial.
- **Using appropriate body language**: This may vary according to audience, but should generally include making frequent eye contact, smiling, avoiding closed body positions (arms folded), and using a persuasive tone of voice.

### ASSERTIVE COMMUNICATION

Assertive communication occurs when the individual expresses opinions directly and actions correlate with words. Assertive communicators are respectful of others and, without bullying, are firm and honest about their opinions. They frequently use "I" statements to make their point: "I would like. . ." Communication usually includes **cooperative statements**, such as "What do you think?" and distinguishes between fact and opinion. Assertive communicators often engender trust

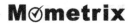

in others because they are consistent, honest, and open in communicating with others. The assertive communicator feels free to express disagreement and anger but does so in a manner that is nonthreatening and respectful of others' feelings. Assertive communication requires a strong sense of self-worth and the belief that personal opinions have value. Assertive communicators tend to have good listening skills because they value the opinions of others and feel comfortable collaborating.

## PASSIVE COMMUNICATION

Passive communication occurs when the individual does not express an opinion directly or verbally but may communicate in a non-direct or nonverbal manner. The passive communicator may be non-committal and submissive, often contributing little to a conversation and unwilling to take sides in a conflict. The person may believe that personal opinions are not important and may avoid direct eye contact and appear nervous and fidgety if confronted. The individual may show signs of anxiety, such as wringing hands and crossing the arms. The passive communicator may respond inappropriately when angry, such as by laughing, and may believe that disagreeing with another person will be upsetting to that person or result in conflict, which the communicator wants to avoid. The passive communicator benefits by rarely being blamed for failures (since the person took little part in decision making) and by avoiding conflict (at least short-term).

## AGGRESSIVE COMMUNICATION

Aggressive communication has some of the same characteristics as assertive communication but lacks a respect for others. The aggressive communicator expresses opinions directly and forcefully but does not want to hear the opinions of others and may denigrate those who speak up or disagree. The aggressive communicator often bullies others into agreement but is usually disliked, and this can increase social anxiety and resentment, leading to further aggression. The aggressive communicator may use sarcasms or insults and may frequently interrupt or talk over other speakers and may intrude on others' personal space. They often believe they are superior to or more intelligent than others and may take an aggressive stance (standing upright, feet apart, hands on hips). Hand gestures may include making fists and pointing fingers at others. Benefits of aggressive communication are being in control, getting one's own way, and feeling powerful.

## PASSIVE-AGGRESSIVE COMMUNICATION

A key aspect of passive-aggressive communication is negativity, which influences people's thoughts and communication strategies. These communicators often appear quite passive but are angry and resentful. They may appear to be in agreement or cooperating while obstructing or undermining communication efforts. They often complain to others about what someone has said or done but fail to confront that person directly; however, they tend to be loners with few friends, and this results in increasing feelings of powerlessness. Passive aggressive communicators attempt to get their way indirectly by convincing others to support their positions. Facial expressions may be at odds with words, and they may make sarcastic comments meant to belittle the other person. If others don't agree with their positions, passive-aggressive communicators may resort to sabotage but often deny there is a problem and cannot acknowledge their underlying anger.

## CULTURAL ASPECTS OF COMMUNICATION

Cultural aspects of communication include the following:

| Hmong | • The eldest male in the family makes the decisions for the family and is deferred to by other family members, so the nurse should ask who should receive information about the patient.<br>• Communication should be polite and respectful, avoiding direct eye contact, which is considered rude.<br>• Disagreeing is considered rude so "Yes" may mean "I hear you" but not necessarily, "I agree with you." |
|---|---|
| Mexican | • Mexican culture perceives time with more **flexibility** than American, so if patients/family need to be present at a particular time, the nurse should specify the exact time (1:30 PM) and explain the reason rather than saying something vaguer, such as "after lunch."<br>• People may appear to be unassertive or unable to make decisions when they are simply showing respect to the nurse by being **deferent**.<br>• In traditional families, the **males** make decisions, so a woman may wait for the husband or other males in the family to make decisions about treatment or care. |
| Middle Eastern | • In Middle Eastern countries, males make decisions, so issues for discussion or decision should be directed to males, such as the spouse or son, and males may be direct in stating what they want, sometimes appearing demanding.<br>• Middle Easterners often require less personal space and may stand very close.<br>• If a male nurse must care for a female patient, then the family should be advised that personal care (such as bathing) will be done by a female while the medical treatments will be done by the male nurse. |
| Asian | • Asian families may expect the nurse to remain **authoritative** and to give directions, and may not ask questions if they are confused.<br>• **Disagreeing** is considered impolite. "Yes" may only mean that the person is heard, not that they agree with the person. When asked if they understand, they may indicate that they do even when they clearly do not, so as not to offend the nurse.<br>• Asians may avoid **eye contact** as an indication of respect. |

## WRITTEN COMMUNICATION

Written communication includes a wide range of choices in which the written word can be utilized. Written communication is most often used for formal proposals, advertisements, brochures, and letters. Contracts are almost always completed in hardcopy written form. However, email messages and documents are now often taking the place of hardcopy written documents because of less cost and more rapid communication. When utilizing written communication, the writer must consider the purpose of the communication, the structure of the document, and the style in which is it written. Templates may be used for structure, but style and content depend on the writer. The information should be well organized with key points clearly outlined and supporting facts included. The introduction should create interest and the conclusion should provide a summary or suggestion for the future. The style of the writing should be appropriate for the recipient and may range from very formal to very informal. Paragraphs should be short, especially for online communications.

## SCRIPTING

Scripting (a pre-written message) is a method used to ensure that communication is consistent among different individuals, such as when staff members are orienting patients. When creating a script, the first step is to determine the purpose and the message the script should convey. Generally, the first words of the script will focus on the topic and the purpose, "Mrs. Smith, we need to review your preparation for the colonoscopy." The script may explain the value to the individual and end with a summary. Scripts are particularly helpful for telephone triage or when responding to customer service requests. In most cases, the script should serve as a guideline rather than a narrative that should be memorized and recited verbatim or read although script users should practice and engage in roleplaying in order to become adept at staying on script as much as possible.

## VERBAL COMMUNICATION

Verbal (spoken) communication can vary from very formal (such as a conference presentation) to very informal (such as a chat with a friend), but every aspect of the communication process has meaning—the words, the posture, the tone of voice, the expression on the face, the use of silence, and the general appearance. The communication of the same words will be very different if heard over the phone, read in an email, or heard face-to-face. In any professional communication, formal or informal, the individual should come prepared and should have some idea of what to say although memorizing word-for-word is not advisable because communication should appear spontaneous even when it is not. The average person speaks about 200 words per minute and each sentence is a new creation. Without planning, the message can easily become muddled. For formal presentations, brief outline notes or presentation software may be helpful to keep focused on the topic.

## SELECTING THE VEHICLE OF COMMUNICATION

The vehicle of communication should best meet the communication needs:

- **Mail**: Use to add a personal touch to messages and to deliver documents securely. Mailings can reach large populations although cost may be relatively high.
- **Email**: Allows for fast communication and mass mailings at little cost, but emails are often screened and may be ignored if the receiver doesn't know or recognize the sender. Documents can be easily transmitted through email as text or PDF files.
- **Telephones** (Landline): Use when interaction and discussion is needed or for personal appeals. The system should include voice mail. This is a relatively inexpensive form of communication, but the ubiquitous use of voice mail often means delays in actual communication.
- **Smartphones**: Use when rapid communication by phone, email, or messaging is needed as well as internet access. This is especially useful when the person is mobile.
- **Video/Web conferencing**: This is valuable when participants cannot otherwise meet face to face and can save money associated with travel expenses. This vehicle allows participants to communicate both verbally and nonverbally.
- **Internet/Webpages**: Internet communication can be synchronous or asynchronous and allows for the presentation of information (such as on a webpage) as well as verbal communication (such as with messaging).

- **Social media**: These provide the opportunity to share professional or organizational information (such as with LinkedIn and Facebook). Twitter may be used to communicate short messages, which should contain hashtags so they can easily be found by users.
- **FAX**: This allows transfer of documents or images quickly and may be used, for example, to send an agenda prior to a meeting or to send documents that must be reviewed. Almost any type of document can be scanned and faxed.

## NONVERBAL COMMUNICATION

Nonverbal interpersonal communication can convey as much information as verbal communication, both on the nurse's part and the patient's. Nonverbal communication is used for a number of purposes, such as expressing feelings and attitudes, and may be a barrier to communication or a facilitator. While there are cultural differences, interpretation of nonverbal communication can help the nurse to better understand and promote communication:

- **Eye contact**: Making eye contact provides a connection and shows caring and involvement in the communication. In many western cultures, avoiding eye contact may indicate someone is not telling the truth or is uncomfortable, fearful, ashamed, or hiding something.
- **Tone**: The manner in which words are spoken (patiently, cheerfully, somberly) affects the listener, and a tone that is inconsistent with the message can interfere with communication. A high-pitched tone of voice may indicate nervousness or stress.

Additional elements of **nonverbal interpersonal communication** include:

- **Touch**: Reaching out to touch an adult's hand or pat a shoulder during communication is reassuring but hugging or excessive touching can make people feel uncomfortable. People may touch themselves (lick lips, pick at skin, scratch) if they are anxious.
- **Gestures**: Using the hands to emphasize meaning is common and may be particularly helpful during explanations, but excessive gesturing can be distracting. Some gestures alone convey a message, such as a wave goodbye or pointing. Tapping of the foot, moving the legs, or fidgeting may indicate nervousness. Rubbing the hands together is sometimes a self-comforting measure. Some gestures, such as handshakes, are part of social ritual. Mixed messages, such as fidgeting but speaking with a calm voice may indicate uncertainty or anxiety.
- **Posture**: Slumping can indicate a lack of interest or withdrawal. Leaning toward the opposite person while talking indicates interest and facilitates interaction.

## SELECTING COMMUNICATION METHOD BASED ON AUDIENCE AND SITUATION
### EMAIL

While emails tend to be more informal than other written forms of communication, business emails should not contain overly informal language, slang, swearwords, emoticons, or abbreviations. The writer should never include confidential information in an email and should limit emails to 5 or 6 sentences and one topic only per email. If a longer document must be sent, it should be sent as an attachment. Email **format**:

- **Email address**: Avoid using personal email accounts for business purposes.
- **Subject line**: Short and succinct, such as "Re: Grant proposal."
- **Opening greeting and pleasantry**: "Good morning, Joan. I appreciate your hard work in ..."
- **Purpose**: "I'm emailing you to..."
- **Request**: "Could you...?" It's less intimidating to phrase requests in question form.

- **Closing**: "Thank you," "I'm looking forward to your response," "Let me know if you have any questions."
- **Signature**: "Sincerely," "Gratefully," "Thank you," and sign full name instead of relying on the reader to note the name in the email address.

## ROLE-PLAYING

Role-playing, a form of simulation, is used often in medical education to teach participants about communication and to help them to practice communication skills. Role-playing activities can be carried out in different manners:

- **Fully scripted**: All participants are presented with a script to follow verbatim.
- **Partially scripted**: Participants are given beginning lines only.
- **One-sided**: One participant is given a script, but other participants are not.
- **Scenario only**: Participants are provided a scenario that briefly describes their roles and the situation.
- **Replay**: Participants act out experiences that they have previously had in reality.

In role-playing, participants may explore choices in the provision of care and communication strategies. When facilitating role-playing, the leader may begin by participating in a demonstration, especially if the participants are nervous or uncomfortable. The leader should also give positive reinforcement to the participants rather than focusing on negative elements.

## REPORTS

A number of issues must be considered in the **design and delivery of reports**:

- **Purpose**: The purpose of the report is primary and should be determined first. For example, the purpose may be to update recipients, gain support, indicate problems, or show progress.
- **Recipients**: Those who need to receive the report must be identified and grouped according to discipline or needs as different individuals or groups may need different reports, some more complex and detailed than others.
- **Delivery mode**: This is the method of delivery, which may include paper document, email, electronic document, spreadsheet, or PDF file.
- **Format**: The format may vary from detailed narratives to simplified graphs and illustrations or some combination. Whenever possible, templates should be utilized. Format should include such considerations as color, font, font-size, and white space.
- **Size**: This refers primarily to the length (pages, kilobytes, megabytes) of the report.
- **Frequency**: Reports may be issued at different frequency, depending on the recipient and the purpose.

## STAFF MEETINGS

Staff meetings are frequently required in healthcare settings, and preparation for the meeting depends on the type of meeting. The most common types of meetings include: **information dissemination**, **opinion solicitation**, and **problem solving**. The agenda will vary depending on the meeting focus. Most staff meetings are semi-formal. That is, the leader prepares an agenda (which should be distributed prior to the meeting), but all members usually contribute with free flow of questions and answers. Staff meetings vary in size, but a group of 4 to 7 participants is ideal. The larger the group, usually the more formal the meeting. Meetings should start on time in an environment conducive to discussion, such as sitting around a table. The leader should give an overview of the purpose of the meeting, ask for input or reports from staff members, and then address the primary purpose of the meeting. Most staff meetings last from 60 to 90 minutes, and the leader should monitor the time and keep the discussions on track.

### ORGANIZATION OF INFORMATION

The organization of information for **meetings** should be given consideration because the information provides an opportunity to not only inform but to involve those receiving the information:

- **Agenda**: This should be prepared and disseminated (electronically if possible) to all interested parties 2-3 days prior to a meeting. The agenda should be itemized and should include receiving and/or giving reports. Approximate times for discussion of each item may be included on the agenda, especially if there are many agenda items. The agenda for reports to upper management or the governing board should include a summary of results of performance improvement. A dashboard may be utilized for this summary.
- **Reports**: These should be scheduled early in the meeting to allow for discussion as they may relate to other agenda items. Electronic projection of information (slide show presentations, overhead projection) may aid in presenting complex summaries.
- **Minutes**: These should be prepared and disseminated within 2-3 days of the meeting and should include brief summaries of each agenda item.

## BOARD MEETINGS

When giving a presentation at board meetings, the nurse executive should have a clear understanding of why the board requested the presentation. Prior to the meeting, the nurse executive should gather data, organize the presentation, and practice presenting so that the information can be presented in a clear, concise, and interesting manner. The nurse should maintain a professional demeanor and dress appropriately for the meeting. During the presentation, the nurse executive should include visuals of various types. If using presentation software, only one concept should be presented per slide and illustrations should be easily visible throughout the room. The nurse executive should never read the material on a slide. If giving a written report as part of the presentation, an ideal size is 5 pages or fewer. The nurse executive should follow the format of the presentation but be open to questions, as board members often want to clarify information during a presentation rather than when it is completed.

## ONE-ON-ONE CONVERSATIONS

One-on-one conversations provide the nurse executive the opportunity to interact directly with individuals. Because one-on-one conversations allow equal exchanges, this type of communication has more parity than most other types of communication. While one-on-one conversations may be casual and completely unplanned, especially in a social context, if conducted as part of a leadership role, the nurse executive often has a goal in mind, such as gaining information about the person or a particular issue, so the conversation may be somewhat structured, as the nurse executive may, to some degree, guide the conversation. However, the nurse executive should engage in active listening in order to encourage the other party to communicate and should be prepared that the responses the other party gives may not be what the nurse executive expected or wanted. One-on-one conversations are relatively easy to schedule compared to group meetings and are more personal.

## PATIENT/FAMILY ADVISORY COUNCILS

The Agency for Healthcare Research and Quality (AHRC) provides tools and guidelines for developing **patient/family advisory councils**, which can provide valuable insight into planning, implementing, and assessing care. Patients and families should be provided literature about the patient/family council and the roles of members. An application form should be used to **screen** applicants regarding why they want to participate and what type of healthcare experiences they have had. An information session should be held in order for applicants to receive an overview of the role of the council. Once council members are selected, they should undergo a more detailed orientation, including the importance of maintaining confidentiality. Additionally, staff members should be educated about the role of the patient/family council and how the council may benefit planning efforts, such as by providing insights into the organization's strengths and weaknesses and feedback on policies.

## CONSUMER FEEDBACK

Consumer feedback is particularly valuable because it assesses the patient's perspective on the healthcare experience. The most commonly used tool for consumer feedback is currently the **Hospital Consumer Assessment of Healthcare Providers and Systems (HCAHPS) survey**, but this survey does not provide data for in-hospital comparisons of one unit with another. However, in-house surveys may also be conducted to obtain such data. Additionally, post-discharge quantitative patient surveys may be used to gather other data as well. These may be conducted through mail, email, or telephone. Another way to obtain consumer feedback is through focus groups in which members of the group respond to a number of questions under the guidance of a facilitator. Patient and family councils can provide valuable insight into the patient/family experience. While these resources can provide valuable data, the best consumer feedback may occur when healthcare providers simply take the time to talk to the patients they are caring for and ask them about their patient experience.

## INTERVIEWING

### INTERVIEWING FOR HIRING PURPOSES

Prior to conducting an interview for hiring purposes, it is important to review the job description and the applicant's work history. Questions should be prepared prior to the interview. In some cases, those hiring are required to ask all applicants the exact same questions although clarification questions may be asked in addition to the core questions. Questions must conform to state and national laws and must be job related. For example, the interviewer cannot ask about the person's age or ethnic background. Interviews should be conducted in a quiet and comfortable setting that ensures privacy. Interviews often begin with background questions that relate to the applicant's work experience and résumé and then move on to specific questions about skills and knowledge related to the position. Typical other questions include those about the individual's greatest strength, greatest weakness, future goals, educational goals, and (if applicable) leadership style.

### MOTIVATIONAL INTERVIEWING

Motivational interviewing (Miller, 1983) aims to help people identify and resolve issues regarding ambivalence toward change and focuses on the role of motivation to bring about change. Motivational interviewing is a collaborative approach in which the interviewer assesses the individual's readiness to accept change and identifies strategies that may be effective with the individual. Elements, principles, and strategies of motivational interviewing include the following:

| Elements | Principles | Strategies |
|---|---|---|
| • **Collaboration rather than confrontation in resolving issues.**<br>• **Evocation (drawing out) of the individual's ideas about change rather than imposition of the interviewer's ideas.**<br>• **Autonomy of the individual in making changes.** | • Expression of empathy: Showing understanding of individual's perceptions.<br>• Support of self-efficacy: Helping individuals realize they are capable of change.<br>• Acceptance of resistance: Avoiding struggles/conflicts with patient.<br>• Examination of discrepancies: Helping individuals see discrepancy between their behavior and goals. | • Avoiding Yes/No questions: Asking informational, open-ended questions.<br>• Providing affirmations: Indicating areas of strength.<br>• Providing reflective listening: Responding to statements.<br>• Providing summaries: Recapping important points of discussion.<br>• Encouraging change talk: Including desire, ability, reason, and need. |

## NEGOTIATION

Negotiating may be a formal process (such as negotiating with administration for increased benefits) or informal process (such as arriving at a team consensus), depending on the purpose and those involved. **Approaches** to negotiation include:

| | |
|---|---|
| **Competition** | In this approach, one party wins and the other loses, such as when parties feel their positions are non-negotiable and are unwilling to compromise. To prevail, one party must remain firm, but this can result in conflict. |
| **Accommodation** | One party concedes to the other, but the losing side may gain little or nothing, so this approach should be used when there is clear benefit to one choice. |
| **Avoidance** | When both parties dislike conflict, they may put off negotiating and resolve nothing so that the problems remain. |
| **Compromise** | Both parties make concessions in order to reach consensus, but this can result in decisions that suit no one, so compromise is not always the ideal solution. |
| **Collaboration** | Both parties receive what they want, a win-win solution, often through creative solutions, but collaboration may be ineffective with highly competitive parties. |

## POSTURES FOR NEGOTIATING

Negotiation is a transaction between two parties to reach a solution to a conflict, such as a contract disagreement. The two primary **postures for negotiating** include:

- **Distributive bargaining**: This is a contentious win-lose focus in which the parties begin with apparently irreconcilable differences. If one party assumes this posture, the other party is likely to follow suit, resulting in prolonged and difficult negotiations. In this situation, the belief is usually that there are limited resources, and each party wants a bigger share than the other. If one wins, the other loses. Parties often overstate demands to have negotiation room.
- **Integrative bargaining**: This is a win-win focus in which the parties' desires are not mutually exclusive, so both parties may be able to achieve objectives to some degree. Parties often collaborate on identifying problems and reaching solutions and tend to be more realistic about demands.

## STRIKES

One of the primary negotiation tactics when parties to a negotiation cannot reach an agreement is for one party (employees) to declare a **strike**, a right protected under the *Landrum-Griffin Act*. Types of strikes include:

- **Unfair labor practice**: With this type of strike in response to unfair labor practices, the NLRB will become involved, and the organization must take care to not interfere with the employees' right to strike. Participants are generally protected from losing employment.
- **Unprotected**: These include sit-down strikes, slow-downs, sickouts, partial walkouts, and strikes in violation of federal law. The law provides no protection, and participants may lose their jobs.
- **Economic**: This involves striking in support of bargaining demands, and the law provides limited protection from loss of jobs.
- **Sympathy**: Strikes in support of other workers who are on strikes. The law may or may not shield the participants from loss of jobs, depending on the circumstances.

# Staffing Fundamentals

## STAFFING MODELS
### PRIMARY CARE NURSING

Primary care nursing is a holistic staffing model in which one nurse is assigned as a primary nurse responsible for 24-hour a day care during the patient's hospitalization with associate nurses providing care when the primary nurse is not there. This model of care developed in the 1960s and 1970s as a method to ensure more holistic care. The primary nurse develops the plan of care with the patient and coordinates all aspects of care, serving much like a case manager. Additionally, the primary care nurse usually provides some direct care while on duty while some tasks are delegated to other nurses or unlicensed assistive personnel (UAP). Because primary care nursing is time-intensive, the caseload needs to be small (usually 3 to 4 patients). If the caseload is too large, then some of patient's needs may not be met. Patients are usually matched with the primary care nurse based on the nurse's skills and the patient's need rather than on geographic proximity on the unit.

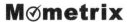

## TEAM NURSING

Team nursing is a staffing model in which a team of workers cares for a group of patients. Team nursing developed in the 1950s in response to a shortage of RNs. The team is led by a team leader, who is generally an RN. The team may include other RNs but is most often comprised of LVNs and UAPs. The team leader provides some care but delegates other aspects of care to members of the team. The duties are delegated according to the skills and expertise of the team members. The team leader remains ultimately responsible for supervision and for the care of the patients. This model of care is more cost-effective than some others because the percentage of RNs in the skill-mix tends to be lower, but RNs in the team other than the team leader may not be able to fully utilize their skills.

## MODULAR NURSING

Modular nursing is a recent staffing model that is an evolution of team nursing. With this model, a group of nurses provides care for a number of patients who are grouped geographically in a modular unit or district so that they are in close proximity. For example, a unit of 40 patients may be divided into 3 or 4 modules with sub-stations so that the team of nurses has easy access to patients. Patients may be placed in modules based on acuity. The same team of nurses is assigned to the same module to provide for consistency of care and development of cohesion as a team. The team is led by an RN but may include other RNs, LVNs, CNAs, and patient care technicians (PCTs) depending on the number of patients in the module. Modular nursing is more cost-effective than primary care nursing and is a response to the shortage of RNs. Hourly rounding is usually a component of modular nursing.

## TOTAL PATIENT CARE

Total patient care is a staffing model that developed in the 1990s. With total patient care, an RN is assigned to a small number of patients and provides care for the patients without assistance of other nursing personnel, such as CNAs, during the time the nurse is on duty. Unlike primary nursing, the nurse is not responsible for the patient 24 hours a day. The nurse is, however, responsible for all aspects of patient care, including administering medications, treatments, bathing, and toileting, during the time the nurse is caring for the patient. Because this staffing model is time-intensive, the nurse-patient ratio is usually quite low. Total patient care is a model often used in ICU and NICU where patients need almost constant attention of the RN, but it is used less frequently in other units because the costs are high, and care tends to focus on current needs rather than future goals.

## FUNCTIONAL NURSING

Functional nursing is one of the first staffing models used in nursing and remained common until the 1960s and is still in use in some facilities. With functional nursing, care is divided into different tasks and different nurses are assigned to these tasks. For example, medications may be passed by one nurse and treatments carried out by another, while bathing and personal care may be done by a CNA. Under this model, nursing care is efficient but impersonal and fragmented with little attempt to gain a holistic understanding of the patient and the patient's needs. Nurses tend to be very task oriented as they have narrow responsibilities. Nurses providing care document separately and report to a head nurse who makes assignments and is usually the individual that communicates with physicians and provides the hand-off reports at the end of shifts, based on input from those providing care, even though the head nurse usually has little actual contact with patients.

31

## PATIENT-CENTERED CARE

Patient-centered care is a staffing model used in acute care. Patients are aggregated not by diagnoses but by a similar need for care and services. Key elements of patient-centered care include the use of protocols or clinical pathways for clinical processes while customizing the nursing care plan according to the patient's needs and wishes. Staffing needs may vary according to the acuity level of the aggregate. Additionally, cross-training of staff is critical to ensure that staff members can assume different roles and have flexibility. While training adds value, it can also be time-consuming and costly, especially initially. All staff members, even housekeeping, are considered caregivers who must consider the needs, goals, and safety of the patient. Therefore, training must extend to all departments. Communication with the patient should be open and honest with the patient having ready access to the health record. The patient (and family) should be actively engaged in decision-making. The elements of patient-centered care include:

- Leadership commitment, including the Board of Directors and physicians
- Patient rounding
- Staff engagement
- Open communication
- Collaboration with patient
- Patient/Family feedback, focus groups, surveys, patient/family advisory councils
- Standards of service with clear outline of expectant behavior and inclusion of patient-centered/family-centered language
- Performance appraisal that includes commitment to patient/family-centered care

## FAMILY-CENTERED CARE

Family-centered care focuses on the needs and desires of the family and is a partnership model in which the family collaborates actively in the plan of care, such as when parents work with healthcare providers to determine the best course of treatment and care for their child or when adult children of a patient with Alzheimer's disease help to develop a plan of care. Important elements of family-centered care include:

- Open communication and sharing of information
- Showing respect for diversity
- Honoring preferences for care
- Working in a collaborative manner
- Recognizing that provision of care can be flexible
- Accommodating psychosocial needs

In the inpatient environment, family-centered rounds should be done at the bedside with both physicians and nurses while the family is present and can contribute. In the outpatient environment, which is quite varied, family should be included in all aspects of care, such as collaborating with the case manager or discussing care options with the emergency department staff.

## "12-BED HOSPITAL"

The "12-bed hospital" is a staffing model that is similar in some ways to modular nursing. Within a larger hospital, smaller 12 to 16-bed "hospitals" are created so that patients feel as though they are in a small hospital even though they have access to diagnostic and therapeutic services often only provided by large hospitals. Staffing includes an RN who serves as patient care facilitator for the mini-hospital and is accountable for patient care 24 hours a day (similar to primary care). Staff members on the interdisciplinary team are generally assigned permanently to the unit in order to provide continuity. The makeup of the team may vary depending on the acuity of the patients. The patient care facilitator serves as a mentor and educator to the interdisciplinary team in the unit in order to meet the performance goals. The patient care facilitator meets regularly with all team members and with patients and families.

## RATIO-BASED STAFFING MODELS

Nurse-patient ratios refer to the number of patients assigned to a nurse. For example, if one nurse is assigned responsibility for 4 patients, the ratio is 1:4. Ratios are an area of concern because studies have consistently shown better outcomes for patients with lower nurse-patient ratios. However, the lower the ratio, the higher the costs. Only the state of California currently has mandated nurse-patient ratios. The California law, often cited as a model, requires a 1:1 ratio in the operating room and for trauma patients in the ER, 1:2 in ICU, NICU, post-anesthesia recovery, labor and delivery, and ICU patients in the ER. Ratios in other areas range from 1:3 to 1:6 (the maximum). A number of other states require staffing committees to establish staffing policies, and some states require public reporting of nurse-patient ratios even though they do not mandate the ratios, so the nurse executive must be familiar with state requirements.

## ACUITY-BASED STAFFING MODELS

In the acuity-based staffing model, patients are assigned acuity levels, often by a point system. Various methods of assigning points are utilized.

- The **nursing workload management system** (NWMS) is a patient classification system (PCS) that provides automated collection of data (based on predetermined criteria) to indicate acuity level. The NWMS evaluates the patient holistically, including symptomology, conditions, coping ability, and adherence.
- The **Patient Intensity for Nursing Index** (PINI) is a classification system that considers both patient acuity and the need for nursing intervention. Each dimension has 10 different items that are scored on a scale of one to four. The acuity system used should facilitate the **five rights of staffing**: (1) right number of staff, (2) right skills, (3) right location, (4) right time, and (5) right patient assignments. Those patients with the highest scores require the most nursing care, so staffing is adjusted to reflect these needs.

Acuity-based staffing may require more flexibility than other models because more nurses may be assigned to serve as float nurses.

> **Review Video: Nurse Staffing Models**
> Visit mometrix.com/academy and enter code: 228282

## STAFFING WORKLOAD

Staffing workload can depend on the numbers of staff and patients, the nursing hours per patient day, the type of unit, and the acuity level of the patients. The nurse-patient ratio will, therefore, vary. For example, the nurse-patient ratio in ICU may be 1:1 or 1:2 but may be 1:5 on a general medical-surgical unit. The skill mix will also affect the workload. If staff is 100% RNs and the model is primary care, then the RN can manage fewer patients than if the skill mix includes LVNs and UAP to whom the RN can delegate tasks. Staffing may be done according to patient acuity. This requires assigning scores to patients based on various factors, including diagnosis, complications, and complexity of care, often using a software program. Patients with higher scores require more intense nursing than those with lower scores so staffing levels on a unit may vary widely, requiring a large group of float nurses.

## SKILL MATRIX

Skill mix is the proportion of RNs providing direct patient care (as opposed to indirect care, such as that of supervision) to total other direct care nursing staff (such as LVN/LPNs and UAP), expressed as a percentage. Skill mix is an important consideration in staffing. If, for example, a unit has 50 FTE staff budgeted with 35 RNs, 8 LVNs, and 7 UAP, the RN skill mix would be 70%:

$$\frac{35}{35 + 8 + 7} = \frac{35}{50} = 70\%$$

If the skill mix is too low, it may have an adverse effect on patient outcomes and nursing and patient satisfaction, but if it is too high, the costs may be prohibitive. Staffers must attempt to provide a skill mix that is appropriate for the needs of the unit. For example, a critical care unit is likely to require a different skill mix than a general post-operative unit.

## RECRUITING STAFF

In a time of nursing shortage, **recruiting staff** can be challenging, so it's important for the recruitment officer to ensure that the organization is competitive. Recruitment considerations include:

- **Emphasis on quality**: Advertisements should stress the organization's efforts at quality improvement and high standards of care.
- **Orientation program**: Extended orientation programs that include mentoring and special programs for new graduates are especially attractive.
- **Partnership with nursing schools**: Graduate nurses often seek employment in hospitals in which they have trained because they know the staff and are familiar with the organizational culture.
- **Welcoming culture**: Engage key stakeholders throughout the organization in providing a supportive environment for new hires.
- **Competitive salary/benefit packages**: Recruitment bonuses may also benefit recruitment efforts.
- **Flexible work schedules**: 8-hour to 12-hour shifts.
- **Role advancement**: Incentive and support should be available for continuing education and career advancement.
- **Employee assistance program**: These programs suggest a caring environment.

## RECOGNIZING STAFF

Recognizing staff for their achievements or expertise is a form of positive reinforcement. While salary increases and job promotions are the primary methods of indicating appreciation for staff, because of the costs involved, these forms of recognition are limited. However, staff recognition can be carried out in a number of other ways:

- Ask staff members to **report on their achievements** to upper management or the Board of Directors
- Provide **acknowledgment** through various means, such as "Employee of the month"
- Establish a staff appreciation program
- **Verbally praise** employees' efforts
- Award certificates of achievement
- Provide a suggestion box
- Ask staff for **nominations** for employee awards
- Write a **letter of appreciation** to worthy employees

- Ask employees to serve on an **advisory or other committee**
- Ask employees with expertise to **mentor** other staff members
- Establish a formal **employee recognition program** with annual awards
- Establish professional **weeks of recognition**, such as "Nurse's Week" in the organization

## RETAINING STAFF

Nursing has been plagued with a shortage of personnel, which poses a risk to patient care, and high rates of turnover with attendant costs in orienting and training new staff. **Retention** is, therefore, a critical concern. Retention estimates can be made through assessing potential retirements and conducting a staff satisfaction survey to identify problem areas. Key elements to staff retention include:

- Providing competitive salaries and benefits
- Establishing thorough orientation program, including mentoring
- Developing support and preceptor programs for new graduate nurses
- Providing flexible work schedules
- Offering health and wellness programs
- Ensuring adequate staffing
- Providing staff training and career development programs
- Hiring recently-retired staff for consultant or part-time work
- Offering educational incentives, such as tuition assistance, to promote advancement and certification
- Encouraging collaboration and team building as well as nursing autonomy and decision-making
- Recognizing professional excellence

## SUCCESSION PLANNING

The first step in succession planning should be to describe the behaviors, skills, and leadership qualities necessary for the role. The next steps include outlining the needs of the organization and developing a formal written succession plan. An organization should have plans in place for both emergency and planned succession. An internal candidate is usually selected for emergency succession because of the need for someone to immediately step into the position and to be familiar with the organizational structure and current demands of the position. The chosen candidate usually fulfills the position on a temporary basis until planned succession can occur. Plans for succession should always be in place so that transitions are not disruptive to the organization. Planned succession may focus on both internal and external candidates, depending on the needs of the organization.

# Employee Performance Management

## JOB DESCRIPTION

A job description should describe the duties, responsibilities, and skills required for a position. The job description usually begins with the job title, place of employment, and a brief description of the position. If appropriate, there may be a statement indicating to whom the person reports and a statement about the scope or territory encompassed in the position. This is followed by a listing of the job responsibilities. When creating the job description, a list of job duties should be created, prioritized, and condensed into 10 to 15 bulleted items. The list should avoid specific targets, such as "reduce infections by 50%." The job description should also include requirements, such as academic preparation and work experience, and benefits (vacation, sick time, retirement plans).

The salary range should be included as well as any collective bargaining agreements. Language should be unbiased (avoiding "he/she"). If the job listing is to be placed online, then including key words is essential.

## NEW OR EXPANDED JOB DESCRIPTIONS

At one time roles changed very little over the years, but with rapid changes in healthcare, this is no longer the case. **New or expanded job descriptions** are commonplace. For example, nurses now must be computer literate in order to utilize electronic health records and other technology. New job descriptions should be developed when there are significant changes in a job while expanded job descriptions may be developed if there are simple additions. New job descriptions are needed when there are changes in the skills needed, experience, or qualifications for a position. Those writing the job description should review other job descriptions for comparable internal or external positions and solicit input from key stakeholders, such as unit supervisors and staff members. Accurate job descriptions are essential in order to recruit the best candidates; additionally, job descriptions can be used to guide training, orientation programs, and performance evaluation.

## CREDENTIALING AND PRIVILEGING

Credentialing is the process by which a person's credentials to provide patient care are obtained, verified, and assessed in accordance with organizational bylaws, which may vary from one organization to another. **Privileging** follows the credentialing process and grants the individual authority to practice within the organization. Decisions regarding credentialing and privileging are usually done by members of a credentials committee although some organizations use internet services to verify credentials. Part of credentialing and privileging is to determine what credentials are necessary for different positions, based on the following:

- Professional standards, such as those of the American Nurses Association
- Licensure
- Regulatory guidelines, such as state requirements
- Accreditation guidelines

Other considerations include best practices, economic considerations, malpractice insurance coverage, disciplinary actions, and organizational needs. Policies for privileging should be in place to allow for temporary staff privileges for special circumstances or for emergencies. State regulations may vary from one state to another.

## CORE CRITERIA

There are many considerations for credentialing and privileging. Some of the considerations are internal organizational considerations that do not involve the quality of the applicant. However, some considerations focus only on the applicant. There are four primary **core criteria**:

- **Licensure**: This must be current through the appropriate state board, such as the state board of nursing.
- **Education**: This includes training and experience appropriate for the credential and may include technical training, professional education, residencies, internships, fellowships, doctoral and post-doctoral programs, and board and clinical certifications.
- **Competence**: Evaluations and recommendations by peers regarding clinical competence and judgment provide information about how the person applies knowledge.
- **Performance ability**: The person should have demonstrated ability to perform the duties to which the credentialing/privileging applies.

36

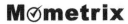

## CERTIFICATION

Certification is a form of professional credentialing that is part of role delineation and is voluntary on the part of the nurse but represents increased education and/or clinical expertise. Certification may be acquired from a large number of different organizations and is monitored by the **American Board of Nursing Specialties**. ANCC, for example, offers a wide range of certificates for nurse practitioners and clinical nurse specialists, such as Adult Care Nurse Practitioner, as well as specialty certifications, such as Ambulatory Care Nursing and Cardiac-Vascular Nursing. Some certification boards provide only one type of certification. For example, the Certification Board of Infection Control and Epidemiology, Inc., provides only the Certification in Infection Control (CIC). Each certification has specific requirements that may include educational preparation/degree, clinical experience, and passing a certifying exam. Certification is for a specified period of time and various requirements are in place for recertification, such as completing continuing nursing education and employment in the area of certification.

## CROSS TRAINING

Cross training is a method employed by many organizations to increase the efficiency and proficiency of staff and to alleviate inadequate staffing resulting from employee absenteeism. When cross training is properly utilized and implemented, staff members are trained to perform more than one job. Generally, staff members who perform similar jobs are trained to cover each other's duties and positions in the event of unexpected illness or vacations. However, knowledge can fossilize, so the manager must rotate staff members to keep them proficient. In the event of an employee termination, cross training empowers the facility to do a thorough search for a new employee while the tasks of the unfilled position are still being completed. The nurse executive often uses an accordion schedule that automatically compresses down to accommodate multiple absences on the unit without compromising essential individual care.

## PERFORMANCE MANAGEMENT

Performance management is the process by which performance is assessed in order to ensure that goals are met effectively. Performance management may be directed at an individual, group, or the organization as a whole. There are three primary steps to performance management:

- **Developing a performance plan**: Review the job description with the individuals and develop 3 to 5 goals with the expected outcomes, measurements, and timeframes delineated.
- **Coaching**: This includes providing ongoing feedback, both positive and negative, to help guide goal attainment. Coaching requirements may vary widely among different individuals, but a coaching plan should include the frequency of required meetings. Coaching should focus on priorities, behaviors, and work, and corrections should be provided in a positive manner.
- **Assessing**: Assessment depends on the performance plan and the coaching but should be carried out at least annually with all items in the assessment completed jointly with the individual being assessed.

## MENTORING

The most common **model for mentoring** is that of a partnership with the mentor providing the expertise and with the mentee utilizing this expertise through learning, action, and reflection. There are a number of steps involved in the mentor-mentee relationship:

1. **Mentor selection**: In some cases, a formal mentor program may be in effect at an institution, but in other cases the mentee may need to identify a candidate for mentor, based on mutual respect. Generally, a mentor should not be a direct supervisor as this can present conflicts. The mentor may be a peer or a nurse in an advanced position.
2. **Determine expectations**: Ground rules should be established, such as when and how frequently to meet.
3. **Competency development**: The mentee works toward specific goals in learning with the guidance of the mentor.
4. **Guidance gives way to consultation**: As the mentee gains confidence and skills, the mentor provides assistance on request, providing the mentee more independence.
5. **Mentorship resolves**.

## PRECEPTING

The nurse is often in the position of having many roles in clinical practice, including educating others and serving as a **preceptor** for graduate students who are studying to enter the field. While mentoring may entail a long-term relationship, precepting is usually a time-limited arrangement related to a term of study, such as a semester, orientation period, or a clinical rotation. The nurse must balance responsibilities and ensure that he or she is able to provide adequate clinical supervision and guidance to the student on a daily basis. This may require coordinating schedules and planning carefully to ensure all responsibilities can be met. The nurse preceptor helps the student to understand his or her impact on the spheres of influence (individual/client, nurse and nurse practice, and organization/system) by including the student in all nursing activities. The preceptor may engage in shared care as well as direct supervision in order to improve the student's skills.

## COACHING

Coaching is an important part of precepting. Coaching can include specific training, providing career information, and confronting issues of concern. While individual safety is the primary consideration, coaching should be done in a manner that increases learner confidence and ability to self-monitor rather than in a punitive or critical manner. The nurse executive must develop confidence in his or her own ability to be assertive and confront issues directly in order to resolve conflicts and promote collaboration. Effective methods of coaching include:

- Giving **positive feedback**, stressing what the student is doing right
- Using **questioning** to help the student recognize problem areas
- Providing **demonstrations** and opportunities for question-and-answer periods
- Providing regular **progress reports** so the student understands areas of concern
- Assisting the student to establish **personal goals** for improvement
- Providing **resources** to help the student master material

## MEASURING CURRENT PERFORMANCE

Measuring current performance requires establishing benchmarks against which progress can be charted. Whatever the process is going to be, the current process must be accurately traced and outlined. A baseline may be established by measuring where an organization is at a point in time or period of time, such as the number of readmissions averaged each month in the previous year. State or national data may also be used to establish benchmarks. Sources for this data include Hospital Compare, Becker's Hospital Review, CMS, AHRQ, Healthcare Effectiveness Data and Information Set (HEDIS), and National Committee for Quality Assurance. Insurance companies may also provide data. A healthcare organization may also use local data, such as from similar hospitals in the same area, to set benchmarks. Once metrics are chosen, the frequency of measurement and the responsibility for measuring must be determined.

## PERFORMANCE APPRAISAL

Performance appraisal is used to confirm hiring, promote, train, or reward staff. It may be done at some point in the first 6 months of employment and on an annual basis and should be primarily based on the person's job description, which should include expectations and goals related to performance. The written appraisal should indicate compliance with performance expectations. The appraisal may include a rating scale, checklist, productivity studies, and narrative. The appraisal should be discussed with the individual so the person is able to respond to the feedback received. As part of the appraisal process, the individual should establish new goals, based on findings from performance improvement measures and related to strategic plans of the organization. Performance appraisal evaluation standards include:

- Clear objective standards
- Criteria for promotions and pay raises
- Conditions for termination
- Time allowed and procedures to correct deficiencies

## PROFESSIONAL DEVELOPMENT

Professional development is essential to keep up with roles based on changing needs in the healthcare environment. The individual needs to identify and prioritize needs, make a plan, carry out the activities outlined in the plan, and evaluate outcomes. Professional development activities may include:

- **Specialized training (task oriented)**: This may include training for specific tasks, such as cardiac monitoring. Specialized training may be conducted in-house through job shadowing and peer training.
- **Continuing nursing education**: Courses may be state mandated or selected according to need and interest to further knowledge and skills.
- **Academic progression**: This may include bridge programs, BSN, MSN, and doctorate in nursing practice or other degree programs, such as management.
- **Certification**: Application for certification usually requires some combination of academic work and experience as well as passing a certification exam.
- **Research**: Active clinical or other research is a valid learning experience. The results of research may be published or presented at conferences.

## CLINICAL STAFF DEVELOPMENT
### PLANNING FOR CLINICAL STAFF DEVELOPMENT

Planning for the development of clinical staff begins with assessment of the current status of staff, including issues such as skill mix, empowerment, diversity, and motivation. The nurse executive must assess the needs of the organization as well in terms of current staffing and levels of education as well as review patient data. The nurse executive should also project future needs in order to determine the focus of staff development. Once a list of needs is compiled, the nurse executive can work with staff development nurses to develop programs that meet those needs. For example, if the skill mix shows a shortage of RNs, the organization may partner with a nursing degree program to provide a bridge program for LVNs/LPNs to advance to BSNs. If patient data show high rates of infection, then training may focus on infection control. Employees should be encouraged to establish personal goals, and staff development should assist the employees in attaining those goals.

## ORIENTATION

When developing an **orientation program**, the nursing professional development specialist should first meet with department administrators to gain valuable insight and information, to show respect for their positions and experience, and to gain cooperation. However, the specialist cannot depend solely on the administrators' suggestions but should follow up with various types of needs assessments, including literature research, observation, interviews, surveys, and reviews of similar orientation programs. Expected outcomes should be identified in the process. Some orientation programs are primarily classroom based with reviews of policies, procedures, and equipment, but many nurses feel overwhelmed when orientation ends, especially new graduates who may lack the experience necessary to work autonomously. For that reason, orientation often includes an ongoing mentoring program to provide support for nurses and the opportunity to benefit and learn from the expertise of others. Formal mentoring programs usually establish one-on-one mentoring relationships rather than the more informal mentoring that occurs when one nurse assists another.

## CONTINUING EDUCATION

Continuing education is that education and training required to remain current in the nursing profession and is an obligation of all those in the field of nursing. Employers may require continuing education for employment and may, in some instances, specify the specific course or type of courses. Continuing education requirements for renewal of an RN license (regardless of the type of program) are established by individual states and vary widely. Some states require no continuing education. Other states require a minimum number of units (one contact hour per unit), often 20-30 units for each licensing period, typically every 2 years. Some states specify certain courses that must be taken for license renewal, such as End-of-Life or HIV/AIDS. Providers of continuing education courses must be approved by state boards of nursing to ensure they meet minimum standards. Continuing education courses may be delivered in traditional classroom settings, via the internet, or with self-study written/video/audio materials.

### EVALUATING CONTINUING EDUCATION CREDITS

When evaluating activities for continuing education credits, the activities should first be evaluated to determine if they meet the ANCC provider design criteria. Continuing education should:

- Address gaps in professional practice
- Include a nurse planner in the planning process
- Be based on needs assessment
- Identify one or more learning outcomes
- Use appropriate teaching strategies
- Base information on evidence-based practice
- Evaluate learning outcomes
- Be free of commercial influence

The nurse planner should determine what the target audience is for the CNE, and develop the learning outcomes. Educational content may be selected by the nurse planner or other presenter, but the nurse planner is responsible for ensuring content is evidence-based and involves learner engagement.

## COMPETENCY VALIDATION

The first task in competency validation is to select the criteria that will be used to determine competency. Criteria may be selected by review of certification requirements, literature, course content, and job descriptions. The nursing professional development specialist should develop a rubric that lists expected competencies and a range of possible scores (such as 1 to 4) indicating the degree of competence with explanations for each score. In some cases, if specific tasks are part of the competency validation, then a checklist should be prepared to guide the individual and to ensure that all tasks are completed as part of the individual's evaluation. Then, the person responsible for completing the competency validation should be selected. In some cases, the individual may be asked to do a self-evaluation; otherwise, the competency validation should be completed in collaboration with the individual.

## PEER REVIEW

Peer review is an intensive process in which an individual practitioner is reviewed by like practitioners. It may be used for an individual practitioner or a group of individuals and often relates to data found as part of root cause analysis, infection control, or other surveillance measures. Peer review is usually conducted within the specified department by a committee. A **ranking system** is usually used to indicate compliance with standards:

1. Care is based on standards and typical of that provided by like practitioners.
2. Variance may occur in care, but outcomes are satisfactory.
3. Care is not consistent with that provided by like practitioners.
4. Variance resulted in negative outcomes.

In some cases, this ranking system is not used and is replaced with a series of questions, with affirmative answers indicating cause for concern.

# Employee Engagement Strategies

## STAFF EMPOWERMENT

Power is the ability to take action even when others are resistant, but **empowerment** refers to a psychological state in which one feels that personal competence is recognized and valued. A person who is empowered is allowed and encouraged to exercise power. Empowerment includes self-determination about aspects of work and recognition by others of competence and the impact of the person's decisions. Empowerment requires that the nurse executive share power to some degree. According to Kanter (1977), the three structures that are essential for empowerment are:

- **Opportunity**: Includes opportunities for advancement and job enrichment.
- **Power**: Derives from access to information, necessary resources, and administrative support.
- **Proportion**: The social composition of the employee workforce, including ethnic minorities.

All employees should have access to education and training that promote empowerment. In the relational approach to empowerment, power is decentralized and authority delegated. In the motivational approach, there is less actual sharing of power, but the focus is on encouraging and training employees to utilize problem-solving approaches and to increase self-efficacy.

## STAFF ADVOCACY

### *ADVOCATING FOR A HEALTHY WORK ENVIRONMENT*

The nurse executive should be a strong **advocate for a healthy work environment**. A healthy work environment is one in which the nurse executive considers both physical and psychological needs.

**Physical considerations** include:

- **Air quality**: No smoking policies and adequate filtering and air exchanges
- **Temperature**: Heating and air-conditioning to maintain safe and comfortable temperature
- **Hazards**: Policies for handling, storing, and disposing of hazardous waste materials
- **Safety**: Lifts to move patients, safety rails, fire alarms and fire extinguishers, adequate maintenance of equipment and facility

**Psychological** considerations include:

- **Fair and equitable treatment of staff**: Equity in pay, fair and adequate scheduling, open-door policy, grievance procedures
- **Protection from lateral violence, bullying**: No tolerance policies in place, staff education
- **Staff empowerment**: Shared decision-making, self-determination, consultation, and collaboration
- **Well-being**: Incentives and rewards, emotional support, employee assistance programs

### *ADVOCATING FOR EQUIPMENT*

Equipment is costly, but staff members must have the equipment they need in order to do their jobs well and safely. For example, lifts should be available to move patients in order to prevent back injuries. There are a number of issues to consider in relation to equipment: cost of equipment, use, life expectancy, and benefits. New equipment and upgrades are constantly available, but the nurse executive must consider if they are simply new or better, and if they are better, in what way? Does the equipment, for example, save time, reduce discomfort, increase safety, or prevent injury? How easy is the equipment to use? How much training is involved? What future costs may be incurred (such as for upgrades and service contracts)? Before a major investment in new equipment, a pilot study should be conducted with the equipment. The nurse executive should consider standardization of equipment whenever possible because that makes training easier and buying in bulk is often a cost-saving measure.

## STAFFING MANAGEMENT ISSUES

Staffing management involves both clinical staff (such as nurses) and nonclinical staff (such as housekeeping staff and office personnel). Issues include:

- Workforce size and distribution, including full-time equivalent staff members (one or a combination of more than one staff member who works 80 hours in 14 days) needed
- Educational resources (training programs), availability of trained personnel (including professional staff and support staff)
- Staff training and ongoing need for staff development and opportunities for certification or advancement
- Demographics: Population (age, economic levels, ethnic backgrounds, lifestyles) affects the need for care
- Incentives for career advancement, including increases in income, promotion, and certification

42

- Staff turnover/burnout and ongoing need for recruitment
- Organizational structure
- Financial resources available
- Cost-effective staffing, billable provision of care
- Reimbursement (Medicare, Medicaid, health insurance, private pay)
- Supervision/feedback
- Strategies for staffing (organization-wide)

## EMPLOYEE ASSISTANCE AND COUNSELING

An employee assistance program (EAP) is part of the benefit package offered employees in many organizations. The purpose of the program is to assist employees with personal or work-related problems that interfere with their ability to carry out their jobs. While EAPs vary, they usually include counseling services and referrals. Supportive services may be available for PTSD, workplace violence, substance abuse, domestic violence, occupational stress, emotional stress, financial issues, legal concerns, and life events (births, deaths, illness, disability). Participation in an employee assistance program is usually voluntary and free of cost (although there may be costs associated with referrals), and participation remains confidential in order to encourage those with problems to take advantage of the program. With some programs, the services are also available to immediate family members. EAPs are available in federal and state agencies as well as in the private sector.

# Team Performance Management

## ORGANIZATIONAL STRUCTURE

### CHAIN OF COMMAND

The Joint Commission has established leadership standards that apply to healthcare organizations and help to establish management's **chain of command** and accountability. Under these standards, leadership comprises the governing body, chief executive officer, nurse executive, and senior managers, department leaders, leaders (both elected and appointed) of staff or departments, and other nurse leaders as well as team members and support staff. The governing body is ultimately responsible for all patient care rendered by all types of practitioners (physicians, nurses, laboratory staff, and support staff) within and under the jurisdiction of the organization, so this governing body must clearly outline the line of authority and accountability for others in management positions. At each level of management, performance standards and performance measurements should be established so that accountability becomes transparent based on data that can be used to drive changes when needed to bring about improved outcomes.

### ORGANIZATIONAL CHART

An organizational chart is a diagram that shows the structure of an organization, indicating the relationship of one unit or department to another and showing the chain of command. The three most common types of organizational charts are hierarchical with the position of power at the top and those below in descending order.

- In the **matrix format**, management may be listed at the top but then each different department or unit is listed on an equal basis.
- The **horizontal format** is similar to the matrix but the chain of command is very limited and department managers are fairly autonomous.

43

- **Committee structure** varies from one organization to another but typically includes an executive committee and a number of subcommittees with responsibility for projects, departments, or concerns.
  - *Ad hoc* **committees** are temporary committees formed to carry out a specific project or task as opposed to standing committees, which are permanent.

## SPAN OF CONTROL

Span of control indicates the number of individuals a person supervises or receives reports from within an organization. This term is most useful in a hierarchical organization with a clear chain of command because the supervisory role is often more difficult to delineate in a nonhierarchical structure, such as one with multiple cross-functional teams.

- A **wide span of control** (large number of subordinates) is common when workers are involved in routine work because the need for supervision is minimal.
- However, with very complex tasks, a **narrow span of control** is usually necessary. The spans of control may vary from department to department in an organization, so viewing the span of control in terms of an average may be misleading.

Factors to consider when determining the span of control include the size of the organization, the skills of the workers, the culture of the organization, and the training and responsibilities of the supervisors.

## INFLUENCE AND POWER

Sources of influence and power within an organization may differ from the chain of command. The different types of power include:

- **Positional**: Most closely corresponds to the chain of command because it refers to legitimate power derived from a supervisory position, but the degree of power varies according to where the person lies in the hierarchy and the number of subordinates.
- **Expert**: Related to an individual with necessary knowledge and skills. This person may wield considerable power if the knowledge and skills are critical, but the power is only within the framework of the person's expertise.
- **Referent**: Based on charisma and the ability to influence others. Those with referent power may wield influence and power far beyond that expected by those in their positions.
- **Coercive**: Based on behavioral tactics, which can include coercion and bullying as well as withholding rewards.
- **Reward**: Associated with the ability to grant rewards, such as salary increases or gifts.

## ORGANIZATIONAL CULTURE

### JUST CULTURE

While it is common practice to blame the individual responsible for committing an error, in a **just culture**, the practice is to look at the bigger picture and to try to determine what characteristics of the system are at fault, leading to the error. For example, there may be inadequate staffing, excessive overtime, unclear orders, mislabeling, or other problems that contribute. A just culture considers the need to change the system rather than the individual and differentiates among the following:

- **Human error**: Inadvertent actions, mistakes, or lapses in proper procedure: Management includes considering processes, procedures, training, and/or design to determine the cause of the error and consoling the person.

- **At-risk behavior**: An unjustified risk or choice. Management includes providing incentives for correct behavior and disincentives for incorrect, and coaching the person.
- **Reckless behavior**: The conscious disregard for proper procedures. Management includes remedial action and/or punitive action.

## TRANSPARENCY

Qualities that are essential to transparency within an organization are information disclosure, clarity, and accuracy. Everyone in the organization should be provided full information and encouraged to have input into what works and what doesn't work within the organization. The administration should welcome questions and reward honesty in those coming forward with concerns. Transparency can include being open about salaries, ownership, and transactions. A transparent organization often has formal shared governance or partnership councils to facilitate sharing of ideas and participation at all levels. Senior administrative support is critical to transparency as mechanisms for dissemination of information must be instituted and leaders prepared to respond to questions. The organization must be open about cost-benefit analyses and return on investment and should provide people with both positive and negative updates. Administrators should conduct employee rounding on a regular basis to encourage participation and may have communication boards to share information readily.

## SHARED GOVERNANCE

Shared governance implies shared decision making, but this can be realized in different ways. A common form of shared governance is for the administration to allow autonomous decision making by specific departments, teams, or groups within an organization regarding issues that apply to them or are within their area of expertise. For example, a unit team may have the authority to establish work schedules for that unit only, and members of a professional development team may be able to make decisions regarding professional development activities. In some cases, shared governance committees communicate with administration and can affect decision-making but do not make the final decision. Members of shared governance teams or groups may be tasked with specific duties, such as developing new policies or procedures related to evidence-based best practices. Shared governance has primarily involved nursing personnel in most organizations.

## PARTNERSHIP

Partnership councils represent an evolution of shared governance, which focuses primarily on nursing. Partnership councils have members from all levels and areas within an organization. Thus, a partnership council may include all disciplines, such as nursing, laboratory, and housekeeping, and all departments. Partnership councils usually exist at different levels in an organization, so there may be department or unit partnership councils as well as a central partnership council that serves as an advisory board and shares decision making with administration. Usually one member (most often a chairperson) of each unit or department partnership council becomes a representative on the central council so that communication moves both horizontally and vertically. This type of sharing of information and ideas helps to promote decision-making that considers the system needs as well as the unit needs.

## PERSONAL ACCOUNTABILITY

Personal accountability is the obligation to assume responsibility for one's own acts. This includes understanding the legal ramifications of actions, including supervision. Accountability is an issue in delegation, because the person who delegates is personally accountable for the appropriateness of delegation and the subsequent supervision of the delegated task. The 5 rights of delegation include:

- **Right task**: The nurse should determine an appropriate task to delegate for a specific individual.
- **Right circumstance**: The nurse has considered the setting, resources, time factors, safety factors, and all other relevant information to determine the appropriateness of delegation.
- **Right person**: The nurse is in the right position to choose the right person (by virtue of education/skills) to perform a task for the right individual.
- **Right direction**: The nurse provides a clear description of the task, the purpose, any limits, and expected outcomes.
- **Right supervision**: The nurse is able to supervise, intervene as needed, and evaluate performance of the task.

## CIVILITY

Civility is treating others with respect and consideration. Lack of civility is an increasing problem in the workplace. Complaints of rudeness, insults, being ignored, and unfair treatment are common between different professional groups (such as physicians and nurses) as well as between members of the same profession (such as nurses) and can result in a toxic work environment and increased staff turnover. Steps to creating a civil organizational culture include:

- **Recognizing the problem**: Observations and surveys may help to discover the perception of the extent of incivility.
- **Establishing clear behavioral and communication codes of conduct** that apply to all members of the organization. Unacceptable behavior (hazing, eye rolling, sarcasm, lateral violence, bullying and other negative behaviors) should be clearly outlined.
- **Modeling civil behavior** from the top down.
- **Training organization members** at all levels in communication strategies and conflict resolution.
- **Addressing offenders**: A zero-tolerance policy should be in place.

## PROFESSIONAL PRACTICE MODELS

### INTERDISCIPLINARY COLLABORATION

Interdisciplinary collaboration is absolutely critical to nursing practice if the needs and best interests of the individuals and families are central. Interdisciplinary practice begins with the nurse and physician but extends to pharmacists, social workers, occupational and physical therapists, nutritionists, and a wide range of allied healthcare providers, all of whom cooperate in diagnosis and treatment. State regulations, however, determine to some degree how much autonomy a nurse can have in diagnosing and treating. While nurses have increasingly gained more legal rights, they have also become more dependent upon collaboration with others for their expertise and for referrals if the individual's needs extend beyond the nurse's ability to provide assistance. Additionally, the prescriptive ability of nurses varies from state to state, with some requiring direct supervision by other disciplines (such as physicians) while others require particular types of supervisory arrangements, depending upon the circumstances.

## MASSACHUSETTS GENERAL HOSPITAL PROFESSIONAL PRACTICE MODEL

The Massachusetts General Hospital professional practice model is a patient-centered model with 9 elements to ensure cohesive and effective interdisciplinary care of the patient:

- **Patient centeredness**: Relationship-based care, stresses the importance of continuity of care and patient advocacy
- **Vision and values**: Direct the provision of care
- **Standards of nursing practice**: State Nurse Practice Act and other national standards serve as guides
- **Narrative culture**: Shared stories
- **Professional nursing development**: Includes thorough orientation and ongoing education as well as internal and external consultation with nurse experts and ready access to clinical reference materials
- **Clinical recognition and role advancement**: Flexible staffing based on acuity and volume, encouragement and support for role advancement and lifelong learning
- **Collaboration** in decision-making
- **Research**
- **Interdisciplinary teams** that demonstrate innovation and entrepreneurship

In this model, the ultimate responsibility and accountability for patient care rests with the RN with standards guided by the state Nurse Practice Act, if applicable, and national standards.

## RELATIONSHIP-BASED CARE MODEL

Relationship-based care (Koloroutis) is a professional practice model that is intended to transform care by focusing on three primary relationships of the nurse or care provider:

- Patients and families
- Self
- Colleagues

This model supports the idea that establishing positive relationships and effective modes of communication can positively affect patient outcomes. Healthcare providers actively engage with and support patients and family members. Patient care is provided by designated healthcare providers (including RN and physician) to ensure continuity of care. Healthcare providers should have the knowledge and tools to handle stress and to recognize their own needs, including finding a good work-life balance. Novice staff members should be mentored in order to improve their skills and level of confidence, and patients and family should participate collaboratively in their plans of care. Open communication and respect among all members of the team are essential for provision of care.

## SYNERGY MODEL

The synergy model of nursing practice, developed by the ACCN for nursing certification, places the needs of the patient as a central focus and defines the relationship between 8 patient characteristics and 8 nurse competencies. These competencies and characteristics are evaluated on a scale (1-5). Patient characteristics include resiliency, vulnerability, stability, complexity, resource availability, participation in care, participation in decision-making, and predictability. Nurse competencies include clinical judgment, advocacy, caring practices, collaboration, systems thinking, response to diversity, clinical inquiry, and facilitation of learning. The system or healthcare environment is the third element of the model. It provides support for the needs of the patients and empowers and nurtures the practice of nursing, caring, and ethical practice. All three of these systems are essential for synergy. The needs of the patient are the driving force for nurse competencies and both are dependent on the healthcare system. When the needs, competencies, and system complement each other, synergy is achieved, and outcomes for the nurse, the patient, and the system are optimized.

## DIFFERENTIATED NURSING PRACTICE

Differentiated nursing practice is a professional practice model in which responsibilities for patient care are differentiated according to level of education, competence, and/or clinical expertise. This model initially promoted the development of associate degree programs of nursing with the concept that the AS-prepared nurse would provide patient care under supervision of a BSN. Most differentiated nursing practice is currently based on **education** alone with a hierarchy that begins with the APN, then to the BSN, to the AS RN, the LPN/LVN, and the UAP. Differentiated nursing practice is in common use even if not stated formally by an organization. Differentiated nursing practice makes the best use of the knowledge and skills of the nurses and can be most cost-effective, but the mindset that "a nurse is a nurse" despite differences in educational preparation has been difficult for the profession to overcome.

## JEAN WATSON'S PHILOSOPHY OF HUMAN CARING

Jean Watson developed the philosophy of human caring in 1979. Watson focused on transpersonal caring, which views the individual holistically from the perspective of the interrelationship among health, sickness, and behavior with a nursing goal to promote health and prevent illness. Watson's theory encompasses 10 **caritas** (methods of caring) the nurse can employ during caring occasions (opportunities to provide care) and caring moments (actions). The 10 caritas include:

- Having loving kindness and equanimity
- Being present and sustaining the spiritual beliefs of individual and self
- Cultivating personal spiritual practice
- Developing and maintaining a caring relationship
- Supporting both negative and positive feelings of the individual
- Being creative in caring
- Providing teaching-learning experiences within the individual's frame of reference
- Creating a physical and spiritual healing environment
- Providing for basic human needs
- Being open to spiritual concepts related to life and death of the self and the individual

## HILDEGARD PEPLAU'S INTERPERSONAL RELATIONS MODEL OF NURSING

Hildegard Peplau developed the interpersonal relations model of nursing in 1952, focusing on the quality of nurse-client interaction. Peplau believed that individuals deserved human care by educated nurses and should be treated with dignity and respect. She also believed that the environment (social, psychosocial, and physical) could affect health in a positive or negative manner. Peplau viewed the nurse as a person who could make a substantial difference for the individual and who acts as a "maturing force." The nurse can focus on the way in which individuals react to their illness and can help individuals to use illness as an opportunity for learning and maturing through the nurse-client interactions. The nurse helps the individual to understand the nature of his/her problem and to find solutions. Peplau's theory stresses the importance of collaboration between the client and the nurse. The nurse-client relationship is viewed as a number of overlapping phases: orientation, identification of problem, explanation of potential solutions, and resolution of problem.

## DOROTHEA OREM'S GENERAL THEORY OF NURSING

Dorothea Orem developed a general theory of nursing in 1959. Orem believed that the goal of nursing was to serve patients and assist them to provide self-care through 3 steps: identifying the reason a patient needs care, planning for delivery of care, and managing care. Within Orem's theory is the concept of the self-care agent (the individual) and the dependent care agent (the caregiver or, in many circumstances, the nurse). Orem's theory is actually a collection of 3 theories:

- **Self-care**: This refers to the ability of the individual to care for their personal needs. There are 3 categories of needs, consisting of universal needs (food, air), developmental needs (from maturation or events), and health needs (from illness, injury).
- **Self-care deficit**: This occurs if the self-care agent cannot provide for his or her own care and requires a dependent care agent. Nursing assists through 5 means: providing care, guiding, instructing, supporting, and adjusting the environment to aid the patient in self-care.
- **Nursing systems**: Actions to meet patient's self-care needs may be completely compensatory (patient is dependent), partly compensatory (patient can provide some self-care), or supportive (patient needs assistance or support to provide self-care).

## IDA JEAN ORLANDO'S NURSING PROCESS THEORY

Ida Jean Orlando developed the nursing process theory of nursing in the late 1950s and published them in 1961 in *The Dynamic Nurse-Patient Relationship*, based on her observations of what comprises good or bad nursing care. She theorized that the nursing process includes:

- **The behavior of the patient**: Behavior is an indication of need, which may be expressed directly or through actions.
- **The nurse's reaction**: The nurse must evaluate the needs of the patient based on their own perception and evaluation of this perception, exploring with the patient the meaning of the patient's behavior.
- **The subsequent nursing actions**: Actions are based on the nurse determining the nature of the patient's real needs (which may be different than expressed) and finding the appropriate action to meet the need. When the patient's needs are met, this decreases the distress of the patient and improves his or her sense of well-being.

## MADELEINE LEININGER'S THEORY OF CULTURE CARE DIVERSITY AND UNIVERSALITY

Madeleine Leininger developed the theory of culture care diversity and universality in 1974, based on anthropological concepts. Transcultural nursing considers cultural issues as central to providing care and promotes study of cultural differences in relation to people's beliefs about illness, behavioral patterns, and caring behavior as well as nursing behavior. Leininger recognized that response to illness is often rooted in cultural beliefs and traditions. Based on research, the goal is to identify and provide care that is both culture-specific (fitting the needs of a specific cultural group based on their belief systems and behavior) and universal (based on belief systems and behavior that hold true for all cultures). Nurses are expected to assess and analyze to determine the most appropriate approach to care, considering not only the needs of ethnic or minority populations but also gender issues. The transcultural theory tries to find ways to accommodate traditional belief systems with modern medicine and to prevent cultural conflict.

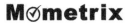

## CRITICAL THINKING SKILLS

Effective critical thinking requires a number of different skills:

| Interpretation | Ability to understand data and explain, knowledge of theories and applications. |
| --- | --- |
| Analysis | Ability to investigate based on objective and subjective data and to consider various methods to solve problems. |
| Evaluation | Ability to assess information obtained regarding reliability, credibility, and validity and to determine if the information is relevant. The person should consider how bias may affect decision-making. |
| Inference | Ability to arrive at a conclusion based on evidence and sound reasoning. |
| Explanation | Ability to explain conclusions and decisions using sound rationale. The person should be able to outline the steps taken to arrive at a conclusion. |
| Self-regulation | Ability to monitor personal thinking and to reflect on processes engaged in to reach conclusions. The person should be able to self-correct errors in thought processes. |

### CRITICAL THINKING STANDARDS

**Paul and Elder** (2001) identified a number of standards that must be applied critical thinking:

- **Clarity**: Reasoning should be transmittable from one medium of communication to another, so concepts must be clearly elaborated.
- **Accuracy**: Data and information must be accurate in order to reach the correct conclusion.
- **Precision**: One should anticipate what information others will need and provide detailed and clear information, proceeding from both the general to specific and specific to general.
- **Relevance**: All pertinent data should be collected and insignificant data omitted.
- **Depth**: One should avoid dealing with issues superficially.
- **Breadth**: Situations and data should be considered from various perspectives.
- **Logic**: Assumptions must be valid and conclusions based on evidence.
- **Significance**: Information should be judged on whether it is significant or peripheral.
- **Fairness**: One should be open to new ideas and viewpoints.

### PROBLEM SOLVING SKILLS

Problem solving to anticipate or prevent recurrences of problems involves arriving at a hypothesis, testing, and assessing the data to determine if the hypothesis holds true. If a problem has arisen, taking steps to resolve the immediate problem is only the first step if recurrence is to be avoided:

- **Define the issue**: Talk with the patient or family and staff to determine if the problem is related to a failure of communication or other issues, such as culture or religion.
- **Collect data**: This may mean interviewing additional staff or reviewing documentation, and gaining a variety of perspectives.
- **Identify important concepts**: Determine if there are issues related to values or beliefs.
- **Consider reasons for actions**: Distinguish between motivation and intention on the part of all parties to determine the reason for the problem.
- **Make a decision**: A decision on how to prevent a recurrence of a problem should be based on advocacy and moral agency, reaching the best solution possible for the patient, family, or staff.

## FACILITATING COLLABORATION

### TEAM BUILDING

Leading, facilitating, and participating in performance improvement teams requires a thorough understanding of the dynamics of **team building**:

- **Initial interactions**: This is the time when members begin to define their roles and develop relationships, determining if they are comfortable in the group.
- **Power issues**: The members observe the leader and determine who controls the meeting and how control is exercised, beginning to form alliances.
- **Organizing**: Methods to achieve work are clarified and team members begin to work together, gaining respect for each other's contributions and working toward a common goal.
- **Team identification**: Interactions often become less formal as members develop rapport, and members are more willing to help and support each other to achieve goals.
- **Excellence**: This develops through a combination of good leadership, committed team members, clear goals, high standards, external recognition, spirit of collaboration, and a shared commitment to the process.

### TEAM STRUCTURE

The appropriate team structure is very important in performance improvement because creating a team does not in itself assure teamwork. The team must be comprised of individuals whose skills complement each other and who have a shared purpose because outcomes will depend on the collaborative efforts of the group rather than individuals within the group. Accordingly, the collective team is accountable for outcomes rather than individuals. When creating teams important elements must be considered:

- **Size**: Teams of fewer than 10 members are most effective.
- **Skills**: Team members should have complementary skills that encompass technical, problem solving, decision making, and interpersonal.
- **Performance goals**: Teams should be allowed a degree of autonomy in producing action plans for performance improvement, based on strategic goals and objectives.
- **Unified approach**: The teams should be created according to the model of performance improvement, but should have some flexibility in working together.
- **Accountability**: The team members are collectively accountable rather than individually.

### PERFORMANCE IMPROVEMENT TEAM

A performance improvement team is a group of people working together to achieve a goal. Performance improvement activities almost always involve a team or teams of staff because of the complexity of healthcare organizations. Rarely is one department solely responsible for outcomes, except in very specialized work. In determining the composition of teams, **tracer methodology**, a method that looks at the continuum of care a patient receives from admission to post-discharge, may be helpful for teams that will be involved in clinical action plans to ensure that all groups that participate in care are represented in the team. Teams require considerable commitment in terms of training and time. Reasons for forming teams include:

- To improve outcomes through common purpose
- To utilize staff expertise and various perspectives
- To facilitate participative management style
- To improve acceptance of processes that impact work practice
- To manage complexity, where many participants are involved in outcomes

- To increase organization-wide acceptance
- To combat resistance

## INTERDISCIPLINARY TEAMS

Interdisciplinary teams (sometimes referred to as cross-functional) comprise individuals from various skill levels or disciplines who work together to accomplish one or more functions. In some cases, interdisciplinary teams may be *ad hoc*, operating for a short time to accomplish specific goals, but other times they become a permanent part of performance improvement. Interdisciplinary teams are most useful when dealing with problems or performance activities that cross disciplines, especially if a broad range of expertise and skills is needed. Selecting team members with the correct mix of abilities is important for success. The roles for the team members should be clearly outlines as well as expected outcomes. Adequate training must be provided to assist cross-functional team members in working together as a unit. Interdisciplinary teams are particularly useful in the following:

- Developing new processes
- Implementing organization-wide performance changes or technology
- Controlling costs and increasing cost-benefit ratio

## GROUP TYPES

Groups can be classified according to **form**:

- **Homogeneous**: Members chosen on a selected basis, such as ED staff
- **Heterogeneous**: An assortment of individuals with different roles, ages, and genders
- **Mixed**: A group that shares some key features, such as the same profession but differs in age or gender
- **Closed**: A group in which new members are excluded
- **Open**: A group in which the members and leaders change

Groups can also be classified according to **purpose**:

- **Task**: Emphasis on achieving a particular assignment.
- **Teaching**: Developed to inform, such as teaching the rules of the unit.
- **Supportive/Therapeutic**: Assisting those who share the same experience to learn mechanisms to cope and to overcome a problem, such as a staff suffering from stress.

## GROUP PROCESS

Phases of the group process are as follows:

1. **Orientation**: The task is identified and members learn mission, depending primarily on the leader in the beginning but beginning to explore their own roles in the group and accept that change can occur.
2. **Organization**: Members make group decisions about rules, limits, criteria, and division of labor. Some resistance or fear of change may occur as members doubt the possibility of change, but members gain confidence as group work becomes better organized.
3. **Flow of information**: Members become more able to express feelings and opinions and accept their roles in the group as interpersonal conflict lessens and group cohesion increases.

4. **Problem solving**: Members have a clear idea of the task and are able to work collaboratively and interdependently. They feel satisfaction with the group and have confidence regarding reaching goals. However, some members or groups may reach an impasse, decide that goals cannot be met, and actively resist change.

## STAGES OF GROUP DEVELOPMENT

**Tuckman's** (1965) group development stages include:

1. **Forming**: The group director takes more of an active role while members take their cues from the leader for structure and approval. The leader lists the goals and rules and encourages communication among the members.
2. **Storming**: This stage involves a divergence of opinions regarding management, power, and authority. Storming may involve increased stress, and resistance may occur as shown by the absence of members, shared silence, and subgroup formation. At this point, the leader should promote and allow healthy expression of anger.
3. **Norming**: It is at this stage where members express positive feelings toward each other and feel deeply attached to the group.
4. **Performing**: The leader's input and direction decreases and mainly consists of keeping the group on course.
5. **Mourning**: This is most deeply felt in closed groups when discontinuation of the group nears and in open groups when the leader or other members leave.

## LEVERAGING DIVERSITY

Leveraging diversity is a win-win proposition for the healthcare industry as the country becomes more diverse and the global economy expands. The healthcare industry must attract a more diverse workforce in the face of changing demographics in order to provide culturally competent care. Nurses entering the profession include older adults, ethnic minorities, and males, and policies and standards should reflect these differences. Studies have shown that a diverse workforce tends to be more innovative because of the variety of perspectives. Diversity is especially important in management because a diverse management is more likely to seek out and attract a diverse workforce. The healthcare organization should develop a strategic plan that specifically addresses issues of diversity, and cultural diversity should be incorporated into training and orientation programs. The nurse executive must ensure that diversity is valued and supported and all workers accorded respect and fair treatment without expecting everyone to conform to the same values.

## CONFLICT MANAGEMENT
### NEGATIVE AND POSITIVE EFFECTS OF CONFLICT

Some type of conflict is usually inevitable in any group of individuals, and it should be viewed as an opportunity for reflection rather than a failing. In fact, there are both negative and positive effects of conflict:

- **Negative**: Conflict can result in impaired communication and resentment and can damage the cohesiveness of a group of individuals, especially if people begin to take sides. Heated disagreements can escalate to fighting and aggressive behavior, and this can hinder performance.
- **Positive**: Conflict can result in new ideas and improved decision-making. Conflict can also result in increased creativity as individuals search for answers to the conflict and may bring about awareness for a need for better communication. Conflict can also result in increased interest and can provide a means of release of tension.

Conflict is best dealt with openly because unresolved conflicts can begin to mushroom into serious problems.

## LEVELS OF CONFLICT

There are two primary levels of conflict:

- **Intrapersonal**: This type of conflict occurs within the individual, often when there are two competing needs or unmet needs. This can occur if a nurse is unhappy with an assignment or feels unable to provide the type of care desired because of job restrictions or inadequate staffing. This can manifest as withdrawal or anger.
- **Interpersonal**: This type of conflict occurs between or among individuals or groups. A typical example is a disagreement between a nurse and a doctor or between two nurses over issues of patient care or personal matters. Subtypes of interpersonal conflict include intragroup, intergroup, and inter-organizational conflicts, such as disagreement between two departments and between nurses and doctors. A group may be splintered by different opinions. Intergroup and inter-organizational conflict may be difficult to resolve, especially if many people are involved, because of competing interests and may require mediation.

## TYPES OF CONFLICT

The three primary types of conflict include:

- **Relationship**: This is characterized by interpersonal conflicts that revolve around personal feelings and discord, such as a disagreement between two individuals. Relationship conflict can have a profoundly negative effect on team satisfaction and function, especially because people tend to become polarized, supporting one position or the other.
- **Task**: This is characterized by differences of opinions in how to accomplish a task, and it can result in heated discussions, but it rarely degenerates into negativity in the same way that relationship conflict does. Resolution should be evidence-based as much as possible.
- **Process**: This is characterized by differences of opinion about who is responsible for accomplishing a task. For example, group members may disagree about who is responsible for ordering supplies. This type of conflict is usually the easiest to resolve by compromise.

## ORGANIZATIONAL CONFLICT

Conflict within an organization can occur for a number of reasons:

- **Power conflicts**: One party holds more power (such as physicians vs nurses, administrators vs staff) and exercises this power, resulting in resentment and/or disagreement.
- **Impaired communication**: Parties may have a misunderstanding or may hold opposing views and are unable to discuss problems dispassionately.
- **Different goals**: Parties may have different goals, especially if the organizational goals are not clearly defined. Parties may have a difference of opinions over general organizational policies.
- **Resource allocation**: Competition for the same or limited resources may lead to ongoing discord, especially if it appears that resources are allocated unfairly.
- **Role conflict**: Parties may suffer from role overload, the feeling that they are burdened with doing jobs that should be done by others. Parties may also have differing ideas about what roles entail.

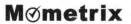

- **Interpersonal conflicts**: Conflicts between individuals over personal matters can have a broad impact. Sometimes, personal behavior by an individual is disturbing or upsetting to others.

## ETHICAL AND CLINICAL CONFLICTS

Ethical and clinical conflicts among patients and their families and healthcare professionals are not uncommon. Issues frequently relate to medications and treatment, religion, concepts of truth telling, lack of respect for patient's autonomy, and limitations of managed care or incompetent care. Additionally, healthcare providers are in a position to easily manipulate patients/families by providing incomplete information to influence decisions, and this can give rise to ethical conflicts. **Facilitation** involves questioning and listening, acknowledging each person's perspective while sharing different viewpoints:

- **Open communication** is critical to solving conflicts. Asking what steps could be taken to resolve the conflict or how it could be handled differently often leads to compromise because it allows for exchange of ideas and validates legitimate concerns. Sharing cultural perspectives can lead to better understanding.
- **Advocacy** for the patients/families must remain at the center of conflict resolution.

## CONFLICT RESOLUTION

Conflict is an almost inevitable product of teamwork, and the leader must assume responsibility for **conflict resolution.** While conflicts can be disruptive, they can produce positive outcomes by forcing team members to listen to different perspectives and opening dialogue. The team should make a plan for dealing with conflict resolution. The best time for conflict resolution is when differences emerge but before open conflict and hardening of positions occur. The leader must pay close attention to the people and problems involved, listen carefully, and reassure those involved that their points of view are understood. Steps to conflict resolution include:

1. Allow both sides to present their side of the conflict without bias, maintaining a focus on opinions rather than individuals.
2. Encourage cooperation through negotiation and compromise.
3. Maintain the focus, providing guidance to keep the discussions on track and avoid arguments.
4. Evaluate the need for renegotiation, a formal resolution process, or a third party.
5. Utilize humor and empathy to diffuse escalating tensions.
6. Summarize the issues, outlining key arguments.
7. Avoid forcing resolution if possible.

## APPROACHES TO CONFLICT RESOLUTION

Approaches to conflict resolution include the following:

| | |
|---|---|
| **Accommodating** | One party ceding to the other, usually when the other has more power |
| **Avoiding** | Taking steps to avoid dealing with the conflict |
| **Collaborating** | Trying to find a solution that pleases both parties |
| **Competing** | One party trying to win at all costs |
| **Compromising** | Each party ceding something in return for harmony |
| **Confronting** | Using "I" messages and assertive problem-solving |
| **Forcing** | One party issuing orders to force a solution |
| **Negotiating** | Similar to collaborating with back-and-forth bargaining |
| **Reassuring** | Attempting to make everyone happy |

| Problem-solving | Trying to find a solution that works for everyone using a step-by-step approach |
|---|---|
| Withdrawing | One party withdrawing from the conflict, leaving the conflict unresolved |

### DEFENSIVE MODE OF CONFLICT MANAGEMENT

The defensive mode of conflict management focuses on avoiding open conflict even though the underlying problem may remain unresolved. Defensive strategies may be used if more proactive strategies (such as compromise) have failed or to initially defuse a situation until other strategies can be employed. Defensive measures include:

- **Separating the parties to the conflict**: This can mean assigning them to different teams or to different shifts or work schedules with different days off in order to avoid contact between those in conflict.
- **Avoiding/Suppressing conflict**: The parties in conflict may choose to avoid discussing the issue or may be advised to do so by supervisory personnel.
- **Ignoring the conflict**: The parties in conflict may agree to disagree and to set the conflict aside and deal with other issues.
- **Providing an indirect solution**: An organizational change may eliminate the basis for the conflict.

### EMOTIONAL INTELLIGENCE

Salovey and Mayer developed the concept of **emotional intelligence** based on ability. Emotional intelligence is the ability to understand and manage one's own emotions as well as the ability to recognize and understand the emotions of others. Emotional intelligence is the understanding of how emotions affect behavior, a valuable skill in leaders. The four types of abilities involved in emotional intelligence include the ability to perceive, use, understand, and manage emotions. Individuals with emotional intelligence know the types of emotions that will be triggered personally by an event and have the ability to manage and use these emotions to enhance decision-making. They also can identify the emotions of others through observation of facial expressions, actions, words, and tone of voice. Individuals with emotional intelligence tend to have better social skills and workplace relationships because they have an innate understanding of how to respond to workers, recognize their concerns, and motivate them.

### GOLEMAN'S CONCEPT OF EMOTIONAL INTELLIGENCE

Goleman expanded on Salovey and Mayer's concept of emotional intelligence and proposed a mixed model (ability and traits). According to Goleman, emotional intelligence requires self-awareness, self-regulation, social skills, empathy, and motivation with each of these characteristics requiring a number of emotional competencies, which Goleman determined were learned rather than innate. Proponents of this view of emotional intelligence promote "**social and emotional learning**" (SEL) beginning in elementary school, where children are encouraged to identify their emotions and understand how these emotions impact their behavior. SEL is one method used to reduce bullying and violence in schools. Concepts of emotional intelligence have been increasingly applied to the field of business, including healthcare, with considerations of emotional intelligence used in hiring, recognizing, and developing leaders in an organization.

### TRAIT MODEL OF EMOTIONAL INTELLIGENCE

The trait model of emotional intelligence (Petrides, 2009) suggests that emotional intelligence is not an ability but rather an aspect of personality that includes emotional traits and emotional self-perceptions. This model does not provide for scientific measures to determine emotional intelligence but depends on personal insight and reporting. Petrides has developed a number of questionnaires, known as TEIQues (adult, child, long-form, short form questions), which cover 15 "facets" or character traits: adaptability, assertiveness, emotion perception (personal, other), emotion expression, emotion management (others), emotion regulation, impulsiveness, relationships, self-motivation, social awareness, stress management, empathy, happiness, and optimism. Individuals score depending on how they perceive themselves in relation to these traits. For example, an individual would score high on adaptability if the responses to questions indicate the person is flexible and able and willing to adapt to changes. The trait model of emotional intelligence suggests that behavior results from personality, which influences beliefs, values, and attitudes.

## THEORY OF MULTIPLE INTELLIGENCES

In the 1980s, Howard Gardner developed the **Theory of Multiple Intelligences**, which states that there are at least seven categories of "intelligences" that people use to comprehend the world about them and to learn. Gardner proposed that teaching that engages multiple intelligences is more effective than teaching focused primarily on linguistic or logical/mathematical intelligences (those most commonly addressed in education). Learners should be assessed to determine their personal intelligence strengths, and teaching should address the learners' preferences:

- **Linguistic**: Ability to use and understand language, written or spoken
- **Logical/mathematical**: Ability to utilize deductive and inductive reasoning, numbers, and abstract thinking
- **Visuospatial**: Ability to visualize and comprehend spatial dimensions
- **Body/kinesthetic**: Ability to control physical action
- **Musical/rhythmic**: Ability to create/appreciate musical forms
- **Interpersonal**: Ability to communicate and establish relationships with others
- **Intrapersonal**: Ability to utilize self-knowledge and to be self-aware

## BUILDING RELATIONSHIPS

### LISTENING

When building effective relationships, listening is more than simply hearing. While listening to the words of others is important, such as in one-on-one conversations, listening to unspoken sentiments is equally important. The nurse executive must be on alert for the undercurrents in an organization that may indicate support or resistance. This means attending to the way in which communication occurs (directly, indirectly) and the tone of the communication. The nurse executive should avoid focusing on internal thoughts when listening to others and should listen without carrying out other tasks because speakers know when the listener is not fully engaged, eroding trust. The nurse should maintain eye contact and engage in active listening. The nurse executive should make time in the work schedule for others, should utilize questioning to encourage others to speak, and should listen to all levels of employees, individually and in groups, so that employees feel valued.

### PRESENCE

Leadership presence is the way in which the leader is perceived by others in the organization, positively or negatively. The nurse executive should use various strategies to convey a positive presence:

- **Remain positive and friendly**: The nurse executive should convey positivity as much as possible to set the tone for the organization. The executive leader can be friendly and approachable while retaining respect.

- **Utilize active listening**: Employees want to feel that their opinions are listened to and acknowledged. The nurse executive should aim to listen about 4 times more than he or she speaks.
- Maintain professional appearance.
- **Share credit**: The nurse executive should make a point of recognizing and rewarding employees for their contributions to the organization.
- **Provide feedback**: Employees should know where they stand and should receive prompt, honest, and fair feedback.
- **Engage in conversations**: The nurse executive should take time occasionally to step out of the leadership role and simply converse with employees.
- **Solve problems**: The nurse executive should assess problems and deal with them promptly.

### COMMUNICATION

Characteristics of communication that should be considered when building relationships include:

- **Process**: Communication is a complex dynamic process that is bi-directional and involves both verbal and nonverbal interactions.
- **Symbolic**: Communication always uses symbols of some type to transmit thoughts and ideas. Almost anything can become a symbol to transmit information: images, words, appearance, color, tone of voice. The same symbol may transmit something very different to different receivers, who translate the symbol received into meaning.
- **Receiver-based**: Communication occurs with the receiver when meaning is attached to the symbol. All behavior communicates whether intended or not.
- **Irreversible**: Once communication occurs, it cannot be withdrawn or reversed. Correction of unintended communication may communicate a different message but the original remains.
- **Unrepeatable**: An original communication can never be repeated in the exact same way because the communication process is dependent on the receiver.

### NETWORKING

Networking, creating a network of contacts throughout the mental health industry and healthcare community, not only helps a nurse to find employment but also provides valuable professional resources. Networking should begin with professors and instructors while still a student through demonstration of competence. The nurse can cooperate with others involved in clinical tasks or research, gaining experience and credibility. Those involved in sales of medications and equipment are resources that can provide the nurse with current trends and changes. One of the most effective ways to network is to become involved in national organizations, such as the American Nurses Association and to participate in conferences through attendance and conference presentations. The nurse executive should make an effort to maintain periodic contact with those in an informal network by telephone, mail, or email.

## Chapter Quiz

Ready to see how well you retained what you just read? Scan the QR code to go directly to the chapter quiz interface for this study guide. If you're using a computer, simply visit the bonus page at **mometrix.com/bonus948/nce** and click the Chapter Quizzes link.

# Quality and Safety

Transform passive reading into active learning! After immersing yourself in this chapter, put your comprehension to the test by taking a quiz. The insights you gained will stay with you longer this way. Scan the QR code to go directly to the chapter quiz interface for this study guide. If you're using a computer, simply visit the bonus page at **mometrix.com/bonus948/nurseexec** and click the Chapter Quizzes link.

## Change Management Frameworks

### PRIMARY FUNCTIONS IN CHANGE MANAGEMENT

The five primary functions in change management include:

- **Making a plan**: This includes determining desired goals and outcomes and deciding who will implement the plan and how those affected by the plan will participate. The change agent should also assess support and resistance to better plan how to proceed with the plan. The plan should be formalized in writing.
- **Organizing**: Decisions must be made about how to achieve goals and reach desired outcomes. Necessary resources must be identified and secured and the cost-benefit analyzed.
- **Implementing**: The change agent should be prepared for the unexpected and modify the plan as indicated, understanding that a change in one part of a system affects all related systems.
- **Assessing**: This is an ongoing process that must continue throughout implementation and after to ensure that the outcomes are achieved.
- **Obtaining feedback**: Both positive and negative feedback should be encouraged.

### CHANGE THEORY
#### ADKAR

ADKAR is the acronym representing the five steps that individuals must go through in order to facilitate change within a group. Change must occur on both the organizational and individual levels. Steps include:

1. **Awareness**: The individuals must understand the need for change based on communication of needs in the organization by the key leaders.
2. **Desire**: The individuals must overcome resistance and fear of change and participate in the process of change with an understanding of how they will benefit.
3. **Knowledge**: The individuals must receive education and hands-on training in order to understand the processes of change once they have achieved awareness and desire for change.
4. **Ability**: Through coaching and practice, the individuals gain the skills necessary to effectively implement change.
5. **Reinforcement**: Feedback, corrections, and recognition help to maintain change and to prevent workers from reverting to previous methods or developing work-arounds.

59

## LEWIN'S CHANGE THEORY

Change theory was developed by Kurt Lewin (a social psychologist) and modified by Edgar Schein. This management theory is based on 3 stages:

1. **Motivation to change (unfreezing)**: Dissatisfaction occurs when goals are not met, but as previous beliefs are brought into question, survival anxiety occurs. Sometimes anxiety about having to learn different strategies causes resistance that can lead to denial, blaming others, and trying to maneuver or bargain without real change.
2. **Desire to change (changing)**: Dissatisfaction is strong enough to override defensive actions and the desire to change is strong but must be coupled with identification of needed changes.
3. **Development of permanent change (refreezing)**: The new behavior that has developed becomes habitual, often requiring a change in perceptions of self and establishment of new relationships.

## FORCE FIELD ANALYSIS

Force field analysis was designed by Kurt Lewin in order to analyze both the driving forces for change and the restraining forces:

- **Driving forces** are those responsible for instigating and promoting change, such as leaders, incentives, and competition.
- **Restraining forces** are those that resist change, such as poor attitudes, hostility, inadequate equipment, or insufficient funds.

Force field analysis is useful when discussing variables related to a proposed change in process. Steps include:

1. List the proposed change at the top and then create two subgroups (driving forces and restraining forces) below, separated by a horizontal line.
2. Brainstorm and list driving forces and opposed restraining forces. (When driving and restraining forces are in balance, this is usually a state of equilibrium or the status quo.)
3. Discuss the value of the proposed change.
4. Develop a plan to diminish or eliminate restraining forces.

## HAVELOCK'S SIX PHASES OF PLANNED CHANGE

Havelock (1973) developed a theory called the **Six Phases of Planned Change** in which he proposed that change can be planned and carried out in a series of sequential phases. Havelock recognized that resistance is an integral part of the change process. The change agents should:

- **Build a relationship with the system**: The change agent must understand the system as it is and the dynamics and organizational culture.
- **Diagnose the problem(s)**: The organization must determine if change is indicated.
- **Obtain necessary resources**: The organization recognizes the need for change and begins to determine the resources needed to carry out the change.
- **Select a solution**: Different options are explored and one or more chosen.
- **Garner acceptance**: Resistance is often a factor at this phase, so careful monitoring of compliance is essential.
- **Stabilize the change and facilitate self-renewal**: Ongoing monitoring is necessary.

## LIPPITT, WATSON AND WESTLEY'S SEVEN PHASES OF PLANNED CHANGE

Lippitt, Watson, and Westley (1958) developed the **seven phases of planned change** in which they proposed that change can be planned and carried out in a series of seven sequential steps:

1. The organization becomes aware of the necessity of change.
2. The change agent and the organization establish a relationship and the organization's motivation and capacity to make changes are assessed.
3. The necessary change is identified and defined, and the change agent's motivation is assessed.
4. The goals are established for bringing about change and options for achieving change are explored.
5. The plan is outlined and implemented, and the role of the change agent is defined.
6. The change is accepted by participants and stabilized across the organization.
7. The parties to the change redefine their relationships based on new dynamics.

## KOTTER'S CHANGE MANAGEMENT THEORY

Kotter's change management theory consists of 8 steps that correspond to three main goals. Because one step needs to be completed before the next, no step can be effectively omitted, and the process can be time-consuming although effective:

**Goal 1: Create a climate in which change is welcome**:

1. Develop a sense of urgency in order to motivate change
2. Create a strong coalition team with a mix of skills
3. Develop a shared vision taking multiple factors into account

**Goal 2: Engage the organization and enabling change**:

4. Communicate the vision and need for change to stakeholders
5. Empower individuals in the organization to enable change
6. Focus on the accomplishment of short-term goals initially

**Goal 3: Implement change and taking steps to ensure sustainability**:

7. Persist in building change
8. Incorporate and institutionalize change

## TRANSTHEORETICAL MODEL

The Transtheoretical Model focuses on changes in behavior based on the individual's (not society's or others') decisions and is used to develop strategies to promote changes in health behavior. This model outlines stages people go through when changing problem behavior and having a positive attitude about change. **Stages of change**:

1. **Precontemplation**: The person is either unaware or under-informed about consequences of a problem behavior and has no intention of changing behavior in the next 6 months.
2. **Contemplation**: The person is aware of costs and benefits of changing behavior and intends to change in the next 6 months but is procrastinating and not ready for action.
3. **Preparation**: The person has a plan and intends to instigate change in the near future (≤1 month) and is ready for action plans.

4. **Action**: The person is implementing behavior modifications that meet a set criterion that prove legitimate changes are being made (such as complete abstinence from drinking).
5. **Maintenance**: The person works to maintain changes and gains confidence that he or she will not relapse.

## 7-S FRAMEWORK

The 7-S Framework (McKenzie) includes 7 different steps to carry out in the process of change, stressing the importance of coordination. The steps are arranged in a circle around shared values (center) rather than a hierarchical arrangement, so a weakness in one area may impact all areas:

- **Strategy** includes a plan and the steps the organization is taking to accomplish future goals. Strategy should be the first step in bringing about change.
- **Structure** refers to how an organization is organized, including the chain of command and other relationships.
- **Systems** include all of the processes in the organization that indicate how work is accomplished.
- **Shared values** of an organization include its overall goal, social missions, and reputation.
- **Style** includes the culture of the organization and codes of conduct.
- **Staff** includes workforce and talents of the organization, models for hiring, and turnover, development.
- **Skills** include both organizational and individual skills that are available or lacking within an organization.

## NUDGE THEORY

Nudge theory (Sunstein and Thaler), originally an ethical concept, depends on "nudging" (inspiring, motivating) individuals in an organization to change. Nudge theory was developed around the idea that leaders should design choices in a way that encourages people to choose wisely and that leads to the change desired, rather than **mandating** change. For example, the organization may provide nutritious snacks rather than high-caloric fast foods in company vending machines to promote better health. Nudge interventions are indirect rather than direct and should be non-judgmental and allow some free choice. Heuristic elements of the theory include:

- **Anchor/Adjust**: Beginning with an anchoring fact that is well-known as a bridge to the unknown
- **Availability**: The perception of how common or familiar something is
- **Representativeness**: The degree to which something is similar to a stereotype
- **Framing**: Positive or negative presentations
- **Mindlessness**: Making of emotional rather than rational decisions
- **Conforming**: Following the lead of others
- **Priming**: Preparation that takes place
- **Temptation**: Greed guiding choices
- **Feedback**: Influences action

## BRIDGE'S TRANSITION MODEL

Bridge's transition model focuses on the transitions that people go through in the process of change and is based on the premise that transitions involve a specific mindset. The stages of transitions that people experience include:

1. **Ending, losing, letting go**: When presented with change, people are often resistive and experience various emotions, such as fear and denial, when they have to face the end of something with which they are familiar and comfortable. It's important to listen and communicate about the changes and how it will affect them.
2. **Neutral zone**: This is the bridge stage during which people may feel anxious and resentful, especially as caseloads may increase or change; however, this is also a time of creative energy. Leaders should provide feedback and encouragement and remind them of goals.
3. **New beginning**: People have begun to accept and feel positive about change and can benefit from rewards and celebration.

## SYSTEMS THEORIES
### BERTALANFFY'S SYSTEMS THEORY

Systems theory, developed by Ludwig von Bertalanffy in the 1940s, is an approach that considers the entire system holistically rather than focusing on component parts. Bertalanffy believed that all of the elements of a system and their interrelations needed to be understood because all interact in order to achieve goals, and change in any one element will impact the other elements and alter outcomes. There are 4 elements in a system:

- **Input**: This is what goes into a system in terms of energy or materials.
- **Processes**: These are the actions that take place in order to transform input.
- **Output**: This is the result of the interrelationship between input and processes.
- **Feedback**: This is information that results and can be used for evaluation of the system.

To achieve desired outcomes, every part of the process must be considered. The individual parts added together do not constitute the whole because viewing the parts separately does not account for the dynamic quality of interaction that takes place.

### NEUMAN'S TOTAL-PERSON SYSTEMS MODEL OF NURSING

**Betty Neuman** developed the total-person systems model of nursing in 1972. The concentric circle of variables (physiological, psychological, sociocultural, spiritual, and developmental) provides defense for the individual and should be considered simultaneously for the individual, who directly interacts with and is influenced by the environment. This model focuses on how the individual reacts to stress through mechanisms of defense and resistance and how this feedback affects that individual's stability. **Stressors** are environmental forces that may provide negative or positive reactions, affecting the individual's stability. Stressors may be intrapersonal, interpersonal, or extrapersonal. The nurse intervenes to help the individual maintain stability and prevent negative effects. **Interventions** include:

- **Primary** (health promotion, education): Preventive steps are taken prior to reaction to the stressor.
- **Secondary**: The goal is to prevent damage of the central core by facilitating internal resistance and by removal of the stressor.
- **Tertiary**: Efforts are made to promote reconstitution and reduce energy needs, supporting the client after secondary interventions.

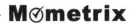

### COMPLEX ADAPTIVE THEORY

According to complex adaptive theory, complex adaptive systems are interdisciplinary systems with multiple components or agents that depend on interaction and adaptation as part of learning. Adaptive systems are open systems that are able to adapt readily to changes and problems. The original adaptive theory referred to biology, but the model has expanded to encompass families, communities, and organizations. Interactions tend to be rich and non-linear with close associates and with much feedback. Interactions are often random rather than planned. Change is often mutual: agents change, causing the system to change, and the system changes, causing the agents to change. Adaptive systems are dynamic by nature with interdependent agents acting together to bring about change. Adaptive systems that are self-adjusting are able to avoid chaos even though changes may bring them to the brink. Adaptive systems tend to favor effectiveness over efficiency and are less rule-governed than non-adaptive systems.

### CONTINGENCY THEORY

Contingency theory is a theory of organizational behavior that states that there is no single best method of organizing a company, corporation, or business but rather, that organization is contingent on a number of factors. In other words, what works in one organization may not work in another. Some common **contingency factors** include the organization size, resources, technology, adaptation to the environment, operations activities, motivating forces, staff education, and managerial assumptions. Contingency theory states that the organization must be designed in such a manner as to fit into the environment. Management should utilize the best approach to achieve tasks. Fielder concluded that leadership should be appropriate for the organizational needs and different organizations require different styles of leadership depending upon contingent factors, such as staff, tasks, and other group variables. Vroom and Yetton concluded that success in decision making is contingent on a number of factors, including information available, acceptance of the decision, agreement or disagreement, and the importance of the decision.

### ORGANIZATIONAL BEHAVIOR THEORIES

Two traditional organizational behavior theories are Frederick Taylor's scientific management theory (1917) and Elton Mayo's motivation theory (1933).

- **Scientific management theory**: Management's role is to plan and control, identifying tasks and then assigning the best person to complete the tasks, utilizing both rewards and punishment as motivating forces. This theory puts the focus on the outcomes rather than on the individuals, but workers are often unmotivated with this structure.
- **Motivation theory**: This theory requires that managers take a more personal interest in the needs of workers. Mayo (in the Hawthorne experiment) found that workers responded positively to changes in the working environment and were motivated by increased managerial interest and involvement, team work, and improved communication between management and staff in which workers are consulted about decisions.

## THEORY X AND THEORY Y

In 1960, Douglas McGregor developed two conflicting theories. He believed that management needed to assemble all needed components (including people) required for the company's economic benefit:

- **Theory X**: The average worker is unmotivated, dislikes work, is resistive to change, is unintelligent, and does not care about the organization. People work because they need the money. In this case, management may become coercive, making threats to control, or may be permissive, trying to placate unhappy workers so they will become more motivated.
- **Theory Y**: Work can be enjoyable, and workers can be motivated to meet goals if they result in feelings of self-fulfillment, causing workers to seek responsibility. People are basically creative and can exercise ingenuity. Management should seek to align organizational and personal goals to motivate workers, delegating, adding responsibilities, encouraging participative management, and allowing workers to set goals and evaluate their success in meeting goals.

## MANAGEMENT STRUCTURES

Stalker and Burns, in *The Management of Innovation* (1961), compared mechanistic and organic systems. Their main focus was that there is more than one way of managing an organization because organizations have different cultures and different contexts and products. According to this theory, different organizations require **different management structures**, and managers should design a system that matches the organizational environment.

| Mechanistic Systems | Organic Systems |
|---|---|
| <ul><li>**Stable conditions.**</li><li>**Tasks are considered distinct and stable.**</li><li>**Tasks differentiated by function.**</li><li>**Tasks defined by supervisors.**</li><li>**Each role has specific responsibilities.**</li><li>**Authority is through hierarchical chain of command.**</li><li>**Communication is vertical.**</li><li>**Loyalty and obedience are valued.**</li></ul> | <ul><li>Changing conditions.</li><li>Tasks are considered as part of the entire situation and change frequently.</li><li>Tasks differentiated by knowledge and experience.</li><li>Tasks defined through interaction.</li><li>Responsibilities are shared.</li><li>Authority is shared and decentralized.</li><li>Communication is lateral.</li><li>Commitment is valued.</li></ul> |

## CREATING A LEARNING ORGANIZATION

A learning organization is one in which the organization is constantly transforming itself and facilitates employee education and training (learning). The learning organization is adaptable to change, but success depends on the members of the organization and their learning and empowerment. Members need to embrace lifelong learning. Five disciplines that are part of a learning organization are:

- **Personal mastery**: The ability of the person to create desired outcomes and to facilitate an environment in which others can do the same.
- **Mental models**: The mindset of an individual affects the person's decisions and actions.
- **Shared vision**: Members share their visions of the future with other members of the group.

- **Team learning**: Members of the organization share knowledge and skills in order to improve the abilities and outcomes of the group as a whole.
- **Systems thinking**: The organization is viewed holistically as an inter-related collection of departments or units rather than unrelated parts.

# Culture of Safety

## HEALTHY WORK ENVIRONMENT

According to the ANA, a **healthy work environment** has three elements:

- **Safety**: This includes not only environmental safety (fire escapes, good air quality, and adequate lighting and heating) but also physical safety and freedom from bullying, violence, and physical and emotional abuse. Healthcare workers should have adequate training in using isolation precautions and the proper equipment, such as lifts.
- **Empowerment**: Healthcare workers should have autonomy commensurate with their position and training and should participate in decision making through some type of shared governance. Leaders should provide opportunities for learning and growth and provide the necessary resources. Training and mentoring programs increase professional development.
- **Satisfaction**: Healthcare workers should have high rates of job satisfaction. Factors that are directly related to job satisfaction include adequate wages, reasonable workload, and good scheduling of work hours. Flexible working schedules and a supportive non-punitive environment contribute to positive attitudes toward work.

## DOCUMENTATION AND REPORTING

### PURPOSES OF DOCUMENTATION

Documentation is a form of communication that provides information about the healthcare individual and confirms that care was provided. Accurate, objective, and complete documentation of individual care is required by both accreditation and reimbursement agencies, including federal and state governments. Purposes of documentation include:

- Carrying out professional responsibility
- Establishing accountability
- Communicating among health professionals
- Educating staff
- Providing information for research
- Satisfying legal and practice standards
- Ensuring reimbursement

While patient documentation focuses on progress notes, there are many other aspects to **charting**. Doctor's orders must be noted, medication administration must be documented on medication sheets, and vital signs must be graphed. Flow sheets must be checked off, filled out, or initialed. Admission assessments may involve primarily checklists or may require extensive documentation. The primary issue in malpractice cases is inaccurate or incomplete documentation. It's better to over-document than under, but effective documentation does neither.

## HAND-OFFS USING SBAR TEMPLATE

The SBAR (situation-background-assessment-recommendation) template is a systematic method of communication that is especially useful during hand-off procedures because it helps the nurse to organize information and present it clearly. Hand-off procedures should be documented and adequate time allowed for communication, including questions from the receiving party. The primary purpose for using the SBAR method for hand-off procedures is to promote patient safety by ensuring that all pertinent information is conveyed during hand-off:

- **Situation**: Name, age, physician, diagnosis
- **Background**: Brief medical history, co-morbidities, review of lab tests, current therapy, IV's, VS, pain, special needs, educational needs, discharge plans
- **Assessment**: Review of systems, lines, tubes, and drains, completed tasks, needed tasks, future procedures
- **Recommendations**: Review plan of care, medications, precautions (restraints, falls), treatments, wound care

Organizations utilizing SBAR should have guidelines that advise staff exactly what should be covered in each element and a template the providers can utilize to organize information.

## BEDSIDE REPORTING

Bedside reporting is done at the end of shift to provide hand-off information to oncoming staff. Patients should be advised about the policy for bedside reporting and encouraged to participate by commenting and asking questions and should be advised that others of their choosing may also be present, such as family members. Bedside reporting should include:

- **Introductions**: The outgoing nurse should introduce the oncoming nurse to the patient.
- Review of **medical record** and update about the patient's condition and treatments. The reporting nurse should use a checklist or the SBAR format to ensure that all pertinent information is covered.
- Review of laboratory and/or imaging findings.
- Review of **medications** administered and scheduled.
- **Physical examination** that includes checking IVs, wounds, dressings, and skin condition.
- **Environmental examination** that checks for safety concerns.
- Questioning the patient about **concerns and personal goals**.

## INCIDENT REPORTING

Incident report review is part of risk management because incidents represent a failure in the system. Incident reports may be filled out by individuals who are involved in the incident or observed the incident. Increasingly, incident reports are generated by electronic data that indicates an error occurred, such as in medication administration. Incident report reviews are less comprehensive and time-consuming and more cost-effective than retrospective medical record reviews but can yield valuable information, so providing staff incentives for reporting and confidentiality are important. Currently, studies indicate that incidents are grossly underreported in healthcare organizations, so one part of review is to determine if incidents are being accurately reported in order to more effectively identify patterns or trends. This may require interviews with physicians and staff. A review looks at the incident in terms of process steps and determines where in the process an error occurred in order to establish a plan for improvement.

## SENTINEL EVENT REPORTING

Sentinel events are defined by the Joint Commission as a death or serious physical injury that is unexpected. This death or injury could be related to many things, including surgery on the wrong body part, suicide, or infection. An infection is considered a sentinel event if it is determined that the death or injury would not have occurred without the infection. Each case must be dealt with individually, and, if defined as sentinel, a root cause analysis is done to gather evidence to identify what contributed to the problem. Once a root cause has been determined, an action plan that identifies all the different elements that contributed to the problem is recommended and instituted. The theory is that finding the root cause can eliminate the problem rather than just treating it. Thus, finding the source of an infection would be more important than just treating the infection. Reporting sentinel events to the Joint Commission is recommended but not required. When reported, the event is added to the Joint Commission's Sentinel Event Database.

## PATIENT SAFETY TECHNOLOGIES
### BARCODE MEDICATION ADMINISTRATION

Barcode medication administration (BCMA) utilizes wireless mobile units at the point of care to scan the barcode on each unit of medication or blood component before it is dispensed. Scanning ensures the correct medication and dosage is given to the correct patient, eliminating most point of administration medication errors. The BCMA system can also be utilized for specimen collection. This system requires monitoring and input from the pharmacy, as each new barcode must be entered into the system. Additionally, some medications are received in bulk, so when they are dispensed in unit doses, barcodes must be individually attached. Staff must be trained to ensure that BCMA is utilized properly and consistently. The FDA has required that drug supplies provide barcodes on the labels of medications and other biological products. BCMA increases safety for patients, integrates with the medication administration record, and incorporates the information system of the organization, providing data for assessment of performance and performance improvement measures.

### RADIO FREQUENCY IDENTIFICATION

Radio frequency identification (RFI) is an automatic system for identification that employs embedded digital memory chips, with unique codes, to track individuals, medical devices, medications, and staff. A chip can carry multiple types of data, such as expiration dates, individual's allergies, and blood types. A chip/tag may, for example, be embedded in the identification bracelet of the individual and all medications for the individual tagged with the same chip. Chips have the ability to both read and write data, so they are more flexible than bar coding. The data on the chips can be read by sensors from a distance or through materials, such as clothes, although tags don't apply or read well on metal or in fluids. There are two types of RFIs:

- **Active**: Continuous signals are transmitted between the chips and sensors
- **Passive**: Signals are transmitted when in close proximity to a sensor

Thus, a passive system may be adequate for administration of medications, but an active system would be needed to track movements of staff, equipment, or individuals.

## PATIENT SAFETY PROGRAM

Each healthcare organization has unique needs and challenges to face in developing a patient safety program although many components are universally needed. Facilitating the development of a **patient safety program** requires planning and taking the following steps:

1. Identifying a quality **professional or interdisciplinary group** to manage the safety program.
2. Defining the **scope** of the program, including risk identification and management as well as response to adverse events.
3. Providing mechanisms to integrate **all aspects** of the program into functions organization-wide.
4. Establishing procedures for **rapid response** to medical errors or adverse events.
5. Establishing procedures for both **internal and external reporting** of medical errors.
6. Defining and disseminating **intervention strategies** such as risk reduction, tracking of risks, and root cause analysis.
7. Outlining mechanisms for **staff support** related to involvement in sentinel events.
8. Establishing procedures and responsibilities for **reporting to the governing board**.

### COMPONENTS

A quality patient safety program must include a number of different **components**:

- Functional infrastructure with a leader, safety officer, teams, and software for tracking and measures
- Linkage of program goals with strategic goals of the organization
- Establishment of policies and procedures to reduce and control risk and supportive educational training
- Reporting system to identify adverse events or incidents
- Participation in national patient safety initiatives, such as NPSGs, IPSG, IHI 5 Million Lives, and Leapfrog
- Rapid response procedures to deal with medical errors and sentinel events
- Adequate data collection procedures to ensure performance measurement, tracking, and data analysis
- Performance improvement activities directed at specific goals
- Documentation of all processes and procedures as well as reporting procedures and timelines

### EVALUATION OF HAZARDS AND RISKS

Development of a patient safety program must include evaluation and management of **environmental safety hazards and risks**. Environmental safety steps include:

- Preparing a **written plan** that clearly outlines environmental safety concerns, policies, and procedures
- Identifying **security risks**, such as infant/child abduction and establishing processes to increase security, such as the use of alarms, identification badges, locks, better lighting, and security officers
- Evaluating **power/utility requirements**, including emergency power, and maintaining, testing, and inspecting utilities
- Establishing an **interdisciplinary team** to identify opportunities for improvement and facilitate performance improvement processes

- Completing **risk assessment** of the physical site, including buildings, grounds, equipment, and related systems, such as electrical, lighting, IT, ventilation, and plumbing
- Establishing a plan for **emergency preparedness**, including evaluation of areas of vulnerability, preparedness, response, and recovery

A patient safety program must include evaluation and management of **environmental safety hazards and risks**:

- Establishing organization-wide safety policies and procedures, including no smoking policies
- **Maintaining** the physical site and **monitoring** and **responding** to product recalls
- **Handling, storing, and disposing of hazardous wastes**, including identifying wastes that are corrosive, ignitable, reactive, or toxic and following state and EPA regulations and educating staff
- Conducting **fire safety drills** and checking equipment and buildings for fire dangers.
- **Monitoring medical equipment**, including ensuring routine maintenance, testing and regular inspection
- Establishing a **safe environment** for staff and patients, including fall prevention strategies, such as installing handrails, contrast strips on stairways, and analyzing work flow to facilitate functions
- Designating individuals to monitor and coordinate **environmental safety management** and to develop procedures for dealing with threats/problems

## CULTURE OF SAFETY
### *EMPLOYEE ENGAGEMENT*

Employee engagement in a culture of safety begins with education about the current status of safety issues, the need for safety, and the benefits to patients and staff from a focus on safety. The nurse executive and others in leadership positions must be committed to change, must allocate adequate resources, and must encourage and reward staff members who report safety concerns or adverse events so that staff are not concerned about reprisals. The nurse executive should acknowledge that healthcare is high-risk because of the nature of the work involved. Steps to engaging employees include:

- Routinely doing safety rounds
- Developing a system of reporting concerns
- Carrying out simulations of adverse events and safety problems
- Sharing safety reports at shift changes
- Conducting routine safety briefings
- Assigning one person on each unit to monitor and report safety concerns
- Educating staff about safety concerns
- Developing a response team to respond quickly to safety concerns

### *EMPLOYEE LIFTING POLICIES*

The concept of a culture of safety is often viewed as protecting the patient, but the **employees** should be an equal concern as many accidents and safety problems involve employees. According to the Department of Labor Bureau of Statistics, nursing employees experience greater than 35,000 back injuries each year, usually because they are lifting or moving patients. Manually lifting or moving a patient can almost never be done safely, so it is imperative that healthcare organizations institute a **no lift policy** that requires the use of patient lifts (such as a Hoyer lift). Equipment should be readily available for each unit and in working condition rather than stored in a central location. Staff should be assigned to monitor and service the equipment. Lift teams may be created to assist with the use of lifts but should be able to respond readily when requested. All staff should be trained in the use of lift equipment.

## ACCOUNTABILITY

The nurse has an obligation to **report** ethical and standards of care violations and to **intervene** to ensure safety of the patient. This **accountability** is outlined by state boards of nursing, professional organizations, and accrediting agencies. The nurse must report suspected or observed diversion of drugs, any type of abuse (physical, emotional, sexual, financial), falsification of patient records, neglect of patients, narcotic offenses, and arrests, indictments, and/or convictions for criminal offenses. Each facility should have policies in place for reporting, but the usual procedure is to report to the immediate supervisor and file an incident report; however, the nurse can file a complaint directly with the board of nursing, especially if the matter is serious. The written report is essential in the event that the nurse should experience reprisals. After filing a report, the nurse should follow up to determine if action has been taken. With ethical dilemmas, a report may be made to the bioethics committee. Violations may result in disciplinary action, mentoring, or loss of license.

## RISK MANAGEMENT

Risk management is an organized and formal method of decreasing liability, financial loss, and risk of harm to patients, staff, or others by doing an assessment of risk and introducing risk management strategies. Much of risk management has been driven by the insurance industry in order to minimize costs, but quality management utilizes risk management as a method to ensure quality healthcare and process improvement. An organization's risk management program usually comprises a manager and staff with a number of responsibilities:

- **Risk identification** begins with an assessment of processes to identify and prioritize those that require further study to determine risk exposure.
- **Risk analysis** requires a careful documenting of process, utilizing flow charts, with each step in the process assessed for potential risks. This may utilize root cause analysis methods.
- **Risk prevention/avoidance** involves instituting corrective or preventive processes. Responsible individuals or teams are identified and trained.
- **Assessment/evaluation of corrective/preventive processes** is ongoing to determine if they are effective or require modification.

### INTEGRATION OF RISK ASSESSMENT OUTCOMES

Because risk management is concerned with decreasing liability and increasing safety, **integrating the outcomes of risk management assessment** into the performance improvement process requires an organization-wide commitment to reducing risk. The governing board and quality professional must ensure that the risk management assessments are considered when formulating mission and vision statements and strategic goals. During process evaluation and process improvement processes, risk management assessment should be one of the first concerns. An organization-wide early warning system should be in place to screen patients for potential risks and identify the following:

- **Adverse patient occurrences (APOs)**: Those unexpected events that result in a negative impact on the patient's health or welfare.
- **Potentially compensable events (PCEs)**: APOs that may result in claims against the organization because of the negative impact on the patient's health or welfare.

If the organization has set up a method to quickly identify problems, then risks may be minimized.

## RISK STRATIFICATION

Risk stratification involves statistical adjustment to account for confounding and differences in risk factors. Confounding issues are those that confuse the data outcomes, such as trying to compare different populations, different ages, or different genders. For example, if there are two physicians and one has primarily high-risk patients, and the other has primarily low risk patients, the same rate of infection (by raw data) would suggest that the infection risks are equal for both physicians' patients. However, high risk patients are much more prone to infection, so in this case risk stratification to account for this difference would show that the patients of the physician with low-risk patients had a much higher risk of infection, relatively-speaking. Risk stratification is also used to predict outcomes of surgery by accounting for various risk factors (including ASO score, age, and medical conditions). Risk stratification is an important element of data/outcome analysis.

# Continuous Process Improvement

## PERFORMANCE IMPROVEMENT, EBP, AND RESEARCH

**Performance improvement (PI)**: PI is a method in which performance is analyzed, baseline or benchmarks established, and programs or processes established to improve outcomes and performance. Different models of performance improvement include Continuous Quality Improvement (CQI) and Total Quality Management (TQM).

**Evidence-based practice (EBP)**: EBP, on the other hand, is based on the processes that are used to achieve performance improvement. The critical element of evidence-based practice is that the processes that are utilized must be supported by research and evidence that show that they improve outcomes. Information should be synthesized from a number of different studies rather than one study alone and should consider healthcare providers' expertise and patient preferences. Evidence may be external or internal or some combination.

**Research**: Research includes the studies that are carried out to obtain evidence-based guidelines. Research may be qualitative or quantitative with research designs that include randomized control groups considered the most reliable.

## CONTINUOUS QUALITY IMPROVEMENT (CQI)

Continuous Quality Improvement (CQI) emphasizes the organization, rather than individuals, and systems and processes within that organization. It recognizes internal customers (staff) and external customers (patients) and utilizes data to improve processes. CQI assumes the concept that most processes can be improved. CQI uses the scientific method of experimentation to meet needs and improve services and utilizes various tools, such as brainstorming, multivoting, various charts and diagrams, storyboarding, and meetings. Core concepts include:

- Quality and success are defined by meeting or exceeding internal and external customer's needs and expectations.
- Problems relate to processes, and variations in process lead to variations in results.
- Change can be made in small steps.

Steps to CQI include:

1. Forming a knowledgeable team
2. Identifying and defining measures used to determine success
3. Brainstorming strategies for change
4. Planning, collecting, and utilizing data as part of making decisions
5. Testing changes and revising or refining as needed

## TOTAL QUALITY MANAGEMENT (TQM)

Total Quality Management (TQM) is one philosophy of quality management that espouses a commitment to meeting the needs of the customers at all levels within an organization. It promotes not only continuous improvement but also a dedication to quality in all aspects of an organization. Outcomes should include increased customer satisfaction and productivity as well as increased profits through efficiency and reduction in costs. In order to provide TQM, an organization must seek the following:

- Information regarding customer's needs and opinions
- Involvement of staff at all levels in decision making, goal setting, and problem solving
- Commitment of management to empowering staff and being accountable through active leadership and participation
- Institution of teamwork with incentives and rewards for accomplishments

The focus of TQM is on working together to identify and solve problems rather than assigning blame through an organizational culture that focuses on the needs of the customers.

## FOCUS PERFORMANCE IMPROVEMENT MODEL

Find, organize, clarify, uncover, start (FOCUS) is a performance improvement model used to facilitate change:

- **Find**: Identifying a problem by looking at the organization and attempting to determine what isn't working well or what is wrong
- **Organize**: Identifying those people who have an understanding of the problem or process and creating a team to work on improving performance
- **Clarify**: Determining what is involved in solving the problem by utilizing brainstorming techniques, such as the Ishikawa diagram
- **Uncover**: Analyzing the situation to determine the reason the problem has arisen or that a process is unsuccessful
- **Start**: Determining where to begin in the change process

FOCUS, by itself, is an incomplete process and is primarily used as a means to identify a problem rather than a means to find the solution. FOCUS is usually combined with **PDCA** (FOCUS-PDCA), so it becomes a 9-step process, but beginning with FOCUS helps to narrow the impact of improvement, resulting in better outcomes.

## PLAN-DO-CHECK-ACT (PDCA)

Plan-Do-Check-Act (PDCA) (Shewhart cycle) is a method of continuous quality improvement. PDCA is simple and understandable; however, it may be difficult to maintain this cycle consistently because of lack of focus and commitment. PDCA may be more suited to solving specific problems than organization-wide problems:

- **Plan**: The first step consists of identifying, analyzing, and defining the problem, clearly defining it, setting goals, and establishing a process that coordinates with leadership. Extensive brainstorming, including fishbone diagrams, identifies problematic processes and lists current process steps. Data is collected and analyzed and root cause analysis completed.
- **Do**: This step involves generating solutions from which to select one or more and then implementing the solution on a trial basis.
- **Check**: The check step involves gathering and analyzing data to determine the effectiveness of the solution. If it is effective, proceed to *Act*; if not, return to *Plan* and pick a different solution.
- **Act**: The last step consists of identifying changes that need to be done to fully implement the solution, adopting the solution, and continuing to monitor results while picking another improvement project.

## ACCELERATED RAPID-CYCLE CHANGE APPROACH

The accelerated rapid-cycle change approach is a response to rapid changes in healthcare delivery and radical reengineering. There are 4 areas of concern:

- **Models for rapid-cycle change**: The goal is doubling or tripling the rate of quality improvement by modifying and accelerating traditional methods. Teams focus on generating and testing solutions rather than analysis.
- **Pre-work**: Assigned personnel prepare problem statements, graphic demonstrations of data, flowcharts, and literature review. Team members are identified.
- **Team creation**: Rapid action (sometimes called rapid acceleration or rapid achievement) teams (known as RATs) are created to facilitate rapid change.
- **Team meetings and work flow**: Meetings/work are done over 6 weeks:
  o Week 1: Review information, clarification of quality improvement opportunities and identification of key customers, waste, and benchmarks
  o Week 2: Review customer requirements and cost/benefit analysis of solutions with testing of data
  o Week 3: Complete design of solution, plan implementation and pilot tests
  o Weeks 4-5: Test, train, analyze, and make changes as needed
  o Week 6: Implement the program

## JURAN'S QUALITY IMPROVEMENT PROCESS (QIP)

Joseph Juran's quality improvement process (QIP) is a 4-step method, focusing on quality control, which is based on a trilogy of concepts that includes quality planning, control, and improvement. The steps to the QIP process include:

- **Defining** and organizing the project includes listing and prioritizing problems and identifying a team.
- **Diagnosing** includes analyzing problems and then formulating theories related to cause by root cause analysis and test theories.

- **Remediating** includes considering various alternative solutions and then designing and implementing specific solutions and controls while addressing institutional resistance to change. As causes of problems are identified and remediation instituted to remove the problems, the processes should improve.
- **Holding** includes evaluating performance and monitoring the control system in order to maintain gains.

## SIX SIGMA

Six Sigma is a performance improvement model developed by Motorola to improve business practices and increase profits. This model has been adapted to many types of businesses, including healthcare. Six Sigma is a data-driven performance model that aims to eliminate "defects" in processes that involve products or services. The goal is to achieve Six Sigma, meaning no more defects than 3.4 to every one million opportunities. This program focuses on continuous improvement with the customer's perception as key, so that the customer defines that which is "critical to quality" (CTQ). Two different types of improvement projects may be employed: DMAIC (define, measure, analyze, improve, control) for existing processes or products that need improvement and DMADV (define, measure, analyze, design, verify) for development of new high-quality processes or products. Both DMAIC and DMADV utilize trained personnel to execute the plans. These personnel utilize martial arts titles: green belts, black belts (execute programs) and master black belts (supervise programs).

## *DMAIC*

The first model for **Six Sigma is DMAIC** (define, measure, analyze, improve, control), which is used when existing processes or products need improvement and is utilized in healthcare quality:

- **Define** costs and benefits that will be achieved when changes are instituted. Develop list of customer needs based on complaints, requests.
- **Measure** input, process, and output measure, collect baseline data, establish costs, and perform analysis, calculate sigma rating.
- **Analyze** root or other causes of current defects, use data to confirm, and uncover steps in processes that are counterproductive.
- **Improve** by creating potential solutions, develop and pilot plans, implement, and measure results, determining cost savings and other benefits to customers.
- **Control** includes standardizing work processes and monitoring the system by linking performance measures to a balanced scorecard, creating processes for updating procedures, disseminating reports, and recommending future processes.

## LEAN

Lean is a continuous performance improvement model derived from the production system of Toyota. This model focuses on reduction of waste, ensuring that processes are error-proof, and reducing processes and activities that add no value. The types of waste that should be eliminated include: overproducing, waiting time, transportation problems, processes with no added value, excess inventory, motion, and costs of quality. Lean principles include perceiving value of an organization from the perspective of the customer (patient), identifying wasted steps in processes, and identifying the value stream (entire process from beginning to end). Products, services, and processes should be evaluated to determine if they are value-added, non-value added, or non-value added essential (such as required by regulations). The demand for services derives from the customer, and the organization should aim at perfection through constant improvement. In order to achieve the highest level of service and value, this model includes respect for the employees, quality products and services, and a just-in-time philosophy (right product/service, right patient, right time).

## LEAN-SIX SIGMA

Lean-Six Sigma, which combines Six-Sigma with concepts of "lean" thinking, is a method of focusing process improvement on strategic goals rather than on a project-by-project basis. This type of program is driven by strong senior leadership that outlines long term goals and strategies. Physicians are an important part of the process and must be included and engaged. The basis of this program is to reduce error and waste within the organization through continuous learning and rapid change. There are 4 characteristics:

- Long-term goals with strategies in place for periods of 1-3 years.
- Performance improvement is the underlying belief system.
- Cost reduction through quality increase, supported by statistics evaluating the cost of inefficiency.
- Incorporation of improvement methodology, such as DMAIC, PDCA, or other methods.

## FADE

FADE is a quality improvement model that was developed by the Organizational Dynamics Institute. FADE has 4 primary steps:

- **Focusing**: Generating a problem list, prioritizing, choosing one problem, and then writing a statement defining the problem.
- **Analyzing**: Collecting data and determining influencing factors in order to establish baseline data for measuring.
- **Developing**: Solutions are explored, one is chosen, and a plan formulated with an implementation plan that identifies a solution to the problem.
- **Executing/Evaluating**: The plan is executed, and this may involve a pilot program if indicated. The impact and outcomes are assessed and a plan for ongoing evaluation implemented. The organization commits to the plan.

## ROOT CAUSE ANALYSIS (RCA)

Root cause analysis (RCA) provides information about causes of adverse or sentinel events, but analysis requires careful review to determine if the RCA was done correctly. In many cases, an adverse event is the result of a series of errors or system problems rather than one clearly identifiable process failure. Environmental factors, such as staff reduction and poor floor design, can affect outcomes as can poor communication, so factors that contribute in some way to the event (fatigue, poor design, inexperienced staff) but are not the direct cause must be identified in order to formulate action plans that will improve outcomes. Those reviewing the RCA must be objective, without bias that may influence their interpretation, such as assuming human error rather than systemic error is at fault, and must allow adequate time for decision making. In assessing the root cause, it's also important to consider how retrospective information available from the RCA may differ from information available to those involved in the procedure related to the sentinel/adverse event.

## IS/IS NOT METHOD

Is/is not is a method to identify root causes and make decisions by determining what a problem or event is and what it is not. The purpose of is/is not is to keep the team focused on the immediate problem. Steps include creating a table with the problem at the top and columns for "is" and "is not" and filling in the table by doing the following:

- **Identifying what the problem/event is**: Ask what, why, when, where, how, and how much in relation to the process rather than focusing on the people involved. Create a detailed description of the problem/event.
- **Identifying what the problem/event is not**: Ask about which things could have caused the same problem but did not. Evaluate similar processes in which the problem did not occur.
- **Comparing**: The two columns of information are examined to determine what distinguishes them, helping to find potential causes
- **Identifying changes**: Note changes that may have occurred, resulting in the problem, leading to a root cause.

## THE FIVE WHYS

The Five Whys is a method of finding root causes and solving problems that was designed by Taiichi Ohno, of Toyota, Japan. This process requires a team comprised of those who are knowledgeable about the process. Essentially, the team asks "why" in a sequential manner, usually at least five times, as an exercise to narrow the focus and arrive at a consensus about the cause of an event. Steps include:

- **Outlining** the process in detail with each event ordered in the sequence of events described.
- Asking **"why" questions** about each step in the sequence of events to try to determine cause. For example:
  - Why did the patient return to the emergency department? Because the doctor failed initially to order an x-ray of the injured hand.
  - Why did the doctor fail to order an x-ray of the injured hand? Because the x-ray department was understaffed and there was a two-hour delay.
- Reaching consensus and proposing solutions to improve performance.

## FAILURE MODE AND EFFECTS ANALYSIS (FMEA)

Failure mode and effects analysis (FMEA) is a team-based prospective analysis method that attempts to identify and correct failures in a process before utilization to ensure positive outcomes. Steps in the process include:

| Step | Process |
|------|---------|
| 1 | Definition: Describe process and scope. |
| 2 | Team creation |
| 3 | Description: Flowchart with each step in the process numbered consecutively and substeps lettered consecutively. |
| 4 | Brainstorming each step for potential failure modes. |
| 5 | Identification of potential causes of failures: Root cause analysis. |
| 6 | Listing potential adverse outcomes (to patients). |

| Step | Process |
|------|---------|
| 7 | Assignment of severity rating: Adverse outcomes rated on a 1 to 10 scale for severity of failure |
| 8 | Assignment of frequency/occurrence rating: Potential failures rated on a 1 to 10 scale for probability of failure in the prescribed time period. |
| 9 | Assignment of detection rating: Potential failures rated on a 1 to 10 scale for the probability that they will be identified before their occurrence. |
| 10 | Calculation of risk priority number (RPN): severity, occurrence, and detection ($S \times O \times D$) to find the RPN. |
| 11 | Reduction of potential failures: Brainstorming. |
| 12 | Identification of performance measures. |

## TRACER METHODOLOGY

Tracer methodology is a method that looks at the continuum of care a patient receives from admission to post-discharge. A patient is selected to be "traced," and the medical record serves as a guide. Tracer methodology uses the experience of this patient to evaluate the processes in place through documents and interviews. For example, if a patient received physical therapy, surveyors may begin with the following:

- **Physical therapists**: How do they receive the orders and arrange patient transport? How is the therapy administered? How is progress noted?
- **Transport staff**: How do they receive requests? How long does transfer take? What routes do they use? How do they transport patients? How do they clean transport equipment? What do they do if emergency arises during transport?
- **Nursing staff**: How do they notify PT of orders? How do they prepare patients? How do they know the therapy schedule? How do they coordinate PT with the need for other treatments? How do they learn about patient progress?

## CULTURE OF CONTINUOUS PERFORMANCE IMPROVEMENT

Creating a culture of continuous performance improvement requires commitment by the nurse executive and active engagement of all levels of staff in identifying opportunities for performance improvement, which should be a central theme of the organization. The nurse executive should establish a recognition and reward program for those who are active in performance improvement, and should provide continuous feedback about progress, such as through bulletin boards or electronic dashboards. Continuous performance improvement should be **reviewed** in regular monthly meetings, and the staff should be kept apprised of recommended evidence-based practices. **Training** regarding performance improvement and problem solving should be provided to staff and staff members should be encouraged to share their ideas and observations. The nurse executive should identify barriers or constraints and take steps to remedy them and should establish standards of care. Leaders should assume the role of facilitator.

## SELECTING CONTINUOUS PERFORMANCE IMPROVEMENT METHOD

Once performance issues are identified, the organization faces a decision about the form that **continuous performance improvement** will take. Many models, such as Total Quality Management (TQM) and Continuous Quality Improvement (CQI) are long-term solutions that require a basic refocusing of the organization, including its vision. Other models, such as Plan-Do-Check-Act (PDCA), focus primarily on the problem at hand and not the overall organization. The organization must decide whether to focus on one issue alone or on multiple issues and whether small changes or organizational changes are needed. The choice of continuous performance technique will depend on the resources (time, staff, equipment, finances) available, the types of performance issues identified, and the organizational culture. There are similar features to all models for performance improvement, and some pilot testing and small tests of change may be indicated in the decision process.

## ACTION PLANNING

Action planning is the phase of strategic planning in which specific actions in support of goals are identified. Once the major quality issues or goals are outlined, action planning is carried out to clarify what will actually be done to achieve those goals. Action planning includes determining objectives and responsibilities for each goal, metrics, and a timeline for evaluation. Objectives should be realistic and attainable and should be written to include who will carry out the actions, the desired outcomes, the measures, the level of proficiency, and the timelines. Objectives should guide the establishment of priorities, plans, assignments, and the allocation of resources. Action planning should also include a plan for communication that identifies who is responsible for carrying out the communication, who needs to be informed about progress, what information needs to be communicated, how often communication should be carried out, and the manner in which communication will be carried out (emails, reports, presentations).

## EXTERNAL BENCHMARKING AND INTERNAL TRENDING

External benchmarking involves analyzing data from outside an institution, such as monitoring national rates of hospital-acquired infection and comparing them to internal rates. In order for this data to be meaningful, the same definitions must be used as well as the same populations for effective risk stratification. Using national data can be informative, but each institution is different, and relying on external benchmarking to select indicators for infection control or other processes can be misleading. Additionally, benchmarking is a compilation of data that may vary considerably if analyzed individually, further compounded by anonymity that makes comparisons difficult.

**Internal trending** involves comparing internal rates of one area or population with another, such as infection rates in ICU and general surgery, and this can help to pinpoint areas of concern within an institution, but making comparisons is still problematic because of inherent differences. Using a combination of external and internal data can help to identify and select indicators.

## OUTCOME MEASUREMENT

### CLINICAL OUTCOME MEASURES

Choosing the appropriate clinical outcomes for interventions is essential in order to determine progress. Indicators should be quantitative so that data can be analyzed. Data may be acquired through surveys or questions with a Likert scale, direct observation, or the use of instruments that have been previously tested for validity and reliability. The primary factors to consider when determining outcomes include:

- **Patients**: Outcomes should relate to the patient population. The Nursing Outcomes Classification (NOC) can be used as a starting point for the evaluation of nursing interventions.
- **Priorities**: When possible, outcomes should be associated with the organization's mission.
- **Performance improvement implementing and monitoring team**: The makeup of the team may influence the selection of outcomes measures, so an interdisciplinary team can provide differing insights. The team should include an advance practice nurse familiar with the use of data and benchmarks.
- **Mandated reporting**: Data that is required should be a primary concern, and the public reporting of the data may provide benchmarks for measuring outcomes.

## FINANCIAL OUTCOME MEASURES

The financial department of a healthcare organization often contains a wealth of data that can be mined and used when determining baselines and outcome measures. Aside from basic revenue stream (which can provide valuable insight into cost-effectiveness of care provided by an organization and the return on investment for interventions), the financial data contain coding information about diagnoses, treatments, and procedures because this information is utilized in billing. Coding includes ICD-10-CM, ICD-10-PCS, CPT, and MS-DRG. This data can be utilized to determine quantitative outcomes. The data can also provide information about the number of patients, lengths of stay, utilization of services, types of medications and treatments, and readmissions. The data can help to identify co-morbidities and hospital-acquired infections/injuries and may be utilized to determine risk adjustments.

## SAFETY OUTCOME MEASURES

The healthcare organization must conduct a needs assessment to determine which areas of safety (such as staff safety, patient falls, healthcare infections, sentinel events, complications) require intervention. Outcome benchmarks and baseline rates can be obtained from a variety of sources and from internal assessment and data analysis, including review of incident reports. Sources of information regarding **safety benchmarks** include:

- **CMS and Hospital Quality Alliance per Hospital compare**: Readmissions, mortality, complications, care processes, patient experience.
- **AHRQ Hospital Survey on Patient Safety Culture**: Complications, patient safety culture.
- **AHRQ**: Patient safety indicators.
- **HCAHPS**: Patient satisfaction.
- **CDC**: Healthcare-associated infections, access to care.
- **CMS**: Chartbooks (hospital performance reports).
- **The Joint Commission**: Sentinel events, patient safety events.
- **National Coordinating Council for Medication Error Reporting and Prevention**: Medication errors, classifications.
- **National Healthcare Quality and Disparities Report**: Benchmarks for quality hospital measures derived from data from top-performing states as well as estimated benchmarks. State and national data available.

## PATIENT SATISFACTION OUTCOME MEASURES

Outcome measures for **patient satisfaction** can be obtained from a number of different sources:

- **Hospital Consumer Assessment of Healthcare Providers and Systems (HCAHPS)**: This mandated data reporting of patient satisfaction with care can provide insight into areas of concern and can provide a benchmark for performance improvement.
- **Patient surveys**: In-house surveys, such as in response to a particular program, may provide unit/department-specific information that can be utilized.
- **Interviews**: One-on-one interviews with patients and families can provide insight.
- **Call lights**: Monitoring the number and frequency of call lights and the types of requests can help to determine areas of weakness in provision of care.
- **Complaints**: Patient complaints should be quantified according to type of complaint to determine if patterns emerge.

- **Social media**: Social media sites, such as Twitter and Facebook, can be monitored for comments about the organization of provision of care to again determine if patterns emerge.
- **Legal actions**: Any charges of malpractice or negligence should trigger assessment for performance improvement.

## EMPLOYEE SATISFACTION OUTCOME MEASURES

Employee satisfaction is essential to quality healthcare, but direct measurement can be challenging. Different methods of assessing satisfaction include:

- **Surveys**: While these can yield valuable data, some employees are reluctant to express discontent, especially if they are concerned about the confidentiality of the survey.
- **Organizational culture**: Indirect assessment of employee satisfaction may be gleaned from consideration of the culture as a whole and the general attitudes (positive or negative) of staff toward the organization.
- **Retention rates**: High rates of staff turnover are often associated with employee dissatisfaction.
- **Sick-time**: High rates of sick time often indicate employee dissatisfaction or inadequate safety measures.
- **Engagement**: Satisfied employees are often engaged and willing to serve on committees and work toward performance improvement projects while dissatisfied employees are more likely to avoid calling attention to themselves.
- **Complaints/Conflict**: The numbers of complaints and conflicts often directly relate to the degree of satisfaction—the more dissatisfied, the more complaints and conflicts.

# Research and Evidence Based Practice

## PROTECTION OF SUBJECTS

### INSTITUTIONAL REVIEW BOARD (IRB)

An institutional review board (IRB) is a committee within an institution that is charged with reviewing research projects involving human subjects. The IRB reviews research proposals, approves them, monitors progress, and reviews outcomes. The IRB may conduct a risk-benefit analysis as part of assessment to determine if the research is an advantage to the organization. The primary role of the IRB is to ensure that human subjects do not experience psychological or physical harm as the result of the research, that the research is carried out in an ethical manner, that regulatory guidelines are followed, and that subjects have informed consent and understand their rights. IRBs are regulated by the Office of Human Research Protections (OHRP), which is part of the US Department of Health and Human Services (HHS). The IRB is required to register with the OHRP and to obtain a Federal-wide assurance (FWA) before any research is carried out with federal funds.

### HEALTH AND HUMAN SERVICES REGULATIONS

Protection of human subjects is covered in the **Health and Human Services, Title 45 Code of Federal Regulations, part 46**. This provides guidance for institutional review boards (independent groups that monitor research to ensure it is ethical) and those involved in research, outlining requirements. Institutions engaged in non-exempt research must submit an assurance of compliance (document) to the Office of Human Research Protection (OHRP), agreeing to comply with all requirements for research projects. Subjects cannot be used solely as a means to an end, but research should hold the possibility of benefit to the subject. Risks should be minimal, and selection of subjects should be equitable. Some research populations are granted additional protections because of their vulnerability and susceptibility to coercion; this includes children, prisoners, pregnant women, human fetuses and neonates, mentally disabled people, and people who are economically or educationally disadvantaged. When cooperative research projects are conducted involving more than one institution, each must safeguard the rights of subjects, insuring informed consent and privacy.

## FDA REGULATIONS

**The Food and Drug Administration, Code of Federal Regulations, Title 21, Volume 1**, regulates the protection of human subjects and states that any researcher involving patients in research must obtain informed consent in language understandable to the patient or the patient's agent. The elements of this informed consent must include an explanation of the research, the purpose, and the expected duration, as well as a description of any potential risks. Potential benefits and possible alternative treatments must be described. Any compensation to be provided must be outlined. The extent of confidentiality should be clarified. Contact information should be provided in the event the patient/family has questions. The patient must be informed that participation is voluntary and that he/she can discontinue participation at any time without penalty. Informed consent must be documented by a signed, written agreement.

## RESEARCH PROCESS

Steps to the research process include the following:

1. **Formulate problem**: Focus first on a broad topic and then narrow it to a specific question
2. **Conduct literature review**: Review existing research on the topic, including meta-analyses
3. **Develop theoretical framework**: Choose a feasible method of reaching a solution to the problem
4. **Develop hypothesis**: Select a hypothesis that predicts expected outcomes
5. **Identify a research design**: Identify the design as experimental (researcher introduces an intervention) or nonexperimental (researcher collects data)
6. **Specify population**: Specify type, number, and characteristics of population
7. **Manage variables**: Devise methods to identify and measure variables
8. **Conduct pilot study**: Conduct a small-scale study of the major project to improve the project
9. **Select sample**: Use care in selecting a representative sample, using sampling procedures
10. **Collect data**: Train staff to collect data, keeping accurate records
11. **Prepare & analyze data**: Organize data and conduct both qualitative and quantitative analysis of data
12. **Interpret & communicate results**: Critically evaluate findings and prepare research report

## DEVELOPING RESEARCH QUESTIONS USING THE PICOT FORMAT

The **PICOT** format is one method of developing appropriate questions to use in searching quantitative research. This method helps clarify the question and necessary information and to identify key words utilized in searching.

| P | Patient/ Population | List important characteristics: 35-year-old male with low back pain |
|---|---|---|
| I | Intervention/ Indicator | Explain the desired intervention under consideration: Acupuncture |
| C | Comparison/ Control | List other possible interventions or alternatives: Surgery |

| O | Outcome | Provide the desired measurable outcomes: Decreased pain levels (from 6–7 to 1–2) and increased mobility |
|---|---------|--------------------------------------------------------------------------------------------------------|
| T | Time | Timeframe (if appropriate) |

This format is then used to formulate a question:

*In a 35-year-old male with low back pain, how does acupuncture compared with surgery affect pain levels and mobility?*

Based on this question, then the search may be conducted with the following (including synonyms): (Back pain or sciatica) and (acupuncture or surgery) and (pain management or pain-free or pain control).

## DATA COLLECTION

### LITERATURE REVIEWS

When conducting a **review of literature** about a particular topic, the researcher should survey a wide range of sources. A literature review most often starts with a search in a database to obtain journal articles (from juried publications), both those reporting on direct research as well meta-analyses, which combines data and information gleaned from a number of different research projects. Meta-analysis can provide useful insight because research projects often involve small numbers of participants, so the results may not have external validity. The Agency for Healthcare Research and Quality (AHRQ) provides funding for research and publishes results and data in many areas of healthcare. AHRQ also provides the National Guidelines Clearing house, which allows search and links to evidence-based clinical guidelines for healthcare. The Centers for Disease Control and Prevention (CDC) carries out behavioral, diagnostic, vaccine, and biomedical research and issues regular publications showing results.

### LITERATURE RESEARCH

Literature research requires comprehensive evaluation of current (less than or equal to 5 years) and/or historical information. Most literature research begins with an internet search of databases, which providing listings of books, journals, and other materials on specific topics. Databases vary in content and many contain only a reference listing with or without an abstract, so once the listing is obtained, the researcher must do a further search (publisher, library, etc.) to locate the material. Some databases require subscription, but access is often available through educational or healthcare institutions. In order to search effectively, the researcher should begin by writing a brief explanation of the research to help identify possible keywords and synonyms to use as search words:

- **Truncations**: "Finan*" provides all words that begin with those letters, such as "finance," "financial," and "financed."
- **Wildcards**: "m?n" or "m*n" provides "man" and "men."
- **BOOLEAN logic** (AND, OR, NOT):
  - Wound OR infect* OR ulcer
  - Wound OR ulcer AND povidone-iodine
  - Wound AND povidone-iodine NOT antibiotic NOT antimicrobial

## Data Retrieval Using Structured Query Language

Structured query language (SQL) is a fourth-generation programming language (4GL) that differs from 3GLs, such as Java, in that SQL uses syntax similar to human language to access, manipulate, and retrieve data from relational database management systems (RDBMS), which stores data in tables. Both the American National Standards Institute (ANSI) and the International Organization for Standardization (IOS) have adopted SQL as a standard; however, because the language is complex, many vendors do not utilize the complete standard which limits portability between vendors without modifications. Despite many available versions, ANSI standards require that basic commands (UPDATE, DELETE, SELECT, etc.) be supported. Language elements of SQL include:

- **Clauses**: From, where, group by, having, and order by
- **Expressions**: Produce scales and tables
- **Predicates**: 3-valued logic (null, true, false) and Boolean truth values
- **Queries**: The most commonly used SQL operation, requires a SELECT statement
- **Statements**: Includes the semicolon (to terminate a statement)

## Critical Reading

There are a number of steps to **critical reading** to evaluate research:

- **Consider the source** of the material. If it is in the popular press, it may have little validity compared to something published in a juried journal.
- **Review the author's credentials** to determine if the person is an expert in the field of study.
- **Determine thesis**, or the central claim of the research. It should be clearly stated.
- **Examine the organization** of the article, whether it is based on a particular theory, and the type of methodology used.
- **Review the evidence** to determine how it is used to support the main points. Look for statistical evidence and sample size to determine if the findings have wide applicability.
- **Evaluate** the overall article to determine if the information seems credible and useful and should be communicated to administration and/or staff.

## Study Methods

### Quantitative Research

Quantitative research includes experimental designs, which often include randomized controlled trials, though a number of different designs are possible:

- **Two group pretest-posttest**: Includes a randomized experimental group with intervention and observation and a randomized control group with observation. Both groups receive a pretest and posttest.
- **Two group posttest**: Includes randomized experimental group with intervention and randomized control group with posttests only.
- **Solomon four group**: Includes two randomized experimental and two randomized control groups with one experimental group receiving a pretest and intervention and the other receiving intervention only and one control group receiving a pretest. All four groups receive a posttest.
- **Multiple experimental**: Two or more experimental groups with one control group. This allows researchers to test various interventions, such as different methods of pain control.
- **Factorial design**: Experimental design in which there is more than one intervention.

## QUALITATIVE RESEARCH

There are four primary types of **qualitative research design**:

- **Ethnographic**: Used to study cultural behavior, cultural knowledge, and cultural artifacts. Subjects are studied in their natural environments over a period of time. Ethnographic research design includes observations and detailed interviews with key informants carried out over an extended period of time (weeks to months).
- **Grounded theory**: Literature review is limited before research in order to prevent bias. Data to obtain information about a process is carried out primarily through one-on-one interviews or a focus group utilizing open-ended questions. Interviews are usually recorded or extensive notes completed.
- **Historical**: Data is collected from eye-witness accounts or from documentation, such as patient's records. This method may be used to determine historical treatment for conditions, for example.
- **Phenomenological**: Data collection involves fieldwork and one-on-one interviews with those who have experienced the phenomenon (experience) being researched. Information obtained is analyzed for patterns and themes.

## DESCRIPTIVE RESEARCH

Descriptive research is intended to explore and describe people, events, or groups in real life situations in order to develop new information or knowledge about the subjects. Descriptive research is especially useful when researching a subject about which there is little information so that the researchers understand how situations naturally occur. An example would be a study looking at the symptoms of survivors of disasters and the variables that affect outcomes. The design begins by identifying a phenomenon of interest and then selecting a number of variables that may influence the phenomenon. A descriptive research project does not involve intervention or treatment but rather observation. The variables are described and measured. Different methods may be employed, including direct observation, measurements, and questionnaires to obtain information. Descriptive designs may be comparative, examining the differences in variable between two or more groups, and time-dimensional, examining changes or trends over time.

## CORRELATIONAL RESEARCH

Correlational research is intended to predict, test, or describe the relationships among different variables. A representative sample must be selected and the type and strength of the relationship examined rather than differences. Designs vary depending on the purpose. A descriptive correlational model that examines the relationship among variables may be utilized to develop a hypothesis. Predictive designs attempt to determine the effect that independent variables have on a dependent variable in order to predict a causal relationship. In a model-testing correlational design, a concept map is created that identifies all exogenous, endogenous, and residual variables. The three possible correlational outcomes of correlational research include:

- **Positive**: Variables increase or decrease simultaneously. Correlation coefficient is closer to +1.00.
- **Negative**: If one variable increases, the other decreases, and vice versa. Correlation coefficient is closer to -1.00.
- **None**: No correlation exists among variables. Correlation coefficient is closer to 0.

## CASE CONTROL STUDIES

Case control studies compare those with a disease/disorder to a group (controls) without it in order to determine if the affected group has characteristics that are different from the control group. Case control studies are done retrospectively backward from onset of disease/disorder to admission. Usually 2 to 4 controls per case are assessed although the larger the number, the more significant the results. Controls should be chosen at random from the same source population of the cases. Case control studies are relatively inexpensive and can quickly assess risk factors during a possible outbreak, such as potential cause and effect; however, case control studies do not prove causality because there can be confounding variables. While case control studies cannot indicate relative risk, they can be used to calculate the odds ratio, which is the estimate of relative risk. Risk factors indicated by case control studies should be studied more conclusively.

## COHORT STUDIES

A cohort study involves a group that is studied over time. There are a number of subtypes.

**Prospective cohort studies** choose a group of individuals without disease, assess risk factors, and then follow the group over time to determine (prospect for) which ones develop disease. This is typical of general surveillance studies for surgical site infections. Cohort studies take more time but are more reliable statistically than case control studies. In another cohort study, an exposed group and a non-exposed group may be followed to determine how many develop a particular disease. Results are often demonstrated in "2 x 2" tables that show presence of disease and exposure/risk.

|  | Disease | No disease | Totals |
|---|---|---|---|
| **Exposure** | 12 | 28 | 40 |
| **No exposure** | 2 | 58 | 60 |
| **Totals** | 14 | 86 | 100 |

Data is used to calculate relative risk, or risk ratios.

**Retrospective cohort studies** are initiated after illness develops and data is collected retrospectively from medical records to evaluate whether members of the cohort selected had exposure and developed disease.

## CROSS-SECTIONAL STUDY

A cross-sectional study assesses both disease and exposure at the same time in a target population, evaluating the presence of disease at a point in time. For example, a group of people with infections may be assessed for a particular type of exposure or exposures to determine if the exposure(s) are the cause of the disease/disorder. Cross-sectional studies can evaluate the effect of multiple variables and how they relate. Cross-sectional studies can be constructed and analyzed similarly to case control when sampling involves cases and a random selection of controls, yielding prevalence odds ratio. If constructed as a cohort cross-sectional study with an entire group being studied at one time, a 2 x 2 table can be used and calculations would provide a prevalence ratio. Cross-sectional studies often look for the same types of data as cohort studies but require less time and are less expensive.

## QUASI-EXPERIMENTAL RESEARCH

Quasi-experimental research is a form of quantitative research intended to examine relationships and to determine the reason that events happen, examining the causal relationship between selected independent and dependent variables. Quasi-experimental designs are often used when complete control is impossible. Quasi-experimental research lacks random assignment but is otherwise similar to experimental studies in design. One common design is non-equivalent groups in which two non-randomized groups are selected and exposed to different variables (such as two classrooms with different teaching approaches). Another design is regression-discontinuity. With this design, groups are divided according to pre-determined criterion, such as a cutoff score on a test as a requirement for an intervention. Pre-test and post-test design involves identifying a group and administering a pre-test and then providing an intervention, followed by a post-test to determine the efficacy of the intervention.

## EXPERIMENTAL RESEARCH

Experimental research provides the best control because it eliminates or controls factors that influence the dependent variable in order to determine causality. The primary elements of experimental research are randomization, manipulation of the independent variables by the research, and control of the experimental situation. There are many design models, but the classic experimental research design involves two randomized groups—one the experimental group and the other the control group. Both groups take a pretest and then the experimental group undergoes an intervention of some type, and then both groups take a post-test to determine if the intervention had an effect. Another model uses only a post-test. The randomized blocking design follows the classic or post-test only design but involves blocking a variable that may interfere with results. That is, identifying the variable and assigning those with the variable according to severity or other ranking randomly to both groups so that the variable is balanced.

## DATA MANAGEMENT

Evidence-based research can generate large amounts of data, especially qualitative research with extensive field notes. **Data management** includes organizing, reducing, and storing the data. Data must be organized according to type (notes, recordings, records) and content for ease of utilization and analysis. Personal computers and word processing programs as well as spreadsheets may be utilized for data entry, which may involve transcribing and typing notes. These notes then are coded to categorize the data or undergo data reduction during which the notes are "cleaned" and abstracted by selecting or focusing on certain aspects of the data. Data reduction is part of analysis so the researcher must make decisions about what data are important. Data storage may include storing files in file cabinets or storing data in software applications or databases. Data must be secured so that privacy and confidentiality are maintained.

## ANALYSIS OF QUALITATIVE AND QUANTITATIVE DATA

Both qualitative and quantitative data are used for analysis, but the focus is quite different:

- **Qualitative data**: Data are described verbally or graphically, and the results are subjective, depending upon observers to provide information. Interviews may be used as a tool to gather information, and the researcher's interpretation of data is important. Gathering this type of data can be time-intensive, and it can usually not be generalized to a larger population. This type of information gathering is often useful at the beginning of the design process for data collection.
- **Quantitative data**: Data are described in terms of numbers within a statistical format. This type of information gathering is done after the design of data collection is outlined, usually in later stages. Tools may include surveys, questionnaires, or other methods of obtaining numerical data. The researcher's role is objective.

## RESEARCH AND EVIDENCE UTILIZATION
### LEVELS OF EVIDENCE

Levels of evidence are categorized according to the scientific evidence available to support the recommendations the evidence makes, as well as existing state and federal laws. While recommendations are voluntary, they are often used as a basis for state and federal regulations:

- **Category IA** is well supported by evidence from experimental, clinical, or epidemiologic studies and is strongly recommended for implementation.
- **Category IB** has supporting evidence from some studies, has a good theoretical basis, and is strongly recommended for implementation.
- **Category IC** is required by state or federal regulations or is an industry standard
- **Category II** is supported by suggestive clinical or epidemiologic studies, has a theoretical basis, and is suggested for implementation.
- **Category III** is supported by descriptive studies (such as comparisons, correlations, and case studies) and may be useful.
- **Category IV** is obtained from expert opinion or authorities only.
- **Unresolved** means there is no recommendation because of a lack of consensus or evidence.

### INCORPORATING EVIDENCE

Evidence should be incorporated into all **policies, standards, procedures, and guidelines**. Each organization must establish procedures to outline research requirements and the steps necessary to incorporate evidence-based research into all aspects of healthcare and nursing practice. These efforts should be guided by an interdisciplinary team with training in evaluating and integrating research findings. When evaluating policies, standards, procedures, and guidelines, each should be evaluated separately to determine if it is supported by current evidence or requires modification or elimination. Policy and procedure manuals can often contain outdated procedures which lead to confusion and errors. The interdisciplinary team should review literature and current research findings to determine those that are applicable and prepare issue briefs (a review and summary of relevant research findings) for each practice under consideration, including pros and cons as well as cost-effectiveness, to help with informed decision-making.

### LINKING EVIDENCE TO DESIRED OUTCOMES

Linking evidence to desired outcomes requires careful planning. First, the desired outcomes must be identified and prioritized. Then, research projects that accomplished similar outcomes must be reviewed to determine if they are applicable. Issues to consider include the target population studied and how closely it aligns with the current population because, if it does not align, the results of the same intervention may be quite different. Additionally, the methodology must be assessed to determine if it could be replicated. Whether or not the research has external validity is especially important. For example, research conducted at a small rural hospital may yield different outcomes from one conducted at a large urban hospital. If an intervention based on evidence-based research is implemented, then careful assessment must be done to determine if the intervention directly affected the outcomes or if other variables intervened.

### RESEARCH UTILIZATION

Research utilization, using critical thinking skills to evaluate insights gained from research and applying them to practice, requires ongoing efforts on the part of the nurse executive and begins with remaining current by reading research reports and participating in research. Results of research may not be disseminated widely or may not be adopted because healthcare providers feel more comfortable with procedures with which they are more familiar, so the nurse executive must actively seek information, utilizing journals and the internet. The nurse can begin by focusing on areas of interest or need. Utilization varies widely depending on the individuals involved, so research utilization requires education of staff involved so that all members have the same approach to utilization and apply the approach consistently, evaluating outcomes. Additionally, resources must always be considered; for example, utilization of a new procedure that requires added staff when no money is available for staffing is doomed to failure.

## DISSEMINATION OF INFORMATION
### METHODS OF DISSEMINATION

Methods of **disseminating research and evidence-based practice findings** include:

- **Oral/Podium presentations**: These are usually formal presentations based on a prepared outline and presented at conferences or other professional gathering. Oral/Podium presentations often involve the use of presentation software.
- **Panel discussions**: This allows for discussion of various approaches so the pros and cons can be discussed. Remarks may be prepared in advance in some situations.
- **Round table discussions**: These presentations are usually informal and include 6 to 12 participants. Usually up to a half of the time is spent in discussion, so presentation time is limited.
- **Small group/Team/Committee meetings**: EB practice findings may be disseminated during grand rounds and clinical rounds as well as at team meetings. Presentations to committee meetings are usually more formal.
- **Community meetings**: Presentations must be sensitive to cultural issues and consider different levels of health literacy. Presentations should be planned with community members.

Methods of **disseminating research and evidence-based practice findings** include:

- **Visual arts**: Information may be displayed in the form of posters and illustrations in print as well as online.
- **Videos**: Information may be shared through videos with limited or open access (such as on YouTube). Videos should be carefully planned and scripted to ensure information is presented effectively. Videos require knowledge of technology and are most likely to maintain attention if limited to about 15 minutes.
- **Audio/Podcasts**: These can be accessed at any time, so they are convenient but also require knowledge of technology. Podcasts should be limited to about 10 minutes to maintain interest.
- **Journal clubs: These may be virtual or on-site** and are usually led by a clinician with expertise in the area of study.
- **Publishing**: Journal articles (print and online) are one of the most effective means of disseminating findings to professionals.
- **Media**: It's important to consider the audience and their interests. Contacting the media may take time and requires preparation.

## PERFORMANCE PRODUCTIVITY REPORTS

Performance productivity reports are a beginning point in efforts to improve performance. The reports must be analyzed to determine what areas of improvement will have the most impact on meeting goals/outcomes related to strategic goals. After prioritizing needs, the quality professional can use the reports as a basis for improved performance in a number of ways:

- **Education and training**: Staff should be apprised of the results of the reports because often making people aware of how well they are doing and what areas need improvement can provide an impetus for change. Specific training aimed at improving performance according to needs indicated by the reports should be developed.
- **Mentoring**: Staff with strong skills should be identified/trained to mentor and assist others in improving performance.
- **Resources**: Productivity reports often highlight resource needs. Staff must be supplied with the equipment and support they need to achieve performance improvement.

## DASHBOARDS

A dashboard (also called a digital dashboard), like the dashboard in a car, is an easy to access and read computer program that integrates a variety of performance measures or key indicators into one display (usually with graphs or charts) to provide an overview of an organization. It might include data regarding patient satisfaction, infection rates, financial status, or any other measurement that is important to assess performance. The dashboard provides a running picture of the **status** of the department or organization at any point in time, and may be updated as desired: daily, weekly, or monthly. An organization-wide dashboard provides numerous benefits:

- Broad involvement of all departments
- A consistent and easy to understand visual representation of data
- Identification of negative findings or trends so that they can be corrected
- Availability of detailed reports
- Effective measurements that demonstrate the degree of efficiency
- Assistance with making informed decisions

## BALANCED SCORECARDS

The balanced scorecard (designed by Kaplan and Norton) is based on the strategic plan and provides performance measures in relation to the mission statement, vision statement, goals, and objectives. A balanced scorecard includes not only the traditional financial information but also includes data about customers, internal processes, and education/learning. Each organization can select measures that help to determine if the organization is on track to meeting its goals. These measures may include:

- **Customers**: Types of customers and customer satisfaction
- **Finances/business operations**: Financial data may include funding and cost-benefit analysis
- **Clinical outcomes**: Complications, infection rates, inpatient and outpatient data, compliance with regulatory standards
- **Education/learning**: Inservice training, continuing education, assessment of learning and utilization of new skills, research
- **Community**: Ongoing needs
- **Growth**: Innovative programs

If the scorecard is adequately balanced, it will reflect both the needs and priorities of the organization itself and also those of the community and customers.

## DISSEMINATING FINDINGS TO STAKEHOLDERS

There are a number of ways to communicate **evidence-based findings** about policies, procedures, products, or technology to internal and external stakeholders:

- **Presentations to administration** and those in positions of leadership, such as the board of directors, team leaders, and managers, to garner support for incorporating findings into practice
- **Inservice training/education** that focuses on results of research and explains applicability
- **Print distribution** in the form of flyers or newsletters that outline the research findings.
- **Electronic newsletters** or training modules that present the research findings
- **Discussions** with intra- and interdisciplinary team members about the research and ways in which to apply those to the practice of care
- **Presentations to community agencies** and community members about benefits to the population
- **Dashboards** to report ongoing findings and progress
- **Media notices** and information sent to local newspapers, magazines, TV, and radio and giving interviews about evidence-based findings

## IMPLEMENTING INNOVATIONS

### SMALL TESTS OF CHANGE

Small tests of change are done to determine if a change can result in positive outcomes. The key word is *small* because small tests of change should be narrow in scope—such as with one nurse, one patient, one team, or one step in a process. Multiple small tests of change should be carried out in different situations rather than one test only. When planning the test, the plan should include how the data will be collected and a prediction or estimate to be used as a benchmark. Directions for the test should be very clear about what's being tested, who is carrying out the test, and how it will be evaluated. It's best to start testing with those who are interested or committed to the change because people who are resistant may negatively influence outcomes or attempt to undermine the process. Evaluation of an initial test may help to determine if ongoing tests should be modified.

### PILOT PROGRAMS

Instituting a pilot program is often an excellent way to ensure that staff members support changes because many people are resistive to changes. A pilot program initiated on a small scale can provide feedback that can be used to modify or revise the program as needed before instituting the program for the entire organization since new projects are rarely without problems. Those involved in the pilot program can also then serve as mentors to others. Pilot implementation is often used in large organizations or those with multiple locations to essentially "try out" the new system before it is further implemented. This is similar to phased rollout except that it is usually limited to one or few units and extensive evaluation is usually completed during the pilot program, including interviews with users, to determine what faults exist and to assess end-user acceptance so that any alterations or modifications needed can be completed prior to further implementation.

### UTILIZING DIVERSITY

Diversity can be defined in various ways, but it generally refers to integral attributes of a human being, such as race, ethnicity, age, religion, gender, sexual orientation, and family status. While diversity can bring conflicts because of prejudice and stereotyping, diversity can also be leveraged positively by bringing different perspectives to the table. In a growing multicultural society, the healthcare organization can benefit from diversity by taking actions:

- Adding **programs and/or services** that target different diverse populations, such as education programs about living with chronic disease for older adults or Spanish-language health programs.
- Mirroring the community by recruiting and developing **employees** from diverse backgrounds.
- Developing **policies** that help to take advantage of skills and productivity of diverse employees.

**Managing diversity** includes recognizing and valuing diversity, developing support systems, such as mentoring, to promote staff development, and ensuring fair treatment and respect for the individual.

## APPLICATION OF TECHNOLOGY

Technology both in terms of equipment and software applications is developing at a rapid pace, with new technology available almost weekly. When **evaluating and applying technology to support innovation**, a selection committee should include members with expertise in technology as well as clinical staff or others who will utilize the technology. There are a number of steps that should be carried out during evaluation and selection:

- Evaluate existing resources and technology
- Identify areas in which new or upgraded technology may benefit innovation
- Prioritize
- Research available technology to determine which technology is most appropriate
- Identify human resources for implementation
- Estimate training needs in terms of time and costs
- Estimate ongoing costs based on life expectancy of technology and need for upgrades
- Conduct a cost-benefit analysis
- Project return-on-investment in terms of both financial returns and healthcare benefits

## CLINICAL PRACTICE INNOVATION
### DIFFUSION OF INNOVATIONS

The adoption of new ideas and how they spread is referred to as the "**diffusion of innovations**." According to Rogers (2003), innovations spread by stages through an organization, and innovations may be continued if accepted and supported by outcomes or may be rejected. The five stages involved in the diffusion of innovations include:

- **Knowing**: Staff must be exposed to an intervention and understand how it functions. Information may be sought or discovered in various ways, such as journal articles and conference presentations.
- **Persuading**: Steps must be taken to engage and interest staff members and to communicate openly about the innovation in order for them to develop positive attitudes.
- **Decision-making**: The innovation may be adopted as is, adapted to meet organization needs, or rejected.
- **Implementing**: The innovation is put into practice with support of key stakeholders, requiring change in behavior. The innovation must be evaluated and modified if necessary.
- **Confirming**: A final decision, based on evaluation, must be made whether to continue the innovation or discontinue it.

92

## ADOPTION OF INNOVATIONS

One of the biggest barriers to innovation in clinical practice is resistance of staff to changes and failure to rely on evidence-based research to guide change. In fact, studies show that most nurses get information from other nurses and do not rely on research. According to Rogers (2003), individuals in a group tend to adopt innovations at different rates (exemplified by a Bell curve):

- **Innovators**: First to seek and accept innovations and change. Often actively seek new information.
- **Early adopters**: Don't seek out innovations but recognize them and apply to practice. Often effective at communicating the value of innovations.
- **Early majority**: Willing to accept changes that are initiated by others but not an active seeker.
- **Late majority**: Reluctant to accept changes. Often must be pressured to overcome resistance.
- **Laggards**: Most resistant. Feel comfortable with the *status quo.*

## FACTORS INFLUENCING THE SUCCESS OF CLINICAL INNOVATION

According to Rogers (2003), change is a complex process that is dependent on a number of different factors because **clinical innovation** requires staff members who are interested in change and innovations and committed to taking steps to ensure change. Five factors that affect the success of clinical innovations include:

- **Relative advantage**: When staff members evaluate innovations, they consider the degree to which the innovation is better than the *status quo.*
- **Compatibility**: To be successful, innovations must be consistent with the current values of the organization or group.
- **Complexity**: Staff may view innovations according to how complex they are and how difficulty to use or understand.
- **Trialability**: An important consideration is how the innovation can be measured to determine its effectiveness.
- **Observability**: This factor considers whether the results of implementation of the innovation are visible to others.

## IMPLEMENTING CLINICAL PRACTICE GUIDELINES

Evidence-based clinical practice guidelines for such things as standing medicine orders or antibiotic protocols are in common use, but decisions are often made based on studies that lack internal and/or external validity or on expert opinion colored by personal bias, so the process of establishing evidence-based clinical practice guidelines should be done systematically. Including those who are resistive to the process often helps to facilitate the establishment of guidelines, but it's important that decisions be made on solid evidence as much as possible. Simply dispensing evidence-based practice guidelines often does not change practice, so consideration must be given to implementation. Decisions must be made as to whether the use of the guidelines is mandatory as standing orders and to what degree individual practitioners can choose other options. Guidelines that are too rigid may be counter-productive. In some cases, establishing guidelines may affect cost-reimbursement from third-party payers.

## IMPLEMENTING CLINICAL PATHWAYS

Clinical pathways are diagnosis-, procedure-, or condition-specific care plans developed for multi-disciplines, outlining steps in care and expected outcomes. The pathways outline goals in individual care as well as the sequence and time of interventions to achieve those goals. They may be developed for physician care or nursing care. Increasingly clinical pathways are being developed as a method to improve and standardize care and decrease hospital stays. There are two basic types of pathways:

- **Guidelines**: These do not require documentation to verify that the pathway has been followed but serve as guides for individual care. The pathway may be in the form of a flow sheet, with different paths to follow depending upon individual's outcomes.
- **Integrated care plan/pathway**: These require dates, signatures, and documentation to show that the steps have been carried out and to indicate specific outcomes.

Pathways should be based on best practices, and effectiveness should be monitored and evaluated to determine if modifications are needed.

## ADVOCATING FOR RESEARCH

### JOURNAL CLUBS

A journal club comprises a group of professionals who meet on a regularly-scheduled basis (such as once monthly) to read and evaluate articles in scientific and professional journals. Elements of leadership include:

- **Selecting appropriate articles to review**: Articles should contain original research or meta-analysis and should contain a section regarding methods. Articles may focus on one area of concern (such as infection control) or topics may vary, depending on the group purpose and interests.
- **Reviewing the articles completely**, including evaluation of methods, materials, and outcomes and identifying the main points and conclusions of the article. Content summary should include authors, source of funding (to help identify bias), research question, study design, subjects, variables (predictor and outcome), results, and conclusions.
- **Disseminating materials** (such as articles and summaries) to all club members at least a week prior to the meeting so they have time to study them.
- **Leading the discussion**, ensuring that all members participate, and determining the validity of the study and application to evidence-based practice.

### RESEARCH COUNCILS

Research councils are formal groups that promote research and support research efforts in a number of different ways, depending on the council's charter. Members are usually interdisciplinary and are often appointed by administration based on their expertise, interest, and willingness to serve. For example, many universities and healthcare organizations involved in research have research councils with representatives assigned from various departments to review research and grant proposals. Some research councils have funds at their disposal and award grants and funding for projects. Research projects that involve human subjects may also require review by other bodies, such as the Institutional Review Board. Some research councils, such as the National Research Council and the Social Science Research Council are private non-profit organizations that conduct and/or promote research and dissemination of research reports, such as the National Research Council's reports on climate change and sexual assault.

## GRANT WRITING

Finding adequate financial resources is often a problem when upgrading to new and expensive equipment or developing new programs. The initial strategy should be to research **grants** as money may be available from other sources. Even if the nurse executive is only able to gain a grant for part of the needed funds, the board of directors may be more willing to consider funding if the organization does not need to bear the entire cost. The nurse executive may also research other sources of financial support, such as community agencies or corporations. The grant applicant should have a clear idea of the type of research project and begin to collect preliminary data and identify those who will supervise or participate in the project before applying. Steps include:

1. Review all directions and written material and follow the directions exactly.
2. Begin application process early to allow time for revisions.
3. Establish a clear timeline.
4. Provide detailed budget information, including support staff (such as office workers) and supplies, outlining exactly the budget for each year of the project.
5. Provide a comprehensive literature review.
6. Write clearly and proofread to ensure there are no grammatical errors.

## Chapter Quiz

Ready to see how well you retained what you just read? Scan the QR code to go directly to the chapter quiz interface for this study guide. If you're using a computer, simply visit the bonus page at **mometrix.com/bonus948/nce** and click the Chapter Quizzes link.

# Business Management

Transform passive reading into active learning! After immersing yourself in this chapter, put your comprehension to the test by taking a quiz. The insights you gained will stay with you longer this way. Scan the QR code to go directly to the chapter quiz interface for this study guide. If you're using a computer, simply visit the bonus page at **mometrix.com/bonus948/nurseexec** and click the Chapter Quizzes link.

## Reimbursement Methods

### PAYOR SYSTEMS

Payors are those that reimburse for healthcare services and most often include individuals, insurance companies, the government, and employers. Healthcare **payor systems** include:

- **Self-pay**: The individual pays out-of-pocket for care, usually at non-discounted prices.
- **Charity care**: No payment is received.
- **Health maintenance organization (HMO)**: Provides health care on capitation basis with members paying set fees to receive all services.
- **Prospective payment system (PPS)**: Payment according to the specific type of patient.
- **Preferred provider organization (PPO)**: Healthcare services provided to a group of individuals based on a negotiated fee. Patients must usually choose physicians within a network to avoid increased costs.
- **Point-of-service organization (PSO)**: Members can receive lower cost coverage if using in-network providers or may pay more to use out-of-network providers.
- **Medicare/Medicaid**: Includes different options, such as pay-for-performance, prospective payment, PPO, and HMO.

### PAYMENT BUNDLING

Payment bundling is a method of reimbursement in which all healthcare providers engaged in an episode of care are reimbursed through one payment rather than billing separately for services so that the group is essentially responsible for the patient rather than the individual. The CMS Innovation Center developed the Bundled Payments for Care Improvement Initiative as a method to improve care and reduce costs. There are 4 models being tested and two phases of implementation:

- **Model 1**: Medicare pays a discounted rate based on the Inpatient Prospective Payment System (IPPS) but physicians are paid separately for acute hospital stay.
- **Model 2**: Fee-for-service payments are made and then retrospectively reconciled against target costs projected by CMS and additional revenue paid or money recouped for hospitalization and post-acute care for up to 90 days.
- **Model 3**: Payment similar to model 2 but episode of care begins with post-acute care services (including SNF, rehabilitation center, and HHA care) initiated within 30 days of discharge and for up to 90 days.
- **Model 4**: Prospective bundled payment made for acute hospital stay.

## PAY-FOR-PERFORMANCE

Pay-for-performance (P4P) is a general term referring to programs that provide monetary incentives for hospitals and healthcare providers to improve the quality of care. Medicare's value-based purchasing program is an example of a P4P program, but there are also many other private and public P4P programs. Pay-for-performance programs are usually based on four types of quality measures:

- **Performance**: Based on carrying out practices demonstrated to improve health outcomes.
- **Outcomes**: Based on achieving positive outcomes (but does not always consider social or other variables that the healthcare provider cannot control).
- **Patient experience (satisfaction)**: Based on patient's perceptions of care received and their satisfaction.
- **Structures/Technology**: Based on facilities and equipment used for care, and may reward some types of upgrades, such as an upgrade to an electronic health record.

Some pay-for-performance programs focus on cost savings and, for example, reward physicians who lower the cost of care, such as by ordering fewer or less expensive tests.

## VALUE-BASED PURCHASING

Value-based purchasing is CMS's incentive program to improve the quality of care by rewarding acute-care hospitals that demonstrate quality care. Incentive payments are paid each year in addition to fee-based payments based on performance and improvement in different measures. Hospital performance is assessed based on sets of measures in specific domains (such as "Clinical Process of Care"). There are a number of measures (such as "fibrinolytic therapy within 30 minutes of hospital arrival") for each domain. Threshold is the 50% rate for hospitals and benchmark is the mean of the top decile. Improvement on measures is scored as 9 if equal to or above benchmark, 0 if at or below threshold rate, and 0 to 9 if between threshold and benchmark. Consistency is scored similarly but with 20 points if all dimension rates are above benchmarks, 0 if at or below threshold, and 0 to 20 if between threshold and benchmark. These points are totaled to make the total performance score (TPS).

# Financial Management and Budgeting

## FINANCIAL MANAGEMENT

Developing and managing a budget for a department requires an understanding of **financial management**. Management must not only include developing and assigning budget items but monitoring expenditures, analyzing, and reporting. Financial planning is a part of strategic planning in which the department demonstrates how resources will be allocated, usually for a one-year period. Financial planning should be based on the best utilization of costs in relation to revenues/outcomes. Objectives include:

- Developing a quantitative **record** of plans.
- Allowing for evaluation of **financial performance**.
- Controlling **costs**.
- Providing information to increase **cost awareness**.

The budget should be linked to daily operations and integrated with strategic vision, mission, goals, and objectives. Those with vested interests in the budget should participate in planning. Monitoring should be ongoing to allow for feedback and modifications as necessary.

## BUDGET MANAGEMENT

Once a budget is developed and established, **budget management** must be conducted on an ongoing basis to ensure that financial targets are met in relation to strategic goals. Management includes:

- **Accountability**: The budget team should include management/directors with an expectation of excellence.
- **Controlling expenses**: This is especially important for departments that do not produce income directly.
- **Monitoring costs in relation to best practice benchmark**: One goal of budget management should be to strive to match benchmarks.
- **Developing corrective action plans**: Any variances in the budget should be accounted for within a week and corrective actions taken.
- **Utilizing a balanced scorecard**: Various measurements, both quantitative and qualitative, should be used to manage cost containment strategies.
- **Recognizing quality**: Rewards for achieving benchmarks should be built in to the budgeting process. In some cases, this may be a bonus.

## REVENUE CYCLE MANAGEMENT

The revenue cycle begins with patient admission and ends with receipt of revenue, and **revenue cycle management** includes all those processes involved in capture (assigning a billable cost) and reimbursement for services provided. The revenue cycle process includes:

- **Pre-registration/Registration**: Information is gathered regarding responsible parties, such as Medicare, the insurance company, and the individual. The patient is assigned an identifier.
- **Billable services**: Services are provided to the patient.
- **Coding**: Services are assigned the appropriate diagnostic and billing codes. Accurate coding is essential and is dependent on documentation of the healthcare provider.
- **Chargemaster**: This must be updated routinely so that the charges are accurate and appropriate.
- **Capture**: Charges documented into billable form.
- **Submission**: Claims are submitted to insurance companies or individuals for collection.
- **Appeals/Resubmissions**: Claims that are denied are reviewed, corrected, and resubmitted as appropriate.
- **Remittance**: Payment is received and posted.
- **Collection**: Unpaid bills are referred for collection.

## SUPPLY AND LABOR EXPENSES

### INVENTORY

Inventory is the stock of materials or equipment on hand. Inventories should be done at least once a year or more often. In many cases, reordering is done when inventory of a particular item drops to a certain pre-established count. Just-in-time ordering, however, waits until inventory stock is almost depleted as a cost saving measure. These types of automatic reordering of supplies are easier with computerized inventories. In some cases, departments have open accounts that can be used for small purchases without bidding. For larger purchases (especially in public institutions), the nurse should state exactly (including brand names when appropriate) those items to be purchased on a bid form. Then, the bids are sent to prospective bidders (at least 3) in a competitive bid process. Organizations vary in what bids are acceptable. Some only accept the low bid, others the best bid (such as those supplying brand names rather than substituting with generic). Many organizations have private purchase plans that allow them to purchase directly without bids or lease equipment, which is less expensive initially.

## OVERTIME

Overtime is always costly to an employer because the federal *Fair Labor Standards Act* (FLSA) requires that an employee who works more than 40 hours per week be paid 1.5 times his or her regular hourly wage. Therefore, authorizing overtime on a frequent basis may cost the organization more money than if it hires another part-time employee (PTE) or full-time equivalent (FTE). Regularly exceeding the staffing budget increases the likelihood of the manager receiving a poor performance appraisal. Overworked employees are more likely to be injured or produce errors and are often inefficient. To minimize overtime, staff should be large enough to accommodate all of the organization's needs. On-call employees should be designated for unscheduled absences. Job descriptions, quality assurance (QA) analyses, and time-motion studies can be used to accurately estimate task completion times and to properly schedule staff.

## COST ALLOCATION

One type of cost analysis for supply and labor expenses involves **cost allocation**. With almost all expenditures, there are direct costs and indirect costs. A direct cost might be the salary of a team leader while indirect costs are those related to accounting, and human resources. To determine cost allocation, the budget must be formatted to determine unit cost or cost per unit of service, so line-item budget format is used. Direct costs must be determined as well as indirect costs. Generally, direct costs benefit just one department or service while indirect costs are shared costs, such as the cost of custodial services. Thus, a percentage of the indirect cost is allocated, based upon the utilization. For a simplified example, if team leaders represent 5% of total employees, then 5% of indirect employee costs would be allocated to this line item. However, there may be many departments and services involved in indirect costs, and to arrive at a true unit cost, all of these costs must be accounted for.

## RETURN ON INVESTMENT AND DEPRECIATION

Return on investment (ROI) is a method used to determine profitability, expressed as a percentage. The basic formula is net profit divided by total cost of investment. Example:

$$\frac{\$20,000 \text{ (net profit)}}{\$120,000 \text{ (cost of investment)}} = \frac{1}{6} = 16.7\%$$

Hospitals often run a narrow profit margin (2% average). Because of this, projected ROI is often calculated prior to investment. For example, if the hospital is considering investing in new equipment, profits would be projected over the expected life of the equipment, and costs for the equipment, maintenance, training, and upgrades would be estimated to determine if the ROI were favorable.

**Depreciation** is the annual reduced value of fixed assets, such as equipment and materials. Depreciation is used for income tax and accounting purposes and when calculating net income. Depreciation is based on the expected useful life of the asset, the salvage value, and the method used to calculate the depreciation (accelerated or steady over the expected useful life).

## PRODUCTIVITY

Productivity is the measure of output produced using a specific quantity of inputs. While the term is often applied to manufacturing, it can also be applied to healthcare:

- Input/Output = Productivity
- Costs/Work hours = Productivity
- Nursing hours/hospital patient days = Productivity
- Nursing staff/hospital census = Productivity

The production process can include marginal productivity (adding additional input to gain additional output), economies of scale (increasing inputs and volume in order to decrease item/unit cost), and short-run distinctions (times with limited change in inputs), long-run distinctions (times when all inputs change) and substitution (replacing inputs with lower cost inputs). Economic evaluation of productivity is carried out through cost analysis, cost-benefit analysis, cost-effectiveness, and cost utility analysis. An organization's charges (revenue) must exceed costs for the organization to remain viable. Additionally, cost minimization may be carried out to determine which of two alternatives is most effective.

## COST-BENEFIT ANALYSIS

A cost-benefit analysis uses the average cost of an event and the cost of intervention to demonstrate savings. For example, according to the CDC, a surgical site infection caused by *Staphylococcus aureus* results in an average of 12 additional days of hospitalization and costs at least $27,000. (In actuality, the cost may vary widely from one institution to another; so local data may be used.)

For example, if an institution were averaging 10 surgical site infections annually, the cost would be: 10 × $27,000 = $270,000 annually. If the interventions include new software ($10,000) for surveillance, an additional staff person ($65,000), benefits ($15,000) and increased staff education, including materials ($2000), the total intervention cost would be: $10,000 + $65,000 +$15,000 + $2000 = $92,000.00. If the goal were to decrease infections by 50% to 5 infections per year, the savings would be calculated: 5 × $27,000 = $135,000. Subtracting the intervention cost from the savings: $135,000 - $92,000 = $43,000 annual cost benefit.

## BUDGETS

### TYPES OF BUDGETS

A departmental budget is part of a larger organizational budget, so an understanding of the different **types of budgets** utilized in healthcare management is helpful:

- **Operating budget**: This budget is used for daily operations and includes general expenses, such as salaries, education, insurance, maintenance, depreciation, debts, and profit. The budget has three elements: statistics, expenses, and revenue.
- **Capital budget**: This budget determines which capital projects (such as remodeling, repairing, and purchasing of equipment or buildings) will be allocated funding for the year. These capital expenditures are usually based on cost-benefit analysis and prioritization of needs.
- **Cash balance budget**: This type of budget projects cash balances for a specific future time period, including all operating and capital budget items.
- **Master budget**: This budget combines operating, capital, and cash balance budgets as well as any specialized or area-specific budgets.

## OPERATIONAL BUDGETS

Most departmental budgets will be **operational**, but there are a number of different approaches to operational budgets that can be used:

- **Fixed/Forecast**: Revenue and expenses are forecasted for the entire budget period and budget items are fixed.
- **Flexible**: Estimates are made regarding anticipated changes in revenue and expenses, and both fixed and variable costs are identified.
- **Zero-based**: All cost centers are re-evaluated each budget period to determine if they should be funded or eliminated, partially or completely.
- **Responsibility center**: Budgeting is for a cost center (department) or centers with one person holding overall responsibility.
- **Program**: Organizational programs are identified, and revenues and costs for each program are budgeted.
- **Appropriations**: Government funds are requested and dispersed through this process.
- **Continuous/rolling**: Periodic updates to the budget including revenues, costs, and volume are done prior to the next budget cycle.

## CAPITAL BUDGETS

Capital budgets are dependent on the strategic plan of the healthcare organization, which usually outlines goals for about a 5-year period. These goals should include capital projects that have been proposed and approved. Capital projects include land and other long-term assets, such as buildings, IT systems, vehicles, remodeling, and major equipment purchases. The strategic plan should outline sources of funding and total projected costs as the costs are the basis for budget development. Part of developing a capital budget is to determine if the projected project is cost-effective and will generate adequate return on investment. Important considerations include possible alternatives, available resources, risk factors, and data regarding costs and benefits. Different from operational budgets (which are usually annual), capital budgets may last for the duration of a project, and this in some cases can be 3 to 4 years or even longer.

## BUDGET VARIANCE

Budget variance is the difference between the budgeted expense or revenue and the actual expense or revenue, and this can result in cost overruns that are prohibitive, so planning must consider all possible scenarios, such as increased equipment, supply, insurance, and labor costs. Budget variance analysis is done for both capital and operational budgets. In budgeting, a positive variance is usually indicated by the letter F (favorable) and a negative variance by the letter U (unfavorable) or A (adverse). Cost variance may relate to materials, labor, sales, or production overhead. Analyses may include:

- **Net present value** (difference between inflow and outflow): Determines if the projected revenue exceeds projected costs.
- **Throughput analysis**: Assesses the ability of a project to increase throughput through bottlenecks in the organization.
- **Discounted cash flow** (Future cash flows estimated and discounted to present time value): Evaluates initial and ongoing costs as well as revenue.
- **Payback**: Assesses how long it will take to recoup expenses (initial costs/average yearly revenue).
- **Internal rate of return**: Assessment of the cash flow stream.

## CONTRACTUAL AGREEMENTS AND OUTSOURCING

Increasingly, healthcare organizations have been using **contractual agreements** and **outsourcing** as a method of cost cutting. Outsourcing has been commonly used for services unrelated to direct patient care, such as food services, housekeeping, and supply management. As the emphasis on data collection has increased along with the change to electronic health records, healthcare organizations have begun to outsource IT services rather than to set up their own departments and hire staff because outsourcing requires less capital expenditure. More recently, outsourcing has moved into areas of direct patient care, such as emergency department physicians, anesthesiologists, hospitalists, imaging services, and dialysis services. When providing services to a hospital, these healthcare providers work for the agency that assigned them rather than for the hospital. These services are often vital to the organization but do not involve positions in which a long-term relationship with a patient is important (such as with primary care physicians).

### VENDORS

Vendors should produce evidence of effective implementation of programs with similar organizations, should provide a product history that includes the frequency of upgrades and the compatibility with previous equipment/software versions, and should provide product, maintenance, and service upgrades. A request for information may be sent to vendors initially to facilitate comparison. Internet searches, networking, and conference attendance may also provide information. In some cases, writing a Request for Proposal (RFP), which outlines the needs of the organization, can be given to a vendor, but most vendors will no longer provide a customized response: however, the evaluation team should prepare such an outline to use as a guide and checklist during the evaluation process. A number of vendor contracts should be reviewed prior to completing the contract and legal advice sought. Contracts should include provisions for delivery and installation, training, support, liabilities, prices, payment terms, program modifications, and confidentiality.

### MATERIALS AND SUPPLIES

Cost-cutting measures are critical to the survival of healthcare organizations, as reimbursements have fallen while expenses have increased. Healthcare organizations have utilized various strategies to decrease the costs of **materials and supplies** obtained through contractual agreements. About three-quarters of purchases by hospitals for materials and supplies are now done through contracts with group purchasing organizations (GPOs). These GPOs aggregate purchase orders in order to buy in large volumes that are lower in cost with savings to healthcare organizations usually ranging from 10 to 15%. GPOs do not directly purchase materials but negotiate the contracts under which the healthcare organizations purchase. Contracting with a GPO also reduces the number of staff and time needed for purchasing, resulting in further cost savings. Healthcare organizations often also use other strategies, such as conducting price comparisons to determine the most cost-effective choice, limiting the number of vendors with whom they contract for materials, and limiting brand names to increase purchase volume.

### STAFFING

Contract employees are employed for a specified period of time, sometimes as short as one day. Generally, they are contracted through an employment agency when a hospital or healthcare organization is short-staffed. In some cases, a hospital may contract with an individual directly for a specific short-term or long-term project.

**Traveler workers** include nurses, physicians, and therapists. Travel nurse agencies have proliferated, and costs are usually higher than when hiring locally. Typically, a traveling healthcare provider works under contract for a limited period of time, such as 4 to 12 weeks although some assignments may last up to 2 years. Most agencies require 1 to 2 years nursing experience for hire as an RN. Nurses may have to relicense if moving to another state unless it is part of the Nurse Licensure Compact. The hospital pays the agency, which in turn pays the nurse, so the nurse is not an actual employee of the hospital and not eligible for benefits provided direct employees.

## HOURS PER PATIENT DAY

Nursing hours per patient day reflect the amount of nursing care necessary per patient in a 24-hour period. The first calculation is the average patient census, which is usually based on the midnight census and historical and current trends. Nursing hours per patient day calculates only productive hours (those in which the nurse is available for patient care) rather than nonproductive hours (such as sick days). For example, if there are 20 average patients on a unit and 6 staff members during the day shift, 4 in the afternoon, and 4 in the night shift for a total of 14 staff members each working 8 hours, this equals 112 productive hours per day:

$$\frac{112 \text{ hr}}{20 \text{ patients}} = 5.6 \text{ nursing hours per patient day}$$

**Productive hours** may vary depending on the benefits package, but it is usually about 80%. So, if an FTE nurse is paid for 2080 hours but has only 80% productive hours, the person is only actually available for patient care for 1664 hours:

$$2080 \times 80\% = 1664$$

## FULL-TIME EQUIVALENCY (FTE)

The Health Care Reform law has established a method of determining **full-time equivalency** (FTE) for employees as part of the determination for tax credits. Employers and accrediting agencies also use FTE when reviewing staffing levels and cost-effectiveness. FTE hours are 2080 annually (40 hours × 52), so to determine the number of FTE employees, the hours of all employees are totaled and then divided by 2080, excluding seasonal workers who work fewer than 120 days during the year (although this usually does not apply to healthcare). Note that only 2080 hours may be counted for any one employee, so hours exceeding this limit are eliminated. For example, if 1 employee worked 2200 hours, 4 employees worked 2080 hours each, 4 worked 1040 hours each, and 1 worked 800 hours, the calculation is:

$$5 \times 2,080 = 10,400; \ 4 \times 1,040 = 4,160; \ 1 \times 800 = 800$$

$$10,400 + 4,160 + 800 = 15,360$$

$$\frac{15,360}{2,080} = 7.38$$

Numbers with decimals are rounded down (not up) to the whole number, so this employer has 7 FTE employees. Note: employees working fulltime at 36 hours per week are counted as 0.9 FTEs.

## COMPENSATION

A number of decisions must be made when determining **compensation** for a position, and the extent and cost of benefits must always be considered as part of the compensation package. Salary may be somewhat dependent on supply and demand but should reflect industry and/or geographic standards. The salary should be included in the job description. The four usual choices are:

- **Salary in exact dollar amounts**: This is clear and unbiased but leaves no room for negotiation or reward for experience or special skills.
- **Salary range**: A rubric should clearly outline the requirements for each level of the salary range (such as years of experience, continuing education, special skills) to avoid bias.
- **Incentive compensation**: A bonus at hire or higher than usual salary range may be provided in order to attract candidates when there is a shortage of eligible hires.
- **Negotiable salary**: This can result in wide ranges of salaries for similar positions and can appear biased.

## BENEFITS

Job benefits may vary widely, but are often as important as salary in determining whether a person chooses employment. Benefits can include:

- **Leave time**: May include holiday time (usually 8 to 10 days per year) sick time (usually 8 to 10 days per year) and vacation time (usually 5 to 20 days) or a combination of paid time off that can be utilized for either vacation or sick days
- **Insurance coverage**: An organization may have group insurance policies available that the employees can pay for or may provide all or part of the cost of insurance, and it may include health, dental, eye coverage, and long-term care and may cover only the individual or the individual and immediate family
- **Childcare**: Reimbursement for cost or on-site childcare facility
- **Retirement policy**: May include profit-sharing plans, traditional pensions, 401K plans with employer contribution, stock ownership, and stock bonus plans
- **Student loan forgiveness**: Often offered as hiring incentive
- **Transportation**: May provide transportation to work or transit passes
- **Credit unions**
- **Employee assistance programs**

> **Review Video: Total Rewards and Compensation**
> Visit mometrix.com/academy and enter code: 502662

# Leadership

## LEADERSHIP STYLES

### PERVASIVE LEADERSHIP

Central to the concept of pervasive leadership is the idea that everyone has leadership potential and influence over others to some degree. Pervasive leadership recognizes the power found in groups and allows them a greater degree of autonomy in making decisions and solving problems rather than their having to wait for a central authority to make decisions. Pervasive leadership is also concerned with relationships that occur among fellow workers and how that can strengthen an organization. Pervasive leadership aims to provide all workers with the tools they need to become better leaders through mentoring, role modeling, and training so there is less reliance on the chain of command so that decisions are often made from the bottom up instead of the top down. Leaders actively share power with staff members and freely share data in order to ensure that staff members are well-informed and understand the needs of the organization.

## SERVANT LEADERSHIP

Servant leadership (Greenleaf, 1970) is a form of leadership in which leaders' first priority is to be servants in the sense of serving others rather than simply leaders concerned with profitability. Servant leaders consider the needs of the organization and the individuals and determine how best to meet these needs and encourage growth and wellbeing. These leaders provide support and encouragement to workers and exhibit skills in listening, empathy, and persuasion. The focus is on collaboration and participation at all levels in an organization. The concept of servant leadership can apply to individual leaders or to the organization as a whole. However, applying the principles of servant leadership to an organization often requires an extended period of time and may necessitate changes to the mission, vision, and strategic plan because a change in organizational mindset rarely occurs easily or rapidly.

## SITUATIONAL LEADERSHIP

Situational leadership (Blanchard and Hersey) is a leadership style that is flexible and changes according to the situation and the skills and needs of the workers. The four behavior types of situational leaders are:

- **S1 (Telling)**: Leader in charge with one-way communication.
- **S2 (Selling)**: Leader in charge with two-way communication and provision of social and emotional support.
- **S3 (Participating)**: Leader utilizes shared decision making for aspects of tasks.
- **S4 (Delegating)**: Leader involved but no longer responsible for tasks.

The qualities needed of a situational leader include:

- **Diagnostic ability**: Able to look at a situation and determine what is needed and to understand the people involved, including the amount of direction and supervision needed and readiness to learn.
- **Adaptability**: Able to adapt behavior to the needs of the particular situation and to provide the needed social and emotional support.
- **Communicative ability**: Able to communicate with others in ways that they can understand and relate to, changing the style of communication as needed for different audiences/populations.

## TRANSACTIONAL LEADERSHIP

Transactional leadership is geared toward the management, supervision, and oversight in and of group performance. Status quo is of chief concern, with goals dictating actions, repercussions, and rewards. Because the focus is on meeting goals and benchmarks that have been predetermined, this is often considered a task-oriented leadership style. While this is an effective management technique, it is often seen as insufficient to motivate and inspire positive change in a work force. Its dependence on a punishment and reward system of extrinsic motivation tends to inspire short term commitment that lacks a common vision.

## TRANSFORMATIONAL LEADERSHIP

Transformational leadership is focused on inspiring and motivating members of the team to identify common goals and visions that intrinsically motivate the individual members to contribute. In this model, the leader's duty is to communicate and identify common goals and visions of the unit, address concerns or discrepancies with those visions, and create an environment of joint commitment and direction. The leader must recognize each individual's strengths and encourage the members of the team to utilize those strengths and hone their weaknesses for the sake of the

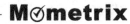

group. Because this leadership style relies on the intrinsic motivation of each member of the team, there is less need of rewards and punishments, as the members are internally motivated to contribute to the maximum of their potential.

## APPRECIATIVE INQUIRY

Appreciative inquiry begins with the premise that there are positive aspects in all individuals and organizations, so the focus is to use questioning to find out what talents and insights individuals have and what in the organization is working well and building from that rather than a focus on identifying what is wrong and problem solving. The five major principles include:

- **Constructionist**: Belief creates reality and interaction constructs situations and organizations.
- **Simultaneity**: Questions themselves promote change.
- **Poetic**: People's words create the life of the organization and cause emotions.
- **Anticipatory**: People act currently in accordance to their beliefs about the future.
- **Positive**: Change necessitates social cohesion and positive sentiments.

The processes involved in appreciative inquiry include discovering (finding processes that are successful), dreaming (imagining processes that will be successful in the future), designing (developing processes that are effective), and deploying (implementing).

## PERSONAL LEADERSHIP EVALUATION

Personal leadership evaluation should involve both self-reflection and assessment with a leadership self-assessment tool. Self-reflection is a method of looking inward and thinking about one's situation to examine thought processes, biases, and motivations. Self-reflection usually involves asking the self a series of questions: "Why did I say that?" "What was my reaction to the response?" "Why did I react that way?" "How could I have handled the situation better?" Self-reflection can be carried out in different ways, such as by internal dialog or by journaling. Honesty is a critical element in self-reflection. Personal leadership evaluation is more structured and formal and often begins with a questionnaire that lists a number of attributes, such as "I am able to articulate the organization's mission and vision statements to others," and then asks the person to rate how true the statement is using a Likert scale.

## INTEGRATION OF DIVERSITY AND SENSITIVITY

The nurse executive's goal of integrating diversity and sensitivity into the work environment should be for employees to be accepting of differences rather than being judgmental or trying to change them. Diversity in the workplace refers to both an increasingly culturally diverse patient population and a culturally diverse workforce. The nurse executive should complete a personal cultural audit in order to better understand personal biases and feelings. The nurse executive must make clear support for embracing diversity by including it in the vision and mission of the organization and should take active leadership in designing services in response to the needs of diverse patients and conducting outreach to attract employees that culturally mirror the population served. The nurse executive should serve as a role model for the staff and should promote educational programs, including mentoring, that outline patient care considerations for different cultural groups so that employees are more sensitive to cultural issues.

## ORGANIZATIONAL COMMITMENT TO DIVERSITY AND SENSITIVITY

Acceptance and responsiveness to diversity requires an organizational commitment with ongoing in-service training to assist staff. This may include:

- **Multicultural advisory committees** with community representatives to provide insight and determine areas for research or outreach to diverse groups.
- **Mentors or consultants** who can provide guidance to staff dealing with issues of diversity.
- Adaptation of **patient/family materials** for diverse groups, including patient information materials and surveys. These should be culturally appropriate and in various languages for those who are not proficient in English.
- Strategies to **hire, retain, and promote** a staff that is diverse and representative of the community.
- Training on how to work with **interpreters**.
- Integrating **cultural content** throughout training curriculum, with specific information about cultural attitudes toward intimacy, sexuality, end-of-life, mental and physical illness, drug use, and health in general. Including representatives of diverse groups for presentations and group or panel discussions is particularly helpful.

## CREATING A CULTURE OF INNOVATION

Innovation is an important element in leadership practice as leaders provide the vision and often initiate and guide change, and the nurse executive should be open to change in leadership practices as well as clinical practices. Steps that encourage innovation and change include:

- **Establishing need**: The nurse executive must not only identify the need for change but articulate the value of change in order to generate support, especially the value to the staff members who will implement change.
- **Facilitating group participation**: The nurse executive should rely on key stakeholders and groups to facilitate change and determine details of change so that they are committed to the process.
- **Providing data**: Data should be complete and reliable.
- **Establishing a reward system**: The nurse executive should motivate staff members through a system of recognition and rewards.
- **Being open and honest**: The nurse executive must ensure to deliver everything promised and to not promise things that cannot be delivered.

# Strategic Planning

## ORGANIZATIONAL STRATEGIC PLANNING

Organization-wide strategic planning requires that an organization look at needs of the organization, community, and customers and establish goals for not only the near future (2-4 years) but into the extended future (10-15 years). Strategic planning must be based on assessments, both internal and external, to determine the present courses of action, needed changes, priorities, and methodologies to effect change. The focus of strategic planning must be on development of services based on identified customer needs and then the marketing of those services. Organization-wide strategic planning includes:

- Collecting data and doing an external analysis of customer needs in relation to regulations and demographics
- Analyzing internal services and functions

- Identifying and understanding key issues, including the strengths and weaknesses of the organization as well as potential opportunities and negative impacts
- Developing revised mission and vision statements that identify core values
- Establishing specific goals and objectives

## ORGANIZATIONAL VISION STATEMENT

An organizational vision statement requires analysis of both internal and external customer-supplier relationships in arriving at a statement about what the organization intends to become. The vision statement is the commitment that the organization is making. The vision statement should include future goals rather than focusing on what has already been achieved. The vision statement is usually stated in one sentence or a short paragraph:

- Hospital X will be the leader in providing sustainable quality patient-centered care to the community to improve the physical and mental health of community members.

The vision statement is often followed by an explanation of terms, so that such concepts as "sustainable" and "patient-centered" are clarified to explain the reason for including the terms in the vision statement. For example, if "sustainable" is part of the vision statement, then the explanation should include the need to function within budget constraints while providing optimum care.

## ORGANIZATIONAL MISSION STATEMENT

The mission statement of an organization usually reflects the current status of the organization and describes, in broad terms, the purpose of the organization and its role in the community. The mission statement should be developed in response to data and program analysis and with input from all members of the organization. The mission statement should identify the organization or program, state its function, and outline the purpose and strategy of the program:

- The mission of X Hospital, a collaborative group of professionals, physicians, administrators, nurses, and support staff, is to promote health and safety of patients, visitors, and staff and provide outstanding quality health care services to the community.

The mission statement should in some way include a commitment to quality and patient care as well as the need to serve the community. In many cases, the mission statement is followed by detailed explanations that may include statements of organizational values, philosophy, and history.

## GOALS AND OBJECTIVES

The development of goals and objectives is done in support of the mission and vision statements and should be completed at the same time to determine if the mission and vision statements can be realized and to explain how that will happen.

- **Goals** should be achievable aims, essentially end results, developed for specific units of the organization or the organization in general, focusing on improving performance. One example of a specific goal is: *Reduction in surgical site infections by 30%.* In healthcare quality management, the goals must be based on knowledge about functions and processes within the organization and prioritized accordingly as part of achieving positive patient outcomes.

108

- **Objectives** are the measurable steps taken to achieve goals. In the case of infections, an example of an objective might include: *Infection control professional will audit antibiotic use, and physician internal medicine committee will establish antibiotic prophylaxis protocol within 6 months.* Objectives should be measurable and should include a timeline and identification of responsibility for achieving the objective.

## SWOT ANALYSIS

SWOT analysis is commonly used to help determine an organization's strengths and weaknesses and as part of strategic planning; however, SWOT analysis can be used for any type of decision-making as it provides a good overview of the organization and helps to provide an outline of different factors affecting decisions. SWOT analysis is often done as part of market planning as preparation for carrying out a marketing program. SWOT analysis considers the strengths and weaknesses of the internal environment and the opportunities and threats of the external environment:

| Internal environment | | External environment | |
|---|---|---|---|
| *Strengths* | *Weaknesses* | *Opportunities* | *Threats* |
| Financial stability | Increasing costs | Increased population | Low reimbursement |
| Programs, services | Outdated equipment | New programs | Regulations |
| Staff persons | Ineffective programs | New markets | Competition |
| Client/Staff satisfaction | Marketing | Stakeholders | Political changes |

## STRATEGIC QUALITY PLANNING

Strategic quality planning to promote performance improvement must begin at the top level of management with a commitment to effecting change at all levels and to providing the financial resources that make these changes possible. This entails beginning with a clear definition of quality as it applies to customers and relating this to mission and vision statements, goals, and objectives. Plans must be made to redesign processes in order to achieve quality and to modify measures of organizational performance to ensure compliance. Total quality management should be at the center of all planning, and an organization-wide model for quality performance should be used that includes at least the following:

- Assessment
- Planning
- Implementation
- Evaluation of continuous improvement

The planning process should be documented with preparation of an action plan that ensures ongoing evaluation of progress.

## MEASURING PATIENT/CUSTOMER SATISFACTION

Patient/customer satisfaction is usually measured with surveys given to patients upon discharge from an institution or on completion of treatment. One problem with analyzing surveys is that establishing benchmarks can be difficult because so many different survey and data collection methods are used that comparison data may be meaningless. Internal benchmarking may be more effective, but the sample rate for surveys may not be sufficient to provide validity. As patients become more knowledgeable and demand for accountability increases, patient satisfaction is being

**109**

used as a guide for performance improvement although patient perceptions of clinical care do not always correlate with outcomes. The results of surveys can provide feedback that makes healthcare providers more aware of customer expectations. Currently, surveys are most often used to evaluate service elements of care rather than clinical elements. Analysis includes:

- Determining the patient/customer's degree of trust.
- Determining the degree of satisfaction with care/treatment.
- Identifying needs that may be unmet.
- Identifying patient/customer priorities.

## ALIGNING NURSING STRATEGIC PLAN WITH ORGANIZATIONAL PLAN

Alignment of nursing's strategic plan with the organizational plan should begin early in the development stage. For example, if part of the organizational plan is to increase labor productivity in order to reduce costs, and the nursing strategic plan includes decreasing the nurse-patient ratio, then the objectives that are developed for the strategic plan should align these two concerns, such as by reducing overtime and/or changing the staffing model in order to compensate for the increased costs of reducing the nurse-patient ratio. The nursing strategic plan cannot be successful if it is at odds with the organizational plan, especially if resources are needed for implementation. The strategic plan should be developed by nursing but in collaboration with organizational leaders, including those from human resources and finance, and should be based on thorough assessment of needs, including gap analysis, surveys, and input from nursing staff at all levels.

## COMMUNICATING AND BUILDING CONSENSUS

If the nurse executive wants to communicate and build consensus and support for the strategic plan, then communication must begin prior to development of the plan. Even though the strategic plan is usually developed at the executive level, all members of an organization should be asked for input to the planning process because the staff members will ultimately determine the success of the plan and are often the most impacted. For example, if expanding services is one of the goals of the plan, then this may require extra responsibilities for existing staff. Benefits to the plan should be stressed as well as concerns. The nurse executive should outline the strategic plan to key stakeholders and department heads and engage them in the process of building support for the plan among all staff members. A reporting system should be in place, such as a dashboard, so that progress can be charted and observed.

# Program Development

## PROPOSALS

When making a proposal for new program development, the first step is to determine whether there is a guide for the proposal format. If so, it must be followed exactly or the proposal may be rejected. In some cases, a letter of inquiry should be submitted prior to the proposal. In general, proposals include an abstract, a narrative proposal, and a budget. The proposal should explain the purpose of the program and the need. The proposal should also outline exactly how the need will be met and by whom and should present an estimated timeline and benchmarks. The proposal should explain how the project management will be carried out and should identify responsible individuals. The projected budget should cover personnel costs (salaries, benefits) and non-personnel costs (contract fees, consultant fees, equipment, travel, and miscellaneous).

## PRO FORMA

A *pro forma* is a financial statement that outlines expenses associated with a new program. The pro forma, usually presented in a spreadsheet, is the projected revenue and expenses for the first year (or beyond) and should include the following:

- **Net Revenue**: Includes total income minus bad debts and discounts (such as for PPOs, HMOs, and third-party carriers).
- **Expenses**: Includes salary expenses (salaries and benefits) and non-salary expenses, such as for clinical supplies, equipment, office supplies, service agreements, insurance, capital expenses (remodeling), telephone, utilities, entertainment, travel, training, rent/lease costs, depreciation, and taxes.
- **Direct expense**: Total of salary and non-salary expenses.
- **Contribution margin**: The total net revenue less the direct expense.
- **Indirect expenses**: Overhead or other costs.
- **Total cost margin**: Contribution margin less the indirect cost.

The **pro forma** should include the **metrics** that will be used for the items in the spreadsheet and should be as accurate as possible using current information as well as future projections.

## BUSINESS PLAN

Elements of a business plan include the following:

| Executive summary | Outline all the key elements to the business proposal, including the customer, product/services, goals, risks, opportunities, costs, management, and timeline. |
| --- | --- |
| Product/Service | Provide a detailed description but avoid being overly technical, including the ways in which this product/service compares to others. Note the need for patents, licenses, or any regulatory requirements. |
| Management | Explain the hierarchy and division of duties, including explanation of professional experience and education. |
| Market Survey | Discuss similar products/services, target groups, and projected market volume. |
| Marketing strategies | Explain placement, promotion, and pricing |
| Organization | Describe structure of business, provide flow charts, and describe production capability, costs, quality assurance methods, and inventory (if appropriate). |
| Timeline | Describe the timeline for implementation from beginning to fully operational business. |
| Risk factors | Describe both opportunities from gain and risk factors that may impact product/sales and methods to deal with risk factors. |
| Appendices | Provide samples of forms and any additional information that is necessary. |

## MARKETING STRATEGY

The first task in the development of a marketing strategy is to determine the objectives and the target market. Market research may involve literature review, surveys, questionnaires, market analysis, and focus groups. The target market may be segmented according to various demographics with each segment requiring a different approach. The marketing plan should include different marketing strategies: advertisements (print, TV, radio), direct marketing, and trade shows/conferences. SWOT analysis is often done to determine the strengths and weaknesses of an organization as part of the marketing plan. If a product is involved, then product research must be conducted. Benchmarking through tracking such as by using web analytics to determine traffic on a website or by list splitting (different versions of a mailer sent to different populations), can help to provide useful data. In some cases, the best initial marketing strategy may be to utilize a market research agency to gather information.

## PROJECT MANAGEMENT
### PROJECT PLAN
**Elements of the project plan** include plans for and management of the following:

- **Purpose**: What will be achieved by the project
- **Scope**: General work to be done, end product, and department involvement/responsibilities
- **Requirements**: Agreed upon documentation, agreements, tracing, and reporting
- **Schedule of activities**: Includes activities, milestones, products, and timeline
- **Finances**: Explanation of budget, financial resources, payroll, and potential unexpected expenses
- **Quality control**: Monitoring, reporting, and correcting for quality issues
- **Resources**: Materials, staff, equipment, finances needed to complete the project and expected utilization of resources
- **Stakeholders**: Identification of stakeholders, prioritizing stakeholders, and methods of communication with and management of stakeholders

**Elements of the project plan** include plans for and management of the following:

- **Risks**: Anticipating and identifying risk factors, methods to manage and respond to risks and reduce liability
- **Communications**: Plans for internal and external communication, including public relations
- **Purchasing**: Vendors, cost-comparison, methods of purchase, timeline for purchase, and inventory
- **Change**: Requirements for and response to change in plans

### GANTT CHART FOR TIMELINE DEVELOPMENT
A Gantt chart is used for developing improvement projects to manage schedules and estimate time needed to complete tasks. It is a bar chart with a horizontal time scale that presents a visual representation of the beginning and end points of time when different steps in a process should be completed. Gantt charts are a component of project management software programs. The Gantt chart is usually created after initial brainstorming, and creation of a time line and action plans. Steps to creation of a Gantt chart include:

1. List the name of the process at the top.
2. Create a chart with a timeline of days, weeks, months (as appropriate for process) horizontally across the top.
3. List tasks vertically on the left of the chart.
4. Draw horizontal lines/bars with from the expected beginning point to the expected end point for each task. These may be color-coded to indicate which individual/team is responsible for completing the task.

Discuss project management to support/achieve the strategic plan: Development of the timeline (Critical path method).

## CRITICAL PATH METHOD FOR TIMELINE DEVELOPMENT

Critical path method is a network diagramming technique used to estimate the total duration of a project. The project manager develops a diagram that shows all of the primary paths with estimated duration of time for each and then identifies the longest path through the network design. This, in turn, provides the latest time by which the project can be completed. Key concepts of timeline development include the following:

- **Slack** or **float** refers to amount of delay time that an activity can be delayed without impacting the overall completion time.
- **Critical chain scheduling** involves identifying constraints and scheduling accordingly. Critical chain scheduling builds in a time buffer for project completion and discourages multitasking, favoring completion of one task before beginning another.
- **Program Evaluation and Review Technique (PERT)** is a technique utilized for project time management. PERT is used to estimate times when the duration of individual activities is uncertain. PERT achieves probabilistic time estimates by taking into consideration optimistic, most likely, and pessimistic time estimates.

## IMPLEMENTATION

Strategic plans begin on paper but are implemented in practice, and **implementation** can often be more difficult than writing the plan because of the complexity of dealing with many different stakeholders. Implementation of a strategic plan involves a series of steps:

1. **Identify goals**: Identify long-term and short-term goals. Determine processes and procedures needed to implement the plan.
2. **Create a guide**: Prioritize and organize processes and procedures and explain how implementation will be coordinated through different departments or units.
3. **Engage staff**: Communicate openly and set performance goals in relation to the strategic plan. Explain benefits as well as problems that may occur.
4. **Align budget to the plan**: Modify budgets as necessary.
5. **Conduct small tests of change/pilot studies**: Practice implementation and test in small increments before rollout.
6. **Roll out**: Prepare and train staff in advance.
7. **Monitor and measure**: This is an ongoing process throughout implementation.
8. **Modify**: Evaluate and modify the plan as indicated.

## MONITORING

Monitoring is an essential part of program evaluation and should be an ongoing process throughout the life of a program. Monitoring principles include:

- Monitoring should compare **current status** with **baseline data**. Baseline data should be used to set targets for improvement.
- Monitoring should determine whether or not **progress** is being made.
- Monitoring should be planned as an integral part of **every program**.
- Monitoring and evaluating should be planned **together** at the same time.
- Information derived from monitoring should be utilized in making **decisions**.
- The **methodology** for monitoring should be clearly outlined and followed consistently.
- Monitoring should be carried out in a manner that protects **confidentiality**.

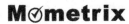

- Monitoring should assess all **primary stakeholders**.
- Monitoring should be scheduled on a **routine basis**.
- A monitoring **matrix** should be developed to facilitate monitoring.
- Resources for monitoring should be **separate** from other program resources.

### PERFORMANCE MEASURES

The purpose of program evaluation is to determine if the program is working effectively by assessing whether objectives are being met. As part of program evaluation, **performance measures** are carried out to evaluate measurable outcomes. Different approaches to program evaluation include:

- **Process**: The purpose is to determine if the program is operating as planned and generally looks at activities and whether the program meets regulatory requirements and professional standards.
- **Outcome**: The purpose is to determine the effectiveness of the program by assessing whether the outputs and outcomes of a program are as intended or whether there are unexpected results.
- **Impact**: The purpose is to attempt to determine the effectiveness of the program by assessing the difference between the outcomes and what would likely have occurred without the program.
- **Cost-benefit/Cost-effectiveness**: Cost-benefit analysis looks at all costs and benefits associated with the program to determine whether or not there is benefit. Cost-effectiveness analysis, on the other hand, looks at the cost effectiveness of individual aspects of the program.

## Chapter Quiz

Ready to see how well you retained what you just read? Scan the QR code to go directly to the chapter quiz interface for this study guide. If you're using a computer, simply visit the bonus page at **mometrix.com/bonus948/nce** and click the Chapter Quizzes link.

# Health Care Delivery

Transform passive reading into active learning! After immersing yourself in this chapter, put your comprehension to the test by taking a quiz. The insights you gained will stay with you longer this way. Scan the QR code to go directly to the chapter quiz interface for this study guide. If you're using a computer, simply visit the bonus page at **mometrix.com/bonus948/nurseexec** and click the Chapter Quizzes link.

## Ethics

### ETHICAL PRINCIPLES

#### AUTONOMY AND JUSTICE

**Autonomy** is the ethical principle that the individual has the right to make decisions about his or her own care. In the case of children, the child cannot make autonomous decisions, so the parents serve as the legal decision maker. The nurse must keep patients and guardians fully informed so that they can exercise their autonomy in informed decision-making.

**Justice** is the ethical principle that relates to the distribution of the limited resources of healthcare benefits to the members of society. These resources must be distributed fairly. This issue may arise if there is only one bed left and two sick patients. Justice comes into play in deciding which patient should stay and which should be transported or otherwise cared for. The decision should be made according to what is best or most just for the patients and not colored by personal bias.

#### BENEFICENCE AND NONMALEFICENCE

**Beneficence** is an ethical principle that involves performing actions that are for the purpose of benefitting another person. In the care of a patient, any procedure or treatment should be done with the ultimate goal of benefitting the patient, and any actions that are not beneficial should be reconsidered. As a patient's condition changes, procedures need to be continually reevaluated to determine if they are still of benefit.

**Nonmaleficence** is an ethical principle that means healthcare workers should provide care in a manner that does not cause direct intentional harm to the patient:

- The actual act must be good or morally neutral.
- The intent must be only for a good effect.
- A bad effect cannot serve as the means to get to a good effect.
- A good effect must have more benefit than a bad effect has harm.

### ETHICAL FRAMEWORKS

An ethical framework may facilitate decision-making in complex healthcare situations:

| Ethical framework | |
|---|---|
| **Identification of issues** | Objectively describe the ethical issue, acknowledging emotional biases. |
| **Values clarification** | Determine if decision-making is impacted by personal values or the values of others and whether there is conflict in these values. |

115

| Ethical framework | |
|---|---|
| **Influences and Barriers** | Consider medical condition, risk factors, socioeconomic status, religion, support systems and barriers, such as conflicts, differing professional assessments, regulations, and control issues. |
| **Principles** | Utilize and apply ethical principles (autonomy, beneficence, nonmaleficence, justice, privacy, confidentiality, veracity, and fidelity). |
| **Alternative solutions** | Explore alternate solutions, considering pros and cons, ethical issues, and outcomes. |
| **Conflict resolution** | Utilize collaboration, compromise, and/or accommodation rather than coercion or avoidance in reaching a solution. |
| **Implementation** | Select and carry out a solution that is defensible as an ethical decision. |
| **Assessment** | Assess the process of reaching an ethical solution and the outcomes. |

## ETHICAL DECISION MAKING

It's important for nurses to avoid making decisions solely based on the belief that they know what is best for individuals. In 1998, Chally and Loriz developed a **model for ethical decision making** for nurses to use when faced with ethical dilemmas or choices. Steps to ethical decision making include:

1. Clarifying the extent/type of **dilemma** and who is ultimately responsible for making the decision.
2. Obtaining more **data**, including information about legal issues, such as the obligation to report.
3. Considering alternative solutions.
4. Arriving at a **decision** after considering risks/benefits and discussing it with the individual.
5. **Acting** on the decision and utilizing collaboration as needed.
6. **Assessing** the outcomes of the decision to determine if the chosen action was effective.

## BIOETHICS

Bioethics is a branch of ethics that involves making sure that the medical treatment given is the most morally correct choice given the different options that might be available and the differences inherent in the varied levels of treatment. In the clinical unit, if the patients, families, and the staff are in agreement when it comes to values and decision-making, then no ethical dilemma exists; however, when there is a difference in value beliefs between the patients/families and the staff, there is a bioethical dilemma that must be resolved. Sometimes, discussion and explanation can resolve differences, but at times the institution's ethics committee must be brought in to resolve the conflict. The primary goal of bioethics is to determine the most morally correct action using the set of circumstances given.

## ENVIRONMENTAL ETHICS

Environmental ethics focus on the belief that human beings have an ethical obligation to the environment and that ethical considerations should be applied to the environment as well as to living things. This includes such things as consideration of the carbon footprint of not only individuals and groups but organizations and governments. Environmental ethics focuses on protection of the environment and prevention of damage and recognizes that all things, living and nonliving, are related and affect each other, negatively or positively. Environmental ethics extends moral standings to animals as well. When applying environmental ethics to healthcare organizations, considerations include:

- Reducing waste and recycling materials
- Reducing heating/cooling use through better construction practices
- Providing appropriate waste management
- Using environmentally friendly materials in construction
- Identifying alternative products to those that contain toxins or harmful substances
- Preventing downstream pollution from medical waste

## PRIVACY

The **Privacy Act** (1974) limits the type of information about employees that federal agencies can collect and keep in personnel files, but non-governmental entities have no such federal restrictions although individual states may have imposed similar restrictions. According to the *Privacy Act* and some state laws, individuals have a right to access their personnel files and letters of reference although the processes for doing so may vary. Information that is collected should be job related only, and information in personnel files should be kept confidential as should all personally identifiable information. Generally, emails, telephone calls, and computer usage in a healthcare organization should have no expectation of privacy, but procedures for monitoring and restrictions of use should be clearly outlined as well as the reasons, such as to prevent workplace harassment, unlawful sharing of information about patients, and liability, as well as to increase productivity.

## ANA NURSING CODE OF ETHICS

The American Nurse Association (ANA) developed the **Nursing Code of Ethics**. There are 9 provisions:

1. The nurse treats all individuals with **respect and consideration**, regardless of social circumstances or health condition.
2. The nurse's primary commitment is to the **individual** regardless of conflicts that may arise.
3. The nurse promotes and **advocates** for the individual's health, safety, and rights, while maintaining privacy and confidentiality and protecting patients from questionable practices or care.
4. The nurse is responsible for his or her **own care practices** and determine appropriate delegation of care.
5. The nurse must retain **respect** for self and his or her own integrity and competence.
6. The nurse participates in ensuring that the healthcare **environment** is conducive to providing good health care and consistent with professional and ethical values.
7. The nurse participates in **education and knowledge development** to advance the profession.
8. The nurse **collaborates** with others to promote efforts to meet health needs.
9. The nursing profession articulates **values** and promotes and maintains the **integrity** of the profession.

# Scope and Standards of Practice

## ANA SCOPE AND STANDARDS

The American Nurses Association (ANA) is a national professional nursing organization that outlines and publishes **Nursing: Scope and Standards of Practice** (2015) and *The Code of Ethics for Nurses*. Nurses are charged with protecting, promoting, and optimizing health and preventing injury and illness as well as alleviating suffering. The scope of practice refers to who, what, when, where, how, and why nursing care is provided. The standards of practice refer to the duties and competencies that all nurses are expected to perform within expected parameters.

The first 6 standards refer to the **nursing process**:

- Assessment
- Diagnosis
- Outcomes identification
- Planning
- Implementation
- Evaluation

The remaining 11 standards refer to **professional performance**:

- Ethics
- Culturally congruent practice
- Communication
- Collaboration
- Leadership
- Education
- Evidence-based practice/research
- Quality of practice
- Professional practice evaluation
- Resource utilization
- Environmental health

## ANA NURSES' BILL OF RIGHTS

The ANA Nurses' Bill of Rights is not a legal document, so it cannot provide legal protection, but it does list expected professional rights that organizations can use as a basis for a sound nursing policy. According to the Nurses' Bill of Rights, nurses have a right to:

- Practice their profession in such a way that allows them to fulfill **societal and patient obligations**.
- Practice in a healthcare environment that permits them to practice in accordance with **professional standards and their scopes of practice**.
- Practice in an **ethical healthcare environment** that supports the *Code of Ethics for Nurses with Interpretive Statements*.
- Serve as **advocates** for themselves and their patients without concern for retribution.
- Receive **fair compensation** commensurate with education, experience, and expertise.
- Practice in a safe work environment.
- Engage in **negotiation** regarding the conditions of employment individually or collectively.

## NURSE PRACTICE ACT

Each state has its own Nurse Practice Act, which is administered by the state Board of Nursing. The Nurse Practice Act outlines requirements for licensure and certification and delineates the scope of practice of nurses, including duties and delegation. Typically, licensure is granted to those who complete an accredited LVN/LPN or RN program and pass the nursing exam (NCLEX) or receive endorsement because of licensure in another state. RN programs may be 3-year hospital-based programs, associate's degree, or bachelor's degree. Foreign-trained nurses may need to meet special requirements that are determined by the state Board of Nursing and included in the *Nurse Practice Act*. The *Nurse Practice Act* of each state provides the requirement for advanced practice certification and the professional designation. Additionally, the Nurse Practice Act outlines the requirements for relicensing or recertification, often including the need for continuing education. The *Nurse Practice Act* also includes provisions for disciplinary action.

## NCSBN MODEL ACT

The National Council of State Boards of Nursing (NCSBN) **Model Act/Rules and Regulations** (2012, 2014) provides an exemplary model act that boards of nursing can use when reviewing and/or updating current state nursing legislation. Because nursing is governed by state legislation, some laws and regulations vary from state to state, and this model is an attempt to help state boards of nursing to develop rules and regulations that are more consistent with other states. The Model Act reflects current best practices. The Model Act outlines the scopes of practice of the RN, LPN/LVN, APRN, and UAP. It also addresses topics related to the authority of state nursing boards, including accountability standards, grounds for discipline, procedures, immunity and protection from retaliation, practice remediation programs, reporting guidelines, and emergency actions.

## TRENDS IN HEALTH CARE

The nurse executive should monitor **key trends** in nursing, health care, and other disciplines and incorporate them into educational programs and activities. Key trends across the disciplines include:

- Use of miniaturized or portable medical devices and robotic-assisted surgical devices
- Social networking, internet access and research, and need for IT specialists
- Nursing involvement in information technology and systems analysis
- Utilization of home health care and decreased length of hospital stay
- Focus on wellness, nutrition, and preventive care
- Focus on sustainability, recycling
- Individualized patient care
- Flexible working hours and cost containment methods
- Specialization, certification, and interprofessional education
- Gender, racial, and ethnic diversity among staff and patients
- Focus on teamwork and interdisciplinary teams
- Focus on patient satisfaction and patient outcomes

# Regulatory Standards

## JOINT COMMISSION

The Joint Commission is the primary accrediting agency for healthcare programs in the United States. The Joint Commission establishes accreditation standards for various types of healthcare programs, establishes general competencies for healthcare practitioners, and issues annual National Patient Safety Goals. Standards for accreditation are, for the most part, performance based and focus on measures of processes and outcomes as well as issues related to patient care and safety. Comparative performance measure data, such as core measures, are integrated into the accreditation process. Most surveyors assess compliance based on the following:

- Document review to validate compliance
- Onsite inspections and observations
- Interviews of staff

- Review of standards implementation measures
- Review of medical records
- Assessment of service and support systems of the organization
- Integration of performance measure data

The surveyors may recommend denial of accreditation if conditions exist that pose a threat to staff, public, or patients, but the organization may request the opportunity to demonstrate compliance through documentation or interviews. In some cases, a second survey may be conducted.

### JOINT COMMISSION NATIONAL PATIENT SAFETY GOALS

The Joint Commission issues **National Patient Safety Goals** annually for different types of healthcare programs, but the hospital goals are fairly representative:

- **Improve accuracy of patient identification**: Two identifiers
- **Improve the effectiveness of communication among caregivers**: Standards for abbreviations, "read back" for verbal or telephone orders, improved timeline for reporting test results
- **Improve the safety of using medications**: Proper labeling, review of drugs with similar names/appearances, reduction in anticoagulation therapy risks
- **Reduce the risk of healthcare-associated infections**: WHO or CDC handwashing guidelines and treating healthcare-associated infections as sentinel events
- **Accurately and completely reconcile medications across the continuum of care**: Accurate listing of patient's medications for patient and other providers
- **Reduce the risk of patient harm from falls**: Fall reduction program
- **Involve patients actively in their own care as a patient safety strategy**: Reporting of safety concerns
- **Identify inherent patient safety risks**: Includes risk of suicide
- **Improve recognition and response to changes in a patient's condition**: Immediate response, consultation

## HIPAA

HIPAA regulations are designed to protect the rights of individuals regarding the privacy of their health information. The nurse must not release any information or documentation about an individual's condition or treatment without consent, as the individual has the right to determine who has access to personal information. Personal information about the individual is considered **protected health information** (PHI), and consists of any identifying or personal information about the individual, such as health history, condition, or treatments in any form, and any documentation, including electronic, verbal, or written. Personal information can be shared with a spouse, legal guardians, those with durable power of attorney for the individual, and those involved in care of the individual, such as physicians, without a specific release, but the individual should always be consulted if personal information is to be discussed with others present to ensure there is no objection. Failure to comply with HIPAA regulations can make a nurse liable for legal action.

## PRIVACY AND SECURITY RULES

HIPAA mandates **privacy and security rules** (CFR, Title 45, part 164) to ensure that health information and individual privacy is protected:

- **Privacy rule**: Protected information includes any information included in the medical record (electronic or paper), conversations between the doctor and other healthcare providers, billing information, and any other form of health information. Procedures must be in place to limit access and disclosures.
- **Security rule**: Any electronic health information must be secure and protected against threats, hazards, or non-permitted disclosures, in compliance with established standards. Implementation specifications must be addressed for any adopted standards. Administrative, physical, and technical safeguards must be in place as well as policies and procedures to comply with standards. **Security requirements** include limiting access to those authorized, use of unique identifiers for each user, automatic logoff, encryption and decryption of protected healthcare information, authentication that healthcare data has not been altered/destroyed, monitoring of logins, authentication, and security of transmission. Access controls must include unique identifier, procedure to access system in emergencies, time out, and encryption/decryption.

| |
|---|
| **Review Video: HIPAA**<br>Visit mometrix.com/academy and enter code: 412009 |

## GENETIC INFORMATION NONDISCRIMINATION ACT

The *Genetic Information Nondiscrimination Act* (2009) prohibits employers from using genetic information (genetic tests of the individual or individual's family members) to make decisions about employing individuals. This act is under the jurisdiction of the Equal Employment Opportunity Commission (EEOC). Covered entities (such as employers, employment agencies, labor-management training programs, and apprenticeship programs) cannot purchase or use genetic information in decision-making. Information obtained indirectly, such as by overhearing comments, cannot be used as well. No genetic information can be used in employment decisions. This act also provides protection for the individual with a genetic disorder by prohibiting any type of harassment, such as making derogatory comments about the individual's disorder. DNA testing for law enforcement is allowed under the act, but the information can only be used for legal proceedings. Covered entities must keep all genetic information confidential regardless of how the information was obtained.

## CENTERS FOR MEDICARE AND MEDICAID SERVICES (CMS)

### ORIGINAL MEDICARE

Medicare, a federal health insurance program for those who have Social Security or bought into Medicare, provides payment to private healthcare providers, such as physicians and hospitals, but limits reimbursement. Physicians receive 80% of usual customary and reasonable (UCR) fees if they accept Medicare assignment. If they do not, they can charge up to 115% of what Medicare allows.

Individuals are responsible for the remaining 20% or up to 115% if the physicians do not accept Medicare. Parts include:

- **Medicare A**: Hospital insurance covers acute hospital, limited nursing home care and/or home health care as well as hospice care for the terminally ill. There is no premium for this part.
- **Medicare B**: Medical insurance covers physicians, CNSs, laboratory, physical and occupational therapy. Individuals must pay an annual deductible as well as monthly payments.
- **Medicare D**: Prescription drug plan covers part of the costs of prescription drugs at participating pharmacies. Medicare D is administered by private insurance companies, so monthly costs and benefits vary somewhat.

## MEDICARE PROGRAMS

Medicare has made a number of modifications to allow Medicare patients to access different types of programs in addition to typical pay-for-service care and managed care through HMOs:

- **Prospective payment system** (PPS) pays a set amount for patient care, depending upon diagnosis (diagnosis-related group or DRG).
- **Preferred provider organization** (PPO) provides discounted rates for those on Medicare who choose healthcare providers from a list of those who have agreed to accept Medicare assignment.
- **Private insurance pay-for-service Medicare plans** are contracted by Medicare and may provide more benefits, but the patient may be required to work individually with the insurance company to determine benefits and may be assessed an additional monthly fee.
- **Specialty plans** are being developed in different areas, some focusing on increased preventive care.

## MEDICAID

Medicaid is a combined federal and state welfare program authorized by Title XIX of the Social Security Act and regulated by the Centers for Medicare and Medicaid Services (CMS) to assist people with low income with payment for medical care. This program provides assistance for all ages, including children. Older adults receiving SSI are eligible as are others who meet state eligibility requirements. The Medicaid programs are administered by the individual states, which establish eligibility and reimbursement guidelines, so benefits vary considerably from one state to another. Older adults with Medicare are eligible for Medicaid as a secondary insurance. Expenses that may be covered for adults include inpatient and outpatient hospital services, physician payments, nursing home care, home health care, and laboratory and radiation services. Adults who are legal resident aliens are ineligible for Medicaid for 5 years after attaining legal resident status. Some states pay for preventive services, such as home and community-based programs aimed at reducing the need for hospitalization.

> **Review Video: Medicare and Medicaid**
> Visit mometrix.com/academy and enter code: 507454

## PUBLIC REPORTING

Public reporting is making performance measures about healthcare providers public. This may be as simple as providing a dashboard in-house so that staff members can assess the quality of care, but public reporting is also supported and mandated by federal and state agencies. About 50% of states require some public reporting. The Centers for Medicare and Medicaid Services (CMS) and the Agency for Healthcare Research and Quality (AHRQ) have both developed quality measures and report on aggregate state and national data. CMS also publishes provider-specific comparative data about hospitals, physicians, HHAs, kidney dialysis centers, and nursing homes. The Hospital Compare website provides measures focusing specifically on the aspect of care in all acute hospitals in the United States and reports data derived from patient surveys. The Affordable Care Act requires public reporting of some performance measures. Additionally, some private agencies and organizations, such as Leapfrog and the National committee for Quality Assurance, also do some public reporting with comparisons based on performance measures.

# Legal Issues

## FRAUD AND ABUSE

Fraud is misrepresentation done for unauthorized self-benefit while **abuse** is conduct that is below acceptable standards and results in fraudulent reimbursement, such as for non-medically necessary services. According to CMS, the types of healthcare fraud include:

- **Theft of medical identity**: Can include misusing another person's medical identity number to obtain services or supplies or stealing a doctor's identifiers to obtain unlawful prescriptions or supplies.
- **Billing for unauthorized or unnecessary materials or services**: States define "medical necessity," and healthcare organizations must meet this definition for billing purposes.
- **Billing for materials or services not actually provided**: This is always a fraudulent act and may involve false records.
- **Upcoding**: Intentional or unintentional coding for materials or services reimbursed at a higher rate.
- **Unbundling**: Billing separately for services/materials that should be bundled in order to gain increased reimbursement.
- **Kickbacks**: Receiving payment for referring patients for healthcare services.

## WHISTLE-BLOWING

A whistleblower is an individual who exposes illegal or unethical practices of an organization in order to facilitate change. The whistleblower may bring forth charges internally, such as by reporting to a supervisor, or externally, such as by reporting to a government agency or the media. Whistleblowers are protected under numerous federal (up to 20 different statutes) and state laws, which are sometimes contradictory and often confusing. Different laws apply to different occupations and subject matter. Depending upon the statute under which a person is acting as a whistleblower, different time limits for filing a complaint exist, so it's imperative that whistleblowers understand the laws that apply to them. In most cases, OSHA's Office of the Whistleblower Protection Program usually enforces statutes as delegated by the Secretary of Labor. Reprisals against whistleblowers, while illegal, are not uncommon, so individuals often risk their jobs and reputations when trying to do the ethical thing.

## CORPORATE COMPLIANCE

Healthcare corporate compliance requires adherence to state and federal regulations, legal standards, and ethical standards. Issues of concern for compliance include:

- **Privacy and security concerns** of HIPAA and HITECH, including conducting audit trails
- **Accountability standards**: Discipline, confidentiality, and privacy policies

- **Regulatory requirements**: Include ADA, CMS, CLIA, EMTLA, OSHA, EEOC, Anti-Kickback Statute, Stark Law (limiting referrals by physicians), Fair Labor Standards Act, Family and Medical Leave Act, and Federal Wage Garnishment Law
- **Record retention** of policies and practices
- **Screening/Employment standards** and practices, including appropriate interviewing (hiring and exit)
- **Third-party due diligence**: Vendors and contractual agreements
- **Communication of regulatory requirements** and education in compliance issues
- **Risk assessment** of organization related to compliance
- **Compliance audits** (internal and external)
- Investigations and disclosures of **non-compliance**
- **Government sanctions lists**: Including country-specific lists as well as terrorism and narcotics sanctions lists and OIG exclusions of individuals
- Organizational **transparency** and culture of **compliance**

## CORPORATE COMPLIANCE PROGRAMS

The federal government establishes annual **corporate compliance programs** for the healthcare industry through the Office of the Inspector General (OIG). The OIG issues corporate compliance guidance for different types of healthcare organizations, such as nursing facilities, hospitals, and hospices, to assist these organizations in complying with applicable statutes and reducing fraud and abuse. The organization must develop an individual compliance plan. Compliance plans are mandated by the Affordable Care Act for those receiving CMS reimbursement. The compliance plan should establish internal controls so that the organization does not violate state or federal rules, laws, or regulations, such as by carrying out fraudulent billing practices. Corporate compliance includes developing written standards of conduct as well as policies and procedures to ensure adherence. A chief compliance officer must be responsible for monitoring compliance. All staff members should be educated about compliance issues, and a process should be in place (such as a hotline) to receive complaints. A system should be in place to respond to any complaints and to ensure confidentiality. Audits and various methods of assessment of compliance should be carried out routinely, and any problems addressed promptly.

## SEXUAL HARASSMENT REGULATIONS

Sexual harassment regulations include:

- The 1964 *Civil Rights Act* (Title VII) prohibited gender discrimination and sexual harassment by employers.
- The 1972 **Education Amendments** (Title IX) extended protection to education institutions.
- The 1980 **Equal Employment Opportunity Commission** (EEOC) defined sexual harassment as quid pro quo (expecting something in return for a favor) or a hostile work environment (unwelcome advances or conduct).
- The 1991 *Civil Rights Act* allowed victims to obtain punitive/compensatory awards if subjected to sexual harassment.
- Additionally, many state laws have requirements regarding sexual harassment, and protection has been extended to **same gender harassment**.

**Sexual harassment** includes unwelcome verbal advances (comments, asking for dates), personal comments (appearance, lifestyle, body), offensive behavior (bullying, leering), offensive materials (jokes, posters, videos, emails), and unwelcome physical contact (touching, hugging, kissing, molesting). Sexual harassment in the healthcare industry is high, with studies showing that offenders are most often physicians, but co-workers, supervisors, and patients also commit sexual harassment. Healthcare providers may be legally and financially liable for harassment.

## MALPRACTICE AND NEGLIGENCE

Advance practice nurses are usually insured for **malpractice** at a higher rate than for registered nurses because their scope of practice is much wider. A nurse may be sued individually or as part of a medical group to which the nurse is associated. Because a suit is a civil matter, loss of judgment may not be reported to the state board of nursing. If a charge of **negligence** is brought to the attention of the board, the board may initiate an investigation and disciplinary action. Negligence may involve a number of failures, such as not referring an individual when needed, incorrect diagnosis, incorrect treatment, and not providing the individual/family with adequate or essential information. Once a nurse has established a duty to an individual—by direct examination or even casual or telephone conversation that involves professional advice—the nurse may be liable for malpractice if he or she does not follow up with adequate care.

### TYPES OF NEGLIGENCE

Risk management must attempt to determine the burden of proof for acts of negligence, including compliance with duty, breaches in procedures, degree of harm, and cause. Negligence indicates that proper care has not been provided, based on established standards. Reasonable care uses rationale for decision-making in relation to providing care. State regulations regarding negligence may vary but all have some statutes of limitation. There are a number of different **types of negligence**:

- **Negligent conduct** indicates that an individual failed to provide reasonable care or to protect/assist another, based on standards and expertise.
- **Gross negligence** is willfully providing inadequate care while disregarding the safety and security of another.
- **Contributory negligence** involves the injured party contributing to his or her own harm.
- **Comparative negligence** attempts to determine what percentage amount of negligence is attributed to each individual involved.

> **Review Video: Medical Negligence**
> Visit mometrix.com/academy and enter code: 928405

## ADDRESSING LEGAL ISSUES
### VIOLATIONS, FRAUD, HARASSMENT, AND WHISTLEBLOWING

Critical to **assessing, addressing, and preventing legal issues**, such as violations, fraud, harassment, and whistleblowing, are the following:

- **Organizational transparency**: The more open an organization is and the more people that have access to monitoring data, the less likely violations will go unnoticed.
- **Compliance monitoring**: Monitoring must be a continual ongoing process that involves all staff members rather than just the compliance officer.
- **Non-punitive reactions to negative reports**: Whistleblowers or those who provide negative reports about legal issues should be rewarded rather than punished to encourage others to come forward.
- **Mechanism for reporting problems**: Confidentiality must be ensured to those reporting problems, and different mechanisms should be provided (hotline, email, reporting forms).
- **Staff education/training**: Staff must be educated about legal issues, such as sexual harassment, as part of orientation programs and then on an annual basis with updates or changes in policies or regulations shared immediately in various forums.

- **Administrative leadership**: Administration must set the standards for the organization.
- **Zero-tolerance policies**: Clear policies regarding sexual harassment, workplace violence and bullying should be in place.

## HIPAA VIOLATIONS

HIPAA Breach Notification Rule requires covered entities to report any breaches in protected health information:

- **Individuals**: Notification by standard mail or email (if the individual has agreed) as soon as possible but no later than 60 days after the breach. If lacking contact information for 10 or more individuals, notice must be placed on the organization's website for 90 days with a tollfree telephone number or notice provided in print or broadcast media. For fewer than 10 individuals, alternate notification, such as by telephone, is permitted. Individual breaches are reported to the HHS Secretary annually.
- **500 or more individuals**: In addition to individual notification, notice must be given in prominent media outlets serving the affected states no later than 60 days after the breach. The HHS Secretary must be notified electronically within 60 days after the breach. If the breach affected fewer than 500 individuals, the HHS Secretary must be notified within 60 days of the end of the calendar year in which the breaches occurred.

## ELECTRONIC ACCESS AND SECURITY BREACHES

The *American Recovery and Reinvestment Act* (2009) (ARRA) included the **Health Information Technology for Economic and Clinical Health Act** (HITECH). Security provisions include:

- Individuals and HHS must be notified of breach in security of personal health information.
- Business partners must meet security regulations or face penalties.
- The sale/marketing of personal health information is restricted.
- Individuals must have access to electronic health information.
- Individuals must be informed of disclosures of personal health information.

HITECH provides incentive payments to Medicare practitioners to adopt EHRs. Additionally, HITECH provides penalties in the form of reduced Medicare payments for those who do not adopt EHRs, unless exempted. HIPAA and the HITECH Act require that clinical data that is to be transmitted over the internet must first be encrypted in order to protect confidentially and protected health information (PHI). Patient health records often contain not only health information but also other identifying information, such as address, telephone number, birthdate, social security number, and sometimes even credit card numbers.

# Community and Consumer Needs

## COMMUNITY HEALTH NEEDS ASSESSMENT

A community health needs assessment evaluates the existing services and need for additional services. Elements include:

- Assessment of **community demographics** to identify underserved populations, such as the homeless, gay or lesbians, or ethnic minorities. This assessment may include review of rates of unemployment to help to determine insurance coverage.
- Assessment of consumer's involvement in **leadership roles** in providing mental health services, such as those on boards, those providing mental health care, and those actively involved in community mental health agencies.

- Assessment of services to determine **availability** (psychiatrists, mental health agencies, outreach programs, half-way houses), **affordability** (fee-based, insurance), and **access** (location, transportation) as well as to identify areas that are inadequate.
- Assessment of **barriers** to people receiving needed care, including child care, lack of insurance, hours of service, language barriers, discrimination, and inadequate training of staff.

## HCAHPS

Hospital Consumer Assessment of Healthcare Providers and Systems (HCAHPS) is a national standardized survey of patients' opinions of their hospital care. HCAHPS (a 32-item survey) was developed by the HCAHPS consortium and the AHRQ and was endorsed by the National Quality Forum. Hospitals that are subject to the Inpatient Prospective Payment System (IPPS) must collect surveys and submit data in order to receive full reimbursement from CMS. Non-IPPS hospitals may voluntarily participate. The Affordable Care Act included HCAHPS as part of payment calculation for Value-Based Purchasing programs. Eleven HCAHPS measures are reported on the *Hospital Compare* website. The surveys are completed by patients who were recently discharged and include questions about how often patients experienced a specific aspect of care and how satisfied they were with the care received. Hospitals may add additional survey questions to the core questions to gather specific data about areas of concern. The surveys can be completed by mail, telephone, mail with telephone follow-up, or interactive voice recognition.

### HEALTHGRADES

Healthgrades is a private company that has amassed information about over 3 million healthcare providers, including hospitals and physicians amongst other healthcare providers. Hospitals are ranked according to mortality and complication rates, and physicians are ranked according to the complication rate at the hospital with which they are affiliated as well as their experience and patient satisfaction. Healthgrades utilizes data from Medicare and other sources, most available to the public. Healthgrades utilizes a star ranking system for healthcare providers with one star indicating quality of care is less than predicted, three stars indicating predicted level of care, and five stars indicating a better level of care than predicted. Consumers can go to the website and search for physicians, hospitals, and dentists and can search by medical specialty. For example, if researching a specific hospital, the link immediately shows the percentage of patients who would "definitely recommend" the hospital with links to the item results of patient surveys.

## Compliance Policy Development

### HEALTH AND PUBLIC POLICY ISSUES

The nurse executive must be informed of **current health and public policy issues** in order to respond effectively and to develop future plans. This requires almost constant review of accreditation and reimbursement guidelines and current trends in order to plan for immediate needs and for at least 3-5 years into the future. Resources include healthcare and government websites, journals, CDC reports, news outlets, and conference presentations. The nurse executive should review demographic statistics, such as aging statistics, and those involving new and developing diseases, such as Zika infections, that may impact healthcare needs. Additionally, the nurse executive should consider global issues, such as outbreaks of COVID-19 and the possible effects of global warming. Planning must also consider workforce issues, such as the shortage of nurses or the need for more flexible working conditions.

## INTEGRATING LEGAL AND REGULATORY REQUIREMENTS INTO POLICY

Legal and regulatory requirements should be integrated into all nursing activities because the provision of medical care is increasingly governed by state, federal, and accreditation regulations and requirements. Healthcare organizations must meet regulatory standards for reimbursement from Medicare and Medicaid. Accreditation agencies, such as the Joint Commission, have had a profound influence on performance standards. Nursing personnel must stay abreast of changes in standards associated with the primary regulatory and accrediting agencies and should have a clear understanding of how these standards relate to quality outcomes. Healthcare providers at all levels must be updated when changes occur, and processes and practices may need to be changed. Documentation requirements may also change, and failure to understand new requirements may adversely affect reimbursement. Additionally, since the Joint Commission now conducts unannounced surveys, nursing staff must be aware of and constantly compliant with accreditation standards.

## POLICY AND PROCEDURE DEVELOPMENT AND MODIFICATION

Policies and procedures should be developed according to the mission statement of the organization.

- A **policy** is a formal guideline that aids in decision-making and promotes consistency in actions. Policies should be written in a way that is understandable and broad and general enough in wording that they can apply to all staff members. Policies should be developed by an interdisciplinary team with input from all stakeholders and then approved by the board. Policies are usually collected in a manual and/or presented online.
- **Procedures**, on the other hand, are detailed step-by-step directions for carrying out a process. Procedures should be developed after research on best practices. Procedures usually begin with a statement of purpose, identification of the persons who will carry out the procedure, and a list of necessary supplies and/or equipment, and the steps to the procedure. Procedures may be specific to one unit, such as the procedure for administering chemotherapy.

## CHANGES IN POLICIES, PROCEDURES, AND WORKING STANDARDS

Changes in policies, procedures, and working standards are common and the nurse executive is responsible for educating the staff about changes, which should be communicated to staff in an effective and timely manner:

- **Policies** are usually changed after a period of discussion and review by administration and staff, so all staff should be made aware of policies under discussion. Preliminary information should be disseminated to staff regarding the issue during meetings or through printed notices.
- **Procedures** may be changed to increase efficiency or improve patient safety often as the result of surveillance and outcomes data. Procedure changes are best communicated in workshops with demonstrations. Posters and handouts should be available as well.
- **Working standards** are often changed because of regulatory or accrediting requirements, and this information should be covered extensively in a variety of different ways (discussions, workshops, handouts) so that the implications are clearly understood.

## MONITORING FOR COMPLIANCE

In order to effectively monitor compliance to administrative policies and procedures, it is first necessary to educate the staff about the policies and procedures to ensure that there is general understanding of their purposes, and administration must clearly state that policies and procedures must be followed. Staff members should be encouraged to notify administration if they feel a policy or procedure needs revision. Compliance monitoring should occur at all levels in the chain of command through observation and both formal and informal interviews and discussions. Compliance monitoring must include steps in dealing with noncompliance, and the staff members should be aware of these steps. Noncompliance is usually initially dealt with through re-education but there should be more serious consequences for continued noncompliance, especially if this noncompliance can increase risk to the organization or patients.

## REVIEWING AND PROVIDING FEEDBACK

**Policies and procedures** should be **reviewed** at least on an annual basis to determine if they still reflect organizational needs and current practice. While policies are usually reviewed by interdisciplinary teams, it's also important to seek feedback from staff members throughout the organization and to engage staff in policy review by keeping them informed of the process and actively soliciting input through postings, meetings, emails, and other means of communication. Review of procedures should begin with research to determine if the current procedures are evidence-based and continue to demonstrate best practices.

**Feedback** (interviews, surveys, questionnaires) should be obtained from those utilizing the procedure, such as staff at a unit level, to determine if the procedure is followed as written, if it has been modified in practice, or if it has been superseded by newer practices for which there is yet no formal written procedure.

# Healthcare Delivery Models

## ACCOUNTABLE CARE ORGANIZATIONS

Accountable care organizations (ACOs), established per the *Affordable Care Act*, are groups of physicians, hospitals, and other healthcare providers who voluntarily establish partnerships or agreements to provide care to Medicare patients. The purpose of ACOs is to improve delivery of quality care while saving healthcare costs. ACOs avoid duplication of services through coordination of care. Medicare shares healthcare savings generated to participating providers. Some of the most common types of ACOs include:

- **Shared savings program**: Payment is made for participants under fee-for-service who meet performance standards while lowering costs.
- **Advance payment model**: This is a supplementary program to the shared savings program. Participants receive monthly upfront payments to invest in staff and infrastructure needs to better meet goals.
- **Pioneer model**: Original model available to those who had already established groups. Shared savings and payments were generally higher than in current plans. No longer accepting applicants.

## PATIENT-CENTERED MEDICAL HOME

A patient-centered medical home (PCMH) is a program of patient care in which initial contact is with a primary physician who coordinates care in partnership with the patient/family and other healthcare providers to ensure that the patient's needs are met. Essential characteristics of a patient-centered medical home include:

- **Access**: The patient is able to make appointments for same-day visits, and extended hours and patient portals are available. Group and e-visits may be options.
- **Comprehensive services**: The patient has access to care for acute and chronic conditions as well as a range of diagnostic, preventive, and therapeutic services.
- **Effective patient care**: The physician is capable of managing needs of the target population.
- **Patient care coordination**: The physician manages coordination of care from all healthcare providers.
- **Team care**: Practice-based care is provided.
- Safe, quality provision of **evidence-based care**.

## NURSE-LED CLINICS

Nurse-led clinics are generally outpatient clinics that are run under the management and supervision of an advanced practice nurse, such as a nurse practitioner or certified nurse specialist. Nurse-led clinics are often part of hospital outpatient services and public-health services but may also be run as independent practices. While state scope of practice laws may vary somewhat, in most cases advance practice nurses may provide some diagnostic and therapeutic services. The focus of care in many nurse-led clinics is management of chronic disease and preventive care. Nurse-led clinics often partner with other healthcare facilities, such as hospitals or laboratories. Some nurse-led clinics also have doctors on call or available at specified times or for referrals. Many nursing schools support nurse-led clinics to provide quality care as well as learning opportunities for student nurses. Nurse-led clinics are especially valuable in areas with a shortage of primary care physicians.

## INPATIENT HEALTHCARE DELIVERY

Inpatient healthcare delivery occurs when a patient is formally admitted to a hospital, such as a general medical-surgical hospital or critical access hospital. Inpatient status is an important consideration for reimbursement by Medicare, Medicaid, and insurance carriers. Patients may be held in the hospital without being admitted, such as when held overnight in the emergency department for observation, but these patients are considered outpatients because they have not been admitted as inpatients. Patient census counts are for 24-hour periods beginning at 12:01 AM. Because census may vary during the day, the hospital designates a specific time for daily census. Each patient counted during census represents one inpatient service day. The bed count days are the number of available inpatient beds in a specified period:

$$\frac{\text{Number of inpatient service days}}{\text{Number of inpatient bed count days over same period}} = \text{Inpatient bed occupancy rate}$$

Length of stay (LOS) is calculated for each patient when the patient is discharged, as LOS is especially important for Medicare reimbursement.

## AMBULATORY CARE

Ambulatory care is healthcare that is delivered to patients on an outpatient basis at a physician's office, clinic, urgent care center, surgery center, dialysis center, or hospital. In most cases, this type of care requires the patient to travel to the site of delivery and to return home without staying the night although some dialysis centers may provide overnight dialysis, and some testing, such as for sleep apnea, may occur during the night. Outpatient services are reimbursed differently from inpatient services and are usually less costly than those provided for inpatients, so the use of ambulatory care is considered a cost-saving method. Primary care physicians often provide ambulatory care in private medical practices or as employees of ambulatory care organizations, such as HMOs. Some hospital-based services are considered part of ambulatory care, including emergency department services, diagnostic and therapeutic services (such as radiation therapy), and outpatient surgical services.

## HOME HEALTH CARE

Home health care is the provision of intermittent care in the patient's home for patients who are essentially homebound. Intermittent care is fewer than 7 days a week or fewer than 8 hours per day over 21 or fewer days during an episode of care, which is 60 days. Most of the care that can be provided in a skilled nursing facility can also be provided by a home health agency. The patient's physician must certify that the patient is in need of services and is homebound but is expected to show improvement with treatment. Services include:

- IV therapy
- Nutritional therapy and counseling
- Social worker services
- Occupational, speech, and physical therapies
- Case management
- Home health aide services for assistance with personal care

Patients with original Medicare receive full reimbursement for HH care but pay 20% of Medicare-approved costs for durable medical equipment. The home health agency must be Medicare-certified.

## ACUTE CARE AND SUB-ACUTE CARE

Acute care is usually provided in a hospital where diagnostic procedures (MRI, CT, lab, X-ray) and the ability to use high technology for monitoring are readily available. Patients admitted to acute care facilities are usually acutely ill and require 8-9 hours of skilled nursing care daily. Physicians and highly skilled nursing staff are available for patients around the clock.

Sub-acute care provides a level of care between that of an acute care hospital and a skilled nursing facility although skilled nurses are available around the clock. Sub-acute patients usually require 4-6 hours of skilled nursing care daily but may receive intensive therapy. In some cases, sub-acute units may be attached to an acute care hospital or SNF, or they may be completely separate facilities. Most sub-acute units do not offer monitoring or sophisticated diagnostic equipment, so patients often have chronic (rather than acute) disorders, such as AIDS, head trauma, and neuromuscular diseases.

## SKILLED NURSING FACILITIES

Skilled nursing facilities (SNF, nursing homes) provide both medical care (medications, treatment) and personal care (bathing, dressing, meals, activities) and are licensed by the state. Patients with insurance or Medicare may be transferred to a skilled nursing facility after acute hospitalization, usually for periods ranging from a few days up to 6 weeks, depending upon condition and progress. SNFs usually provide physical therapy and occupational therapy and may include respiratory therapy as well. The goal of SNF care is to provide transitional care between the hospital and the home environment. In some cases, patients who cannot be cared for at home and require medical care may remain in the SNF until death. Some patients have long-term care insurance that will pay for this although Medicare will not. State Medicaid programs may pay if certain restrictions (income, condition, age) are met. Others pay privately, with costs usually ranging from about $4000-$10,000 monthly.

## REHABILITATION CENTERS

Rehabilitation centers may be separate departments that are part of acute, subacute, or skilled nursing facilities. In some cases, separate rehabilitation centers focus solely on rehabilitation and improving a patient's ability to function and remain as independent as possible. There is a wide variety of rehabilitative programs, including stroke and brain injury programs, cardiac health programs, and physical therapy for those with bone or muscle injuries. For example, older adults may receive rehabilitative physical therapy to strengthen muscles and improve mobility after a hip fracture. Comprehensive rehabilitation programs usually offer speech and occupational therapists. Depending upon the need for rehabilitative care, individual patients may need only a few hours of outpatient care or months of inpatient care. Increasingly, rehabilitative treatment utilizes computerized technology to assist patients. Insurance, Medicare, and Medicaid usually cover the costs of rehabilitative care that is indicated to improve functionality or prevent further deterioration.

## ASSISTED LIVING FACILITIES

Assisted living facilities comprise a wide range of options, from residential care facilities that house 2-3 patients in a home setting to large facilities with dozens or even hundreds of patients. Typically, nurses are not on duty and medical assistance is therefore limited. Services usually offered include staff on duty 24 hours a day to provide assistance if needed, meal service (2-3 meals daily), and sometimes cleaning, activities, and transportation services. Costs vary widely ($500/month to $10,000/month). The goal of assisted living is to allow the patient to remain as independent as possible within his or her physical/cognitive abilities. Residents often have individual apartments. Assisted living is usually limited to those with mild to moderate functional impairment, but licensure varies somewhat from state to state. Those facilities focusing on patients with Alzheimer's disease may have further requirements, such as provision of a safe environment that prevents patients from wandering away from the facility.

### RESIDENTIAL CARE FACILITIES

Residential care facilities (a type of assisted living/group home) vary from state to state, but a typical facility may be a large home with 2-6 or more patients, cared for by a person (often non-medical) licensed by the state. Depending upon the number of patients, nurse aids may be available to assist patients. Residents receive assistance with bathing and dressing as needed and are provided meals and activities. Patients are usually required to be ambulatory, but this may vary according to the facility and the state regulations. Usually, residential care facilities do not provide medical care, so patients needing treatments (other than assistance with taking medications or minor treatments) are seen by home health agency nurses. In some cases, Medicaid may provide payment to house older adults in residential care facilities, but the pay rate is low, so finding a residential care facility that accepts Medicaid can be difficult. Costs range from $500/month to many thousands of dollars for luxury facilities.

## RESPITE CARE

Respite care is provided to serve the caregiver rather than the patient although in some cases, such as with older adults, the caregiver may be an older adult as well. Respite care is provided in a number of different ways. Under Hospice, the patient may be admitted to a skilled nursing facility for up to 5 days, but with other programs, a nurse aide may be provided to stay with the patient for a few hours while the caregiver leaves the home, or the caregiver may be provided money to hire help in the home. Most respite programs are intended for those providing long-term care for those

132

with chronic or terminal diseases or those with dementia, usually related to Alzheimer's disease. Caregivers can easily feel overwhelmed with the constant need to provide care, especially if patients are up at night (as often occurs with Alzheimer patients) or can never be left unattended for safety reasons.

## TELEHEALTH

Telehealth is providing health care and monitoring to individuals at a distance utilizing telecommunications and information technologies. Telehealth may include two-way video conferencing for interviewing, diagnosing, monitoring, and treating. Store-and-forward telehealth technology stores data (such as BP and heart rate) and transmits it electronically at specified times or under specified conditions (such as sending an ECG when tachycardia occurs). The aging population is a reason for the increasing trend of utilizing telehealth technologies as a preventive measure (monitoring patient's conditions) and to reduce the need for hospitalization. Other reasons include the systemic transition to telehealth during the recent outbreak of COVID-19, the increasing cost of healthcare and hospitalization, a more educated populace that wants to be involved in its own healthcare, the shortage of nursing and other healthcare personnel, and the increase (tied to the aging population) of chronic illnesses. If an outpatient facility plans to establish a telehealth program to provide medical consultation and services to multiple states, the first consideration is state laws and regulations, as these may vary considerably.

## ELECTRONIC HEALTH

eHealth (electronic health) is an emerging specialty that refers to the use of information technology in the care and treatment of patients. eHealth is usually associated with the use of the internet but in some cases may only refer to the use of computers and computer systems as definitions vary somewhat. eHealth includes the use of:

- Electronic health records
- CPOE and CDSS systems
- Mobile health applications
- Telemonitoring
- Telehealth services
- Virtual health care
- Integrated networks
- Mobile devices, such as tablets and smart phones

CMS has an eHealth initiative that aligns health IT with industry electronic standards as part of the plan to promote the use of electronic health records throughout the healthcare industry. Health information exchanges (HIEs) are utilized to facilitate the secure exchange of information, always a concern in eHealth. eHealth has shown rapid growth but is impacted by a shortage of trained personnel, high maintenance costs, and budgetary constraints.

# Workflows

## WORKFLOW MAPPING

Workflow includes the actual steps involved in completing a process. These steps may not be those indicated in a procedure manual or even reported. In order to create a **workflow map**, it's necessary to actually observe processes and interview more than one person carrying out the processes because practices may vary somewhat. A workflow map is a flow chart that begins with the first step in the process and ends when the process is completed with arrows connecting the actions. Each step is represented in the chart and labeled with the action and the person carrying out the action (RN, clerk, physician, CNA, laboratory technician). There may be alternate paths in the workflow map. For example, if lab results are positive, actions may be required (such as reporting to the physician) that are not if the results are negative. Workflow mapping is especially useful for performance improvement projects because it helps to identify redundant or time-consuming actions that can be improved.

## WORKFLOW DESIGN

When designing workflows based on the care delivery model and population served, the designer must have a clear understanding of both. Workflow design (or redesign) should begin with the following:

- Observations of staff members engaged in routine activities
- Review of information systems requirements and problems
- Current workflow maps or practices
- Interviews with staff members
- Identification of problems in workflow (from observations and interviews)
- Workarounds in common use
- Patterns of communication and miscommunication, including information transfer
- Response to problems/roadblocks

Once all the data has been gathered, workflow mapping can begin. The first areas to concentrate on are reducing redundancies (which can be time-consuming and expensive), reducing workarounds (which can be safety concerns), and finding solutions to problems and roadblocks. Workflow design may begin with simple sketches and diagrams done manually, but workflow design software applications are usually used for workflow mapping.

## WORKFLOW THROUGHPUT

Throughput is almost always a concern when designing workflow. **Throughput** refers to the maximum amount of data, information, or materials that can pass through a process or system. The term has been most commonly used to refer to data processing, and this use applies to the efficiency of the electronic health record, CPOE, CDSS, and other data processing and storage systems. Additionally, the term has evolved to include other healthcare processes. In order to accurately measure throughput, a baseline or benchmark must be established for the sake of comparison. This benchmark may be internal or external, depending on the process. Reference to throughput is often made when setting goals and targets. For example, a goal may be to increase utilization of an outpatient clinic in order to maximize return on investment and to target an increased throughput of 15% with the benchmark being the average number of patients in the previous months.

## UTILIZATION OF INTERDISCIPLINARY TEAMS

Interdisciplinary teams, teams comprised of representatives from various departments, are an integral part of healthcare delivery; so effective workflow is an important factor in their effectiveness. Issues to consider when designing or redesigning workflow include:

- **The purpose of the interdisciplinary team**: Can include direct patient care, leadership, peer review, information management, and assessment
- **The composition of the teams**: The number of individuals and the departments represented
- **The number of teams**: One or many

- **Status differences** (such as physician and housekeeper): How this affects power, roles, interactions, and decision-making
- **Communication links and patterns**: How members communicate with each other and with those outside of the team (face-to-face, telephone, email)
- **Team leadership**: Collaborative, status-based, or rotating
- **Responsibilities**: Individual and team responsibilities and the way in which they are delegated and managed
- **Approach to responsibilities**: Collaborative, sequential, or parallel
- **Conflicts**: Disagreements, resentments, and discontents

## CASE MANAGEMENT

The case manager supervises and manages all aspects of care to ensure continuity. Within an acute, sub-acute, or skilled nursing facility, the case manager may chair the interdisciplinary team to ensure that the needs of the patient are communicated and that all members of the team are focused on similar goals. The case manager is responsible for screening patients from the time of admission (or before admission in some cases) and assisting with planning for discharge. As the patient moves back into the community, the case manager needs to consider the social support services (home health care, transportation, meals-on-wheels) that are needed for the person to remain as independent as possible and to function safely. Case managers are involved in all aspects of patient care, across many disciplines:

- Assessing plan of care
- Coordinating treatment and providing continuity
- Providing continuous assessment includes evaluating for variances to critical pathways
- Completing evaluation and discharge planning
- Doing post-discharge assessment

### MODELS FOR CASE MANAGEMENT

There are a number of **models for case management** that can be utilized to integrate the outcome of utilization management assessment into the performance improvement process:

- **Type of provider care**: Includes self-care (patient provides own care), primary care (patient and primary care physician), episodic care (patient, primary care physician, and specialist as well as the case manager), and brokered care (involves community, government, or private services).
- **Focus of care**: The focus may be on cost containment, common to managed care programs, where service depends upon the program's benefits and criteria for medical necessity and there is little or no direct contact with patient or family. The focus may also be on coordination of care, which involves direct patient and family contact and individualized assessment and intervention.
- **Professional discipline**: Case management may be done by nurses, social workers, psychiatrists, or other specific disciplines, depending upon the goals of case management.

## DISEASE MANAGEMENT

Disease management can become quite complex in terms of services required. For example, if a patient comes to the emergency department with a fractured hip, by the time the patient has been discharged, the patient may have used the following services: ED, imaging, laboratory, admissions, anesthesiology, surgery, pharmacy, nursing, physical therapy, occupational therapy, nutritional services, transportation services, case management, and discharge planning. Disease management in terms of care of chronic diseases poses similar concerns, but services may include those available in the community and the focus may be on maintenance and prevention. Part of workflow design is to determine how these different services interrelate and how to effectively coordinate services while preventing roadblocks that interfere with throughput. A major problem when multiple services are utilized is that redundancies are common, so identifying these is essential to improving cost-effectiveness and throughput.

## STAFFING ASSIGNMENT AND SCHEDULING

Staffing assignment and scheduling can be quite complex. A number of factors must be considered:

- Mix of part-time and full-time staff.
- Hours: 8 hours a day / 40 hours a week, 12 hours a day / 36 hours a week, 10 hours a day / 40 hours a week, or some mixture.
- Staffing model, such as acuity-based, primary care, total-patient care.
- Nurse-patient ratios for different departments.
- Specific requests and limitations, such as the inability to work certain days or a desire to work only weekends.
- Shifts: five traditional 8-hour shifts, three 12-hour shifts, four 10-hour shifts.

Most work schedules cover a 4- to 6-week period. Weekly predictable work schedules (such as Monday through Friday) repeat the same pattern of shift hours and days, but they can be problematic when factoring in vacation time or special requests. Rotation schedules in which days vary to accommodate rotating weekend coverage may entail different workdays over a two- to four-week period, which then repeats. When building the schedule, inflexible scheduling (requested days off, requested workdays) should be attended to first.

## MODELS OF SCHEDULING

There are three common models of scheduling:

- **Decentralized**: In this case, the schedule is developed by each unit manager, separate from all of the other units. This model depends on a stable list of employees for each unit and is problematic with acuity-based patient care that requires increased floating and different levels of staffing depending on needs.
- **Self-scheduling**: Each nurse develops his or her own schedule, often in cooperation and consultation with other staff members to ensure adequate coverage. This scheduling encourages autonomy, but issues can arise if, for example, weekend coverage is inadequate or if those with seniority always want first choice.
- **Centralized**: The advantage to centralized scheduling is that the coordinator can look at the whole picture and assign staff as needed, often with the help of software programs. The disadvantage is that the coordinator may not always understand the distinct needs of each unit and staff members may feel they have little or no input.

# Emergency Preparedness

## DISASTER/EMERGENCY RESPONSE PLANS

Disaster/emergency response plans should be in place for the facility based on the Hospital Emergency Incident Command System (HEICS), which provides a model for management, responsibilities, and communication. Disasters can include a multi-casualty influx of individuals from a community emergency, such as a train accident, an epidemic, a fire, an internal hospital problem requiring evacuation, or inadequate staffing to safely treat ED individuals. Plans should include/address:

- Readily available **information** and disaster preparedness **drills**.
- **Activation** of the plan, including the individual(s) responsible.
- Chain of command.
- **Facility damage assessment**, usually conducted by a plant safety officer.
- **Hospital/ED capacity** to receive individuals.
- **Triage**, including in community and in the ED.
- **Transfer protocols** for distributing individuals to other facilities.
- **Staffing**, including telephone tree to notify staff to report to facility.
- **Intra- and Inter-facility communication** and communication with pre-hospital EMS personnel.
- **Supplies** on hand and methods to obtain added supplies.
- **Delineation** of receiving and treatment areas.

## DISASTER PLANNING

Disaster planning should include plans for both internal and external disasters. Critical elements of preparation include:

- **Communication plans**: Includes phone trees or other notification systems and external notification of community agencies/resources.
- **Essential supplies**: IVs, dressing supplies, and essential medications should be stockpiled.
- **Staff roles and responsibilities**: Staff members should be trained in disaster preparedness and understand their roles and responsibilities.
- **Power/Utilities**: Backup systems should provide power for up to 96 hours.
- **Clinical patient care**: Plans for provision of care under varying circumstances, including alternate plans.

**Internal disasters**, such as fires, flooding, storm damage, and terrorist attacks, often result in the evacuation of patients and the need for transportation services to transfer patients. **External disasters**, such as hurricanes, tornadoes, terrorist attacks, floods, pandemics, and transportation disasters, more often result in a large influx of patients and the need to discharge non-critical patients to make room for new patients.

> **Review Video: Emergency Response, Business Continuity, and Disaster Planning**
> Visit mometrix.com/academy and enter code: 678024

# Facilitation of Patient Experience

## PATIENTS' BILL OF RIGHTS

Patients' and residents' Bill of Rights in relation to what they should expect from a healthcare organization are outlined in both standards of the Joint Commission and National Committee for Quality Assurance. Rights include:

- **Respect** for the patient, including personal dignity and psychosocial, spiritual, and cultural considerations
- **Response** to needs related to access and pain control

- Ability to make **decisions** about care, including informed consent, advance directives, and end of life care
- Procedure for registering **complaints or grievances**
- Protection of confidentiality and **privacy**
- **Freedom from abuse** or neglect
- **Protection** during research and information related to ethical issues of research
- Appraisal of **outcomes**, including unexpected outcomes
- **Information** about organization, services, and practitioners
- **Appeal procedures** for decisions regarding benefits and quality of care
- Organizational **code of ethical behavior**
- Procedures for **donating and procuring** organs/tissue

## ACCESS TO CARE

Challenges facing patients in regard to healthcare include quality issues, costs of care, and **access to care**. Two primary issues related to access are:

- **Insurance coverage**: Even with the Affordable Care Act, many people remain uninsured or underinsured. Employer-provided insurance coverage is becoming less common as the costs switch to the employees. While insurance companies and CMS negotiate fees, private individuals without insurance are usually billed full price—although in many cases healthcare providers are not able to collect.
- **Geographic location**: Access is more readily available in urban areas than in rural and in wealthy areas than in poor. People may have to travel long distances for medical facilities, healthcare providers, and medical services.

Expanding insurance coverage is one answer, but access can still be limited. Another answer is the development of increased numbers of nurse-managed health centers and decentralized disease-specific ambulatory care centers (sometimes mobile).

## MEDICAL DEVICE SAFETY

The FDA maintains and regulates procedures and recalls regarding contaminated equipment and supplies on a website entitled **MedWatch** (http://www.fda.gov/medwatch/index.html) to provide safety information for drugs and medical equipment. MedWatch provides electronic listing service to medical professionals and facilities for the following:

- Medical product safety alerts
- Information about drugs and devices
- Summary of safety alerts with links to detailed information

The *Safe Medical Practices Act* (1990) requires manufacturers and medical device user facilities to report problems with medical devices, including deaths or serious injuries (defined as requiring medical or surgical intervention), within 10 working days. Facilities must also file semiannual reports on January 1 and July 1. User facilities must maintain records for 2 years and must develop written procedures for identification, evaluation, and submission of medical device reports (MDR). MedWatch provides:

- **Reporting forms** (downloadable) for voluntary and mandatory reports
- **Safety information** about recalls, market withdrawals and safety alerts, organized by months and years.

## CUSTOMER SERVICE

### INTERNAL CUSTOMER SERVICE

Internal customer service is directed at those who are members of the healthcare organization rather than those being served by the organization although maintaining good internal customer service can, in turn, affect the quality of external customer services. The goal of internal customer service is to provide the customers with the things they need and want in order to carry out their jobs effectively. Important factors in internal customer service include the following:

- Treat all staff with respect
- Set standards for service
- Educate all levels in the chain of command so they remain up-to-date
- Carry out fair and equitable performance evaluation processes with input from staff members
- Remain available to staff
- Maintain open channels of communication
- Encourage empowerment
- Develop a reward system to acknowledge achievements
- Anticipate needs before they become acute
- Seek feedback from staff members about internal customer service

### EXTERNAL CUSTOMER SERVICE

External customer service involves interpersonal communication with a customer (such as a patient or vendor) to attend to the person's needs. This communication may be face-to-face or via telephone, email, internet chat, or text messaging. For face-to-face and telephone communication, the customer service individual must have strong **verbal communication skills**. For email, internet chat, or text messaging, the individual must also have good **typing and grammar skills**. The customer service individual should be knowledgeable about the needs of customers, have up-to-date information, and understand the level of authority needed to respond to customers' needs. In all cases, the individual must exhibit patience and have a good understanding of behavioral psychology in order to assess the customer's emotional status. It's important for the individual to listen attentively to customers and to use positive language in response. The individual must also have good time management skills in order to avoid wasting time with customers.

### SERVICE RECOVERY

Service recovery is important in healthcare. One patient may have to wait a short period for a procedure (minor problem) while another patient may develop a life-threatening postoperative infection (major problem). In both cases, the goal of service recovery is to retain the goodwill of the patient and to continue the relationship despite the problems that occurred. While patients may not complain directly to the healthcare providers, they often share their discontent with family and friends and increasingly on social media. When a problem occurs, the best course of action is to immediately **acknowledge** the problem and **apologize**. Apologizing is not the same as assuming blame, a concern sometimes expressed by healthcare providers: "I know you had to wait longer than expected, and I'm sorry for your inconvenience." Even if there is no fault, denying a problem or making excuses for it usually only increases resentment. The problem should be rectified if possible and, when appropriate, some type of compensation offered.

# Care Delivery Evaluation

## OUTCOME MEASURING AND MONITORING

Measuring and monitoring of a project are ongoing procedures that evaluate progress toward objectives and indicate any deviations so that corrections can be made. Processes vary according to the knowledge area of the project. For example, costs should be compared to the forecast budget and any change requests to determine if there are cost overruns. Activities on the timeline should be assessed to determine if they are on schedule, ahead of schedule, or behind schedule. Risks should be assessed and managed. Changes should be assessed through integrated change control and all change requests documented as well as their approval or rejection. Quality control measurements should be carried out and any defects noted and corrected. Performance of team members should be monitored. Any changes in the scope of a project should be noted and the project plan updated. Performance reports should be completed as scheduled and disseminated to the proper individuals or agencies.

## NURSE-SENSITIVE INDICATORS

In 1994, American Nurse Association (ANA) began to investigate the impact healthcare restructuring had on patient care, identifying nurse-sensitive indicators. **Nurse-sensitive indicators** are the elements of care—process, outcomes, and structures—related specifically to nursing. Indicators should be able to be tracked and evaluated and may focus on the following:

- **Patient-focused outcomes**: Measurable outcomes, such as rate of urinary tract infections, pressure ulcers, falls, patient injuries, patient satisfaction with care (pain control, nursing response, education). These outcomes should improve with increased quality or quantity of nursing care.
- **Process of care**: Methods used to provide care (such as routine infection control measures) and staff satisfaction. These processes should improve with better education, supervision, mentoring, and feedback.
- **Structure**: Staffing ratios (such as RN to LVN to CNAs), total hours of nursing care per patient per day, nurse turnover, and nursing education and certification. An improvement in structure often requires increased financial and/or time investment and evidence of cost effectiveness.

## IHI BUNDLES

The Institute of Healthcare Improvement (IHI) is a nonprofit organization that promotes better and more cost-effective patient care with the goals of preventing needless deaths, pain and suffering, helplessness, excessive waiting, waste, and lack of care. IHI encourages such measures as the use of rapid response teams and medication reconciliation. IHI has developed bundles, a group of processes based on evidence-based practices that must be carried out in order to improve patient outcomes. Bundles include 3-5 steps, but each step is critical, and all steps should be performed as prescribed, as in the following examples for sepsis (first hour) and central line infection prevention:

| Sepsis First Hour Management | Central Line Infection Prevention |
|---|---|
| • Measure lactate (and remeasure if level is higher than 2 mmol/L).<br>• Collect blood cultures prior to antibiotic administration.<br>• Administer broad-spectrum antibiotics.<br>• For hypotension or lactate >4 mmol/L: Rapid administration of crystalloid fluids (30 mL/kg).<br>• If hypotension continues, initiate vasopressors for MAP goal >65 mmHg. | • Proper hand hygiene<br>• Use of barrier precautions (PPE)<br>• Skin antisepsis with chlorhexidine<br>• Choosing the optimal site for catheter insertion<br>• Daily evaluation of catheter and assessment for potential removal |

## ORYX INDICATORS

ORYX indicators are measurement requirements of the Joint Commission utilized as part of the accreditation process. Large and small acute hospitals must collect and transmit data for at least 6 core measure sets while critical access hospitals must collect and transmit data on 4 core measure sets. **Core measure sets** include: Acute Myocardial Infarction, Children's Asthma Care, Emergency Department, Hospital Outpatient Department, Hospital-Based Inpatient Psychiatric Services, Immunization, Perinatal care, Pneumonia Measures, Stroke, Substance Use, Surgical Care Improvement Project (SCIP), Tobacco Treatment, and Venous Thromboembolism. Hospitals with 300 or more live births must report on perinatal care. New guidelines are issued annually. Data is publicly reported to The Joint Commission's website so that the data can be utilized for state and national comparisons.

## LEAPFROG

Leapfrog is a consortium of healthcare purchasers/employers providing benefits to millions of Americans. The focus initially was on reducing healthcare costs by preventing medical errors and "leaping forward" by rewarding hospitals and healthcare organizations that improve safety and quality of care. Leapfrog provides an annual Hospital and Quality Safety Survey to assess progress, releases regional data, and encourages voluntary public reporting. Leapfrog has instituted the Leapfrog Hospital Rewards Program (LHRP) as a pay-for-performance program to reward organizations for showing improvement in key measures.

### INITIATIVES

Leapfrog has developed a number of **initiatives** to improve safety. These initiatives can be valuable tools in assessing and developing a patient safety culture. Initiatives include:

- **Preventing medical errors** through encouraging patient safety concerns to be reported and by generating Hospital Safety Grades that provide the public with current safety ratings of each hospital
- **Educating** enrollees about patient safety and providing comparative performance data
- **Recognizing and rewarding** healthcare organizations that demonstrate improvement in preventing errors
- Making health plans **accountable** for implementing these principles
- **Advocating** for these principles with clients by utilizing benefits consultants
- Implementation of **computerized physicians order entry** (CPOE) system that includes software to detect and prevent errors with a goal of decreasing prescribing errors by more than 50%

- **Evidence-based hospital referral** requiring referral to hospitals that can demonstrate the best results and experience related to high-risk conditions and surgeries, assessed according to the number of procedures/treatments they do each year and outcomes data with a goal of reducing mortality rates by 40%
- ICU physician staffing requiring specially trained **specialists** (intensivist) with a goal of reducing mortality rates by 40%

Leapfrog Safe Practices Score assesses the progress a healthcare organization is making on 30 safe practices that Leapfrog has identified as reducing the risk of harm to patients.

## MAGNET RECOGNITION PROGRAM

The American Nurse's Credentialing Center, affiliated with the ANA, developed the **Magnet Recognition Program** to reward hospitals that meet a set of criteria related to excellence in nursing and positive patient outcomes associated with high job satisfaction and low staff turnover. Hospitals must apply for Magnet status and undergo extensive review for compliance. Criteria include:

- **Educational requirements**: CNO must have an MS or a doctorate in nursing; 100% of nurse managers must have a degree in nursing (BS or higher).
- Evidence of innovative health care.
- Evidence of **improvement** in meeting the goal of 26% professional certification of nurses by credentialing agencies.
- **Patient outcome data**: Includes falls, pressure ulcers, BSI, UTI, VAP, restraint use, pediatric IV infiltrations, and other nationally benchmarked indicators of specific specialties. Data should outperform the mean of the selected national database.
- **Patient satisfaction surveys and data**: Pain management, education, nursing courtesy and respect, listening, and response time.

## NATIONAL QUALITY CORE MEASURES

The Joint Commission has established **National Quality Core Measures** to determine if healthcare institutions are in compliance with current standards based on CMS quality indicators. The Core Measures involve a series of questions that are answered either "yes" or "no" to indicate if an action was completed. There are now 9 **Core Measure sets**:

- Accountable care organizations/patient centered medical homes/primary care
- Behavioral Health
- Cardiology
- Gastroenterology
- HIV and Hepatitis C
- Medical Oncology
- Neurology
- Obstetrics and Gynecology
- Pediatrics

For each condition, questions relate to whether or not standard care was provided, such as giving an aspirin for those with acute MI. The data are public and provide useful information about these particular standards, but do not necessarily reflect the overall quality of care, so these measurements alone are not adequate performance measures but must be considered along with other indicators.

# Advocating for the Nursing Profession

## PROFESSIONAL ORGANIZATIONS

When advocating for the nursing profession, the nurse executive should become an active member in **professional organizations**, such as the American Organization of Nurse Executives and the American Nurses Association (both national and state organizations). Professional organizations are often leaders in lobbying for laws to support healthcare organizations and the role of nurses. The nurse executive can be active on many levels, from attending conferences in order to gain information to giving presentations to serving on committees and boards of the professional organization. Participation in professional organizations is invaluable in establishing networking systems and becoming more aware of issues affecting nursing practice. As a nursing advocate, the nursing executive should promote the rights of others, facilitate innovative changes to the system, promote self-determination, promote autonomy, leverage diversity, and ensure others are treated with respect.

## PROMOTING EDUCATION

An important aspect of advocating for the nursing profession is **promoting education**. Steps the nurse executive can take to promote education include:

- **Flexible scheduling**: Staff members are more likely to enroll in educational programs if they are allowed to schedule work time around their class schedules so that they don't lose income while studying.
- **Incentives**: Paying staff members for class time, paying tuition, or reimbursing for tuition costs in return for a commitment to remain employed for a specified period of time or after they have done so can encourage education and help retain staff.
- **Rewards**: This can include salary increase and/or public recognition of achievements.
- **Continuing nursing education**: The organization can become a provider of CNEs.
- **Partnerships/Agreements**: The nurse executive can collaborate with institutions of higher learning to establish classes for staff, such as an onsite BSN bridge program.

## LIFE-LONG LEARNING

Life-long learning is the ongoing pursuit of knowledge often simply for the sake of learning. Life-long learning is almost always a voluntary type of education in which the individual utilizes a variety of resources—including books, magazines, workshops, conferences, videos, continuing education courses, and academic classes—to stay current in one or more fields of study or just in general knowledge to keep informed. For example, many universities and adult schools now offer programs geared to the interests of older adults. Planning for academic progression, on the other hand, requires more formal education and involves further academic studies in order to advance in one's career. For example, an RN with an AS degree may enroll in a bridge program to receive a BS in nursing and then may work and apply to graduate school to work toward an MS or a doctorate degree.

## CERTIFICATIONS

Information about **certifications** can be obtained from a number of different sources:

- **State Boards of Nursing**: Each state outlines the type of certifications recognized for advance practice nurses and provides the scope of practice.
- **Books**: Career-related nursing books are widely available regarding all different types of certifications.

- **Journals**: Nursing journals often have career-related articles and/or articles of interest to those with specific certifications. Other journals are aimed at those with certification in a specific field, such as the *Clinical Journal of Oncology Nursing*, and can provide valuable insight into specialized practice.
- **State and national professional organizations**: Organizations, such as the National Nursing Staff Development Organization, provide information about certification programs, including location of programs, professional resources, and requirements.
- **Certification organizations**: Organizations that provide credentialing, such as the American Nurses Credentialing Center (ANCC) provide information about obtaining certification, maintaining, and renewing.

## SUPPORTING CERTIFICATION AND CREDENTIALING

When coordinating activities that support certification and credentialing, the nurse executive must first determine the type of certification and credentialing and the specific requirements of the credentialing organization in order to produce activities that can be counted toward achieving or maintaining certification and credentialing. The nurse must provide oversight to ensure that certification activities are performed effectively and documented as required. Coordinating responsibilities include:

- Providing an adequate support system
- Developing educational programs and activities or assisting and supervising others to do so
- Developing educational materials in support of certification/credentialing
- Collecting data regarding certification/credentialing and maintaining records
- Consulting with professionals (such as doctors and nurse specialists) as needed to facilitate activities
- Managing budget for activities
- Initiating programs for quality performance improvement
- Auditing individual records of educational activities and preparing reports
- Communicating with staff personally or via telephone and/or email to respond to questions regarding activities

# Chapter Quiz

Ready to see how well you retained what you just read? Scan the QR code to go directly to the chapter quiz interface for this study guide. If you're using a computer, simply visit the bonus page at **mometrix.com/bonus948/nce** and click the Chapter Quizzes link.

# Nurse Executive Practice Test #1

Want to take this practice test in an online interactive format?
Check out the bonus page, which includes interactive practice questions and much more: **mometrix.com/bonus948/nurseexec**

**1. Fogging is a communication technique for managing criticism, which allows a person to:**

a.  agree in principle and receive criticism without becoming defensive.
b.  encourage others to communicate assertively.
c.  use distraction to avoid acknowledgment of the criticism.
d.  use intimidation to redirect the conversation.

**2. A nurse executive is most likely to use which of the following decision-making models to implement a nursing program that requires evaluation after implementation?**

a.  Bureaucratic Model.
b.  Collegial Model.
c.  Cybernetic Model.
d.  Garbage Can Model.

**3. All of the following questions would be considered acceptable to ask a prospective employee during an interview EXCEPT:**

a.  have you worked for this hospital in the past under a different name?
b.  do you feel you will be able to perform the duties of this position?
c.  are you authorized to work in the United States?
d.  do you have any children?

**4. Nursing staff in an emergency department labeled a patient as "borderline," "attention seeker," and a "services abuser." Nursing documentation in the patient's record reflects these views, including additional statements, such as the patient "shows up at least once a week with various complaints." On one visit, the patient complained of abdominal pain and vomiting. Minimal treatment was provided, and the patient was discharged. Later, the staff is informed that the patient required surgery at another hospital for an intestinal blockage; litigation is pending. The defense attorneys reviewed all existing nursing documentation. It is likely that the nursing staff in the Emergency Department will be charged with:**

a.  slander.
b.  libel.
c.  harassment.
d.  unintentional tort.

**5. In all 50 states, minors can provide informed consent for:**

a.  HIV testing and treatment.
b.  sexually transmitted disease testing and treatment except for HIV.
c.  contraceptive services.
d.  abortion.

**6. Paternalistic actions are incompatible with nursing ethics because they:**

    a. reduce ethical obligation.
    b. reduce the accountability of the nurse.
    c. decrease the authority of the nurse.
    d. diminish the autonomy of the patient.

**7. The nursing care delivery model in which a nurse holds 24-hour responsibility for a patient from admission through discharge is known as:**

    a. team nursing.
    b. modular nursing.
    c. functional nursing.
    d. primary nursing.

**8. A patient classification system is used to measure:**

    a. customer satisfaction.
    b. acuity level.
    c. performance variations.
    d. patient safety.

**9. The original purpose for the development of diagnosis-related groups was to:**

    a. determine Medicare reimbursement at a fixed-fee.
    b. provide funding for private insurance companies.
    c. determine prescription drug benefits.
    d. provide sliding-scale reimbursement for Medicare beneficiaries.

**10. Medical waste disposal programs are primarily regulated at the:**

    a. federal level.
    b. local level.
    c. state level.
    d. community level.

**11. The Patient Self-Determination Act requires federally funded hospitals to provide:**

    a. written notice to patients regarding their rights to make treatment decisions.
    b. treatment to patients who are uninsured.
    c. reasonable accommodation to patients with disabilities.
    d. protection to patients by making nurses accountable through practice regulations.

**12. The business analysis technique most likely to be used by a nurse executive for strategic planning is known as:**

    a. VPEC-T analysis.
    b. SWOT analysis.
    c. MoSCow analysis.
    d. PC analysis.

**13.** The budget method that requires a comprehensive review and justification of all expenditures before resources are allocated is known as:

    a. incremental budgeting.
    b. priority-based budgeting.
    c. activity-based budgeting.
    d. zero-based budgeting.

**14.** Fifty new hospital beds are required to replace beds with faulty rails on several units. The funds for these new beds are allocated from which type of budget?

    a. Capital budget.
    b. Operational budget.
    c. Labor budget.
    d. Marketing budget.

**15.** A comparison of hospital services to the best practices of other industries with similar services with the goal of establishing higher standards is one example of:

    a. networking.
    b. market research.
    c. quantitative research.
    d. benchmarking.

**16.** Which component of the nursing process may be delegated with supervision?

    a. Assessment.
    b. Planning.
    c. Intervention.
    d. Evaluation.

**17.** Standards of the Occupational Safety and Health Administration require that all new employees who provide direct care must:

    a. be offered the hepatitis B three-injection series vaccination.
    b. have an annual TB test.
    c. accept evaluation by a health care provider in the event of a needle stick.
    d. obtain a titer following hepatitis B three-injection series vaccination.

**18.** Which of the following laws was passed in 2002 to address the nursing shortage through retention and recruitment initiatives?

    a. Model Nursing Practice Act.
    b. America's Partnership for Nursing Education Act.
    c. National Nurse Act.
    d. Nurse Reinvestment Act.

**19. Which of the following statements regarding the privacy rules of the Health Insurance Portability and Accountability Act (HIPAA) is correct?**

    a.  HIPAA privacy rules authorize covered entities to disclose protected health information without an individual's authorization in the event of a public health emergency.

    b.  HIPAA privacy rules authorize covered entities to impose fees for searching and retrieving copies of medical records when copies of records are requested.

    c.  HIPAA privacy rules authorize covered entities to retain tape-recorded information, following transcription of medical information.

    d.  HIPAA privacy rules restrict an individual's access to their medical record, following a clinical trial.

**20. Which quantitative research methodology focuses on the statistical analysis of multiple research studies on a selected topic with the goal of investigating study characteristics and integrating the results?**

    a.  Meta-analysis.

    b.  Survey.

    c.  Needs assessment.

    d.  Methodological study.

**21. Federal regulation regarding Institutional Review Boards has which of the following characteristics?**

    a.  They may consist entirely of members from the same profession.

    b.  They should not include a member whose primary concerns are nonscientific.

    c.  They may invite experts in special areas to vote on complex issues.

    d.  They must include one member who is not affiliated with the institution.

**22. Under the HIPAA Privacy Rule, clinical health records of living adults must be maintained for at least:**

    a.  2 years.

    b.  4 years.

    c.  6 years.

    d.  8 years.

**23. Recently, the nursing staff has been notified that their medical surgical unit will be relocated to another building on campus to allow for the construction of a new intensive care unit. Several of the nurses are complaining about moving to a smaller unit and are verbalizing possibilities of decreases in staffing and compromised patient care. An effective change agent should do which of the following?**

    a.  Hold a department meeting to notify nursing staff that the move is mandatory and not debatable.

    b.  Recommend that staff nurses prepare a formal written complaint, which will be presented to administration.

    c.  Avoid acknowledgment of complaints, and move forward to discourage additional negative communication.

    d.  Involve staff nurses in the move, including staff meetings to provide information and receive feedback.

**24. Which of the following conflict resolution styles includes both parties actively attempting to find solutions that will satisfy goals of both parties?**

a. Avoidance.
b. Accommodation.
c. Compromise.
d. Collaboration.

**25. Under the Fair Labor Standards Act, which of the following statements concerns exempt employees?**

a. They must be paid for 7 holidays a year if working 40 hours a week.
b. They must be paid overtime if they work more than a 40-hour week.
c. They are salaried employees and are not subject to minimum wage.
d. They must receive a minimum of one break period for each 4 hours of work.

**26. Expectations of the Joint Commission's Sentinel Event Policy for accredited hospitals include all the following EXCEPT to:**

a. report all defined sentinel events.
b. conduct a root-cause analysis within 45 days of becoming aware of a reviewable sentinel event.
c. define all events within the hospital that are subject to review under the Sentinel Event Policy.
d. develop an action plan and respond appropriately to defined sentinel events.

**27. Which of the following is an example of a reviewable sentinel event as defined by the Joint Commission's Sentinel Event Policy?**

a. Patient death, following a discharge "against medical advice."
b. Unsuccessful suicide attempt without major loss of permanent function.
c. Employee death, following blood-borne pathogen exposure.
d. Patient fall, resulting in permanent loss of function.

**28. As part of the Joint Commission's National Patient Safety Goal, a list of "do not use" abbreviations, acronyms, and symbols were developed for accredited hospitals to assist in attaining the safety goal. Which of the following is a "do not use" value symbol in medication orders?**

a. 1.0 mg.
b. 1 mg.
c. 0.1 mg.
d. 1 mL.

**29. For a nurse to be held liable for malpractice, all of the following elements must be proven EXCEPT that:**

a. a nurse–patient relationship existed.
b. standards of care were breached by the nurse.
c. injury or damage was suffered by the patient.
d. there was a direct cause between the nurse's actions and the patient's injury.

**30. The Health Insurance Portability and Accountability Act (HIPAA) privacy rule allows the disclosure of protected health information for clinical research under all of the following circumstances EXCEPT:**

    a. the subject has signed valid Privacy Rule Authorization.
    b. a waiver was granted by an Institutional Review Board or Privacy Board.
    c. protected health information has been de-identified.
    d. the subject has signed an informed consent.

**31. Under the Health Insurance Portability and Accountability Act (HIPAA) Privacy Rule, protected health information may be disclosed following de-identification. Which of the following descriptive elements of an individual would not require removal during the de-identifying process?**

    a. Date of birth.
    b. State.
    c. Social security number.
    d. Electronic mail addresses.

**32. The five-stage model called Tuckman's stages, regarding group dynamics, is often used in decision-making groups. In which of the following stages would a leader clarify roles and rules for working collaboratively and team members begin to build a commitment to the team goal?**

    a. Norming.
    b. Storming.
    c. Performing.
    d. Forming.

**33. In which of the following types of leadership power do followers comply, not for rewards or the possibility of negative consequences, but because the leader is perceived to have the authority to direct others?**

    a. Referent power.
    b. Legitimate power.
    c. Expert power.
    d. Coercive power.

**34. A newly licensed nurse accepted a position on a medical unit. As part of the orientation process, he was assigned a preceptor for 4 weeks. Over time, the nurse noticed that his preceptor consistently provided only partial answers to many important questions, often in a condescending tone, and frequently stated "You do not need to know that right now." This type of behavior is known as:**

    a. clinical violence.
    b. verbal abuse.
    c. intimidation.
    d. lateral violence.

**35. A standard Centers for Disease Control case form must be completed for which of the following notifiable infectious diseases?**

   a. Campylobacteriosis.
   b. Listeriosis.
   c. Histoplasmosis.
   d. Leptospirosis.

**36. The Department of Health and Human Services division responsible for investigating Medicare fraud is the office of:**

   a. Medicare Hearings and Appeals.
   b. Global Health Affairs.
   c. Inspector General.
   d. Intergovernmental Affairs.

**37. The American Nurses Association Principals for Nurse Staffing questions the usefulness of which of the following factors when determining staffing plans?**

   a. Nursing hours per patient day.
   b. Number of patients.
   c. Available technology.
   d. Staff experience and skill level.

**38. An example of centralized decision-making is:**

   a. staff members participate in self-scheduling.
   b. the nurse manager approves all new hires through the nurse executive.
   c. nurses provide care based on the Primary Nursing Model.
   d. a committee of nurses is formed to engage in quality-improvement initiatives.

**39. A unit manager notifies the nurse executive of her intent to resign because she is unable meet the recently reduced expectations for staff budgeting. The cognitive distortion of the nurse manager is known as:**

   a. fortune telling.
   b. disqualifying the positive.
   c. catastrophizing.
   d. all-or-nothing thinking.

**40. Which of the following statements best describes the Belmont Report?**

   a. It makes specific recommendations for Health and Human Services (HHS) administrative action, regarding unethical treatment of human subjects in research.
   b. It defines regulations for human subject protection during research.
   c. It is based on the ethical principles of justice, autonomy, and respect.
   d. It identifies ethical principles, which form the basis of the HHS human subject protection regulations.

**41.** The U.S. Equal Employment Opportunity Commission (EEOC) enforces federal laws against discrimination in the workplace. Which of the following statements best describes what is least likely to be prohibited by the EEOC employment laws and regulations?

    a. Advertising for employment, seeking female staff only.
    b. Recruiting by word-of-mouth, resulting in an almost entirely similar workforce.
    c. Reducing benefits for older workers if the reduction results in matching the cost of the benefits to the cost of those for younger workers.
    d. Requesting a photograph of an applicant during the initial hiring process.

**42.** The overall goal of Healthy People 2030 is to:

    a. promote health and prevent disease for all Americans.
    b. track national disease data over 10 years.
    c. educate public health workers on leading causes of disease.
    d. compile evidence-based literature on public health issues.

**43.** What type of insurance covers employers against litigation as a result of negligence by employees for work-related accidents?

    a. Workers' Compensation Insurance.
    b. Employer's Liability Insurance.
    c. Public Liability Insurance.
    d. Keyman Insurance.

**44.** PHI shared during a telephone call is subject to the HIPAA Security Rule:

    a. in all instances.
    b. if the information is stored in electronic form.
    c. if it involves discussion of diagnosis.
    d. if the information is not stored in electronic form.

**45.** What condition is no longer covered by Medicare under the Deficit Reduction Act?

    a. Urinary tract infection.
    b. Blood administration.
    c. Bypass surgery.
    d. Air embolism.

**46.** To comply with the Occupational Safety and Health Administration requirements for an Exposure Control Plan, all of the following elements must be included in the plan EXCEPT:

    a. an exposure determination, identifying job classifications.
    b. procedures to evaluate exposure events.
    c. implementation of methods of exposure control.
    d. a list of all hazardous chemicals and safety data sheets.

**47.** Which of the following quality-improvement methods is used to identify and prevent potential problems?

    a. Root-cause analysis.
    b. Barrier analysis.
    c. Causal factor analysis.
    d. Failure mode and effects analysis.

**48. Which analysis tool is based on the 80/20 rule (80% of problems are caused by 20% of the causes)?**

a. Pareto chart.
b. Run chart.
c. Gantt chart.
d. Flow chart.

**49. What is the difference between a Gantt chart and the Program Evaluation Review Technique (PERT) chart?**

a. Dependencies between activities in Gantt charts are easier to follow than PERT charts.
b. Gantt charts are usually preferable to PERT charts for large projects.
c. Activity times are represented by arrows between activity nodes in Gantt charts.
d. PERT is a flow chart, and Gantt is a bar chart.

**50. What nonprofit organization accredits health plans, individual physicians, and medical groups and provides additional programs, such as credential verification and a multicultural health care distinction?**

a. Joint Commission.
b. National Nonprofit Accreditation Center.
c. Council on Accreditation.
d. National Committee for Quality Assurance.

**51. According to Healthy People 2030, what is the most preventable cause of disease and death in the United States?**

a. Obesity.
b. Tobacco use.
c. Sexually transmitted diseases.
d. Poor diet and low physical activity.

**52. With the professional practice model of differentiated nursing practice, responsibilities for patient care differentiate according to:**

a. level of education/clinical expertise.
b. patient's acuity level.
c. costs of care.
d. patient DRG.

**53. A person's right to privacy extends:**

a. 10 years following death.
b. 25 years following death.
c. 50 years following death.
d. 75 years following death.

**54. Corporate compliance requires adherence to:**

a. accreditation standards.
b. state and federal regulations and legal and ethical standards.
c. timely billing practices.
d. established organizational goals and objectives.

**55. Which of the following reasons for telephoning a patient would be considered HIPAA noncompliant?**

    a. Appointments and reminders
    b. Lab test results
    c. Post-discharge follow-up
    d. Assessment of patient regarding new health issues

**56. The Consumer Credit Protection Act (Title III) prohibits employers from:**

    a. discharging employees because of wage garnishment.
    b. disclosing information about an employee's salary.
    c. limiting garnishment to 50% of salary.
    d. garnishing wages for creditors.

**57. If an evidence-based intervention has been implemented but outcome measures show that the results are not on par with those experienced by other organizations, the most likely reason is:**

    a. different population.
    b. inadequate measures.
    c. lack of treatment fidelity.
    d. common cause variation.

**58. If a unit supervisor comes to the nurse executive and discusses a problem the supervisor is trying to solve, the nurse executive should:**

    a. give advice.
    b. listen.
    c. provide reassurance.
    d. question.

**59. If a full-time employee who has met eligibility requirements requests unpaid medical leave under the Family Medical Leave Act, the employer may:**

    a. request a medical certificate.
    b. refuse the request.
    c. discharge the employee.
    d. limit time off to six weeks.

**60. The key to leveraging diversity in the workplace is:**

    a. accommodation.
    b. representation.
    c. education.
    d. communication.

**61. If an organizational goal is to decrease the rate of postoperative infections, which method of communication of results is likely the most effective in encouraging ongoing efforts?**

    a. Written report to administration.
    b. Dashboard updates.
    c. Oral report at staff meetings.
    d. Posted paper notices on bulletin boards.

62. Which of the following is likely to be most disruptive to healthcare quality?

    a. Increased regulations.
    b. Social changes.
    c. Increasing costs.
    d. Ethnic diversity.

63. Before facilitating change in a healthcare organization, it's especially important to have an understanding of the organizational:

    a. service population.
    b. financial status.
    c. structure.
    d. culture.

64. The most effective method of establishing a professional network is to:

    a. associate with nurses from other departments.
    b. become active in professional organizations.
    c. utilize social media to interact with others.
    d. socialize with other staff in off-hours.

65. Which of the following questions should be asked when authenticating a patient?

    a. "Is your name John Brown?"
    b. "Is your telephone number still 409-6214-3752?"
    c. "Has your insurance number changed?"
    d. "What is your address?"

66. Which of the following is a nursing sensitive quality indicator?

    a. Patient readmission rate.
    b. Patient acuity classification.
    c. Skill mix of nursing staff.
    d. Cost of care.

67. In patient care delivery, a nurse accessed the wrong EHR and retrieved an incorrect medication for a patient. While preparing the drug for administration, the nurse noticed the incorrect medication and returned it immediately. This would be classified as a(n):

    a. negligent act.
    b. adverse patient occurrence.
    c. close-call event.
    d. potentially compensable event.

68. According the Change Theory (Lewin, Schein), the first stage, motivation to change (unfreezing), may be characterized by:

    a. overriding of defensive actions.
    b. a change in perceptions of self and relationships.
    c. identification of needed changes.
    d. survival anxiety and learning anxiety.

**69. Emergency planning should begin with:**
    a.  hazard vulnerability analysis.
    b.  survey of other institutions' policies.
    c.  review of past emergencies.
    d.  cost assessment.

**70. If the organization's overall staff turnover rate exceeds the benchmark (<6%) set by the organization, the next step should be to:**
    a.  analyze the rate by job class.
    b.  survey all staff regarding job satisfaction.
    c.  develop a strategy for retention.
    d.  carry out a salary comparison study.

**71. If censuses in the oncology unit and medical-surgical unit fluctuate widely, often resulting in overstaffing or understaffing, the best solution is to:**
    a.  reassign staff to other units.
    b.  lay-off some members of the staff.
    c.  cross train staff members.
    d.  use temporary nursing staff to resolve understaffing.

**72. The nurse executive wants to increase patient engagement, realizing that according to the Patient Activation Measure (Hibbard et.al., 2004), the first stage of patient engagement is:**
    a.  having the ability (resources) to take action.
    b.  persisting even in the face of stress.
    c.  taking action to improve health.
    d.  believing in the importance of the patient's role.

**73. In order to improve relations between physicians and nurses, the nurse executive stresses support for the "platinum rule" associated with interdisciplinary collaboration. The "platinum rule" states:**
    a.  treat others as they want to be treated.
    b.  treat others as you want to be treated.
    c.  treat everyone the same.
    d.  treat everyone differently.

**74. If a union is organizing employees, what percentage of employees must sign union authorization cards before the union requests that the organization voluntarily recognize the union as the bargaining agent for the employees?**
    a.  20%.
    b.  30%.
    c.  40%.
    d.  50%.

**75. According to force field analysis (Lewin), the two forces that must be considered for change include:**

   a.  costs and benefits.
   b.  time and effort.
   c.  staff and administration.
   d.  driving and restraining.

**76. Which of the following strategies for change reflects the normative reeducative approach?**

   a.  Using power to coerce change.
   b.  Using data to influence others.
   c.  Focusing on the need to get along with others.
   d.  Setting arbitrary standards.

**77. Once an emergency operations plan is developed for a healthcare organization, the most important next step is to:**

   a.  carry out drills.
   b.  educate the staff.
   c.  gather resources.
   d.  develop partnerships.

**78. Training output estimating is used primarily to:**

   a.  estimate the supply of health practitioners.
   b.  evaluate clinical application of training.
   c.  determine the need for additional training.
   d.  estimate outcomes associated with training.

**79. To ensure that new hires are correctly licensed and credentialed, it is necessary to:**

   a.  ask the individual for detailed information.
   b.  require presentation of licenses and credentials.
   c.  contact previous employers.
   d.  carry out a primary source verification.

**80. What are the 4 core criteria for credentialing and privileging?**

   a.  Licensure, performance ability, recommendation, necessity.
   b.  Education, licensure, necessity, and recommendation.
   c.  Licensure, education, competence, performance ability.
   d.  Recommendation, education, licensure, experience.

**81. Before instituting organization-wide utilization of SBAR for hand-offs and transitions of care, the nurse executive should initially:**

   a.  survey the staff.
   b.  provide guidelines and training.
   c.  mandate a date for implementation.
   d.  advise staff to research SBAR.

**82. What four types of quality measures are pay-for-performance programs usually based on?**

    a.  Costs, outcomes, timeliness, and best practices.
    b.  Performance, costs, outcomes, and patient experience.
    c.  Performance, outcomes, patient experience, and structure/technology.
    d.  Patient experience, outcomes, costs, and timeliness.

**83. According to the general systems theory, which of the following would be classified as an output?**

    a.  Changed behavior.
    b.  Praise.
    c.  Facts.
    d.  Lived experience.

**84. The nurse executive appears to have staff support for proposed changes as no one voices opposition, but anonymous surveys indicate widespread opposition. The type of power that the nurse executive is likely utilizing is:**

    a.  expert.
    b.  informative.
    c.  legitimate.
    d.  coercive.

**85. After selecting a number of possible vendors for a complex upgrade of equipment and services, the next step is to develop a:**

    a.  business plan.
    b.  request for proposal.
    c.  request for quotation.
    d.  budget allowance.

**86. According to the Joint Commission, the first element of the six critical areas of emergency response to be addressed is:**

    a.  resources and assets.
    b.  safety and security.
    c.  staff responsibilities.
    d.  communication.

**87. If a hospital has instituted a just culture to encourage staff to report incidents and unsafe practices, a nurse who misread a medication order and administered an incorrect dosage to a patient should be:**

    a.  placed on probation.
    b.  provided a coach and further training.
    c.  fired for incompetence.
    d.  consoled and supported.

**88. Once an evidence-based change has been implemented, the next critical element is to:**

    a.  measure outcomes.
    b.  survey staff.
    c.  assess costs.
    d.  punish non-compliance.

**89. If the hospital has a high turnover rate and difficulty recruiting staff, which strategy is most likely to increase retention?**

a. Providing on-site childcare.
b. Providing career ladders.
c. Providing educational benefits.
d. Providing employee lounges.

**90. The hospital has begun developing a transitional care model for at-risk patients. The patients' care is generally coordinated by a(n):**

a. family physician.
b. team of healthcare providers.
c. trained family member.
d. advanced practice nurse.

**91. When estimating employment costs (salary plus benefits), benefits account for approximately what percentage of the total costs?**

a. 10%.
b. 20%.
c. 30%.
d. 40%.

**92. Which of the following is an example of a mass casualty event, as opposed to a mass effect event?**

a. Hurricane
b. Pandemic
c. Flood
d. Earthquake

**93. The four leadership styles (Hersey, 2008) associated with situational leadership are:**

a. telling, selling, participating, and delegating.
b. forming, norming, storming, and performing.
c. separating, conflicting, confronting, and asserting.
d. self-disclosure, trust, listening, and feedback.

**94. The hospital is considering hiring additional fulltime staff in order to reduce overtime costs. Which of the following types of analysis would use the average cost of overtime and the cost of hiring fulltime staff to demonstrate savings?**

a. Efficacy study.
b. Cost-effective analysis.
c. Cost-utility analysis.
d. Cost-benefit analysis.

**95. The first step in planning continuing education opportunities for staff members is to:**

a. survey staff preferences.
b. conduct a needs assessment.
c. define objectives.
d. select a pilot group.

96. Which of the following patient assessment instruments must inpatient rehabilitation facilities submit in order to receive reimbursement from Medicare and Medicaid?

    a. OASIS.
    b. MDS.
    c. IRF-PAI.
    d. IRF-OASIS.

97. If a nurse executive avoids hiring nurses in their mid-20s because of the belief that they will require family leave to have and/or care for children, what type of discrimination does this represent?

    a. Statistical discrimination.
    b. Illegal discrimination.
    c. Gender discrimination.
    d. Retaliation.

98. If the nurse executive wants to reassure staff members that internal whistleblowing will be dealt with anonymously and without repercussions, the best method(s) for reporting is:

    a. telephone.
    b. in person.
    c. written complaint.
    d. multiple methods.

99. When developing disaster preparedness plans, which of the following agencies provides the Disaster Technical Assistance Center (DTAC) to deal with behavioral health problems?

    a. OSHA
    b. CDC
    c. SAMHSA
    d. FEMA

100. If the hospital has a limited marketing budget but needs to attract more patients to services, the most effective approach is probably:

    a. alliance marketing.
    b. brand marketing.
    c. targeted marketing.
    d. above-the-line mass marking.

101. According to Kotter and Cohen's theory of change (2002), the first step in bringing about change is:

    a. creating a sense of urgency.
    b. building a team to guide change.
    c. removing barriers to change.
    d. communicating the need for change.

102. For performance appraisal, which method is likely to provide the most equitable measure?

    a. Forced ranking.
    b. Behavioral anchored rating scale.
    c. Graphic rating.
    d. Self-appraisal.

**103. For staffing purposes, a staff nurse who works 20 hours a week throughout the year would be considered:**

    a.  2.0 FTEs.

    b.  1.0 FTE.

    c.  0.5 FTE.

    d.  0.2 FTE.

**104. The affirmative action plan for the organization must:**

    a.  provide equal hiring opportunities for qualified individuals.

    b.  establish a quota system for hiring.

    c.  outline steps to retain minority staff members.

    d.  provide justification for current hiring practices.

**105. All of the following are types of bargaining that are utilized in the negotiation process EXCEPT:**

    a.  distributive.

    b.  integrative.

    c.  collaborative.

    d.  mixed.

**106. A hospital is located in a flood zone and water in a nearby river is rising, resulting in the activation of the Disaster Preparedness Plan. Which of the following elements of the plan is initially the most critical?**

    a.  Food supplies

    b.  Medication supplies

    c.  Evacuation plans

    d.  Staffing plans

**107. Under hospital 501(r) requirements for not-for-profit hospitals, hospitals must perform a community health needs assessment (CHNA) at least every:**

    a.  year.

    b.  2 years.

    c.  3 years.

    d.  5 years.

**108. Which of the following websites provides information and star ratings about the quality of hospitals, dentists, and doctors in the area for consumers and allows an "experience match" so that profiles can match the criteria used for searching?**

    a.  Hospital Compare.

    b.  HealthGrades.

    c.  RateMDs.

    d.  WebMD.

**109. What is the most important element of a disaster/emergency preparedness plan?**

    a.  Readily available information and practice drills.

    b.  Transfer protocols established.

    c.  Triage protocols for handling injuries.

    d.  Chain of command clearly outlined.

**110. When collecting clinical outcomes data, primary consideration should be given to:**

    a. patient population and mandated reporting requirements.

    b. costs of care and patient diagnoses.

    c. organization's mission and vision statements.

    d. length of stay and complications.

**111. Utilizing the worst-case scenario method of decision-making is most indicated for:**

    a. everyday decisions.

    b. financial decisions.

    c. decisions that pose risks.

    d. personnel decisions.

**112. According to Provision 1 of the ANA Code of Ethics, the nurse must respect the rights of the patient. When the patient's choices are risky or self-destructive, the nurse's best approach is to:**

    a. remain supportive but express concern.

    b. address the behavior and offer resources.

    c. say nothing out of respect for patient's rights.

    d. criticize the patient's behavior and point out problems.

**113. A physician at hospital A is able to access patient information from hospital B and another physician. The system that allows this exchange of information is a(n):**

    a. EHR.

    b. CDSS.

    c. CPOE.

    d. HIE.

**114. The primary protection included in the Patient's Bill of Rights under the Affordable Care Act is:**

    a. insurance coverage for pre-existing conditions.

    b. limits of deductibles insurance companies can charge.

    c. right to see a physician of choice.

    d. extending insurance coverage of dependents to age 21.

**115. To meet ORYX® quarterly reporting requirements for hospitals with a daily census greater than 10, how many chart-extracted electronic clinical quality measures (eCQMs) must the hospital report?**

    a. 5.

    b. 6.

    c. 9.

    d. 13.

**116. The four criteria used to classify accountability measures (formerly core measures) are:**

    a. readiness, education, complications, and interventions.

    b. evidence, intervention, results, complications.

    c. plan, do, study, act.

    d. research, proximity, accuracy, and adverse effects.

**117. A nurse executive who promotes pervasive leadership will:**

a. assume responsibility for all decision making.
b. encourage decision making by others.
c. constantly check up on subordinates.
d. create a hierarchical system with many layers.

**118. When evacuation of a facility is necessary because of storm damage, which of the following groups of patients should be dealt with first?**

a. ICU patients
b. Patients who can be discharged early
c. NICU and infant nursery patients
d. PACU patients

**119. A group of nurses on the staff have expressed interest in researching evidence-based practice but admit to having limited time to do so and ask the nurse executive for advice. The best suggestion is:**

a. forming a journal club.
b. telling staff members to make time.
c. using paid time off to research.
d. researching during slow times on duty.

**120. With appreciative inquiry, which principle suggests that people's actions are associated with what they believe?**

a. Principle of simultaneity.
b. Positive principle.
c. Constructionist principle.
d. Anticipatory principle.

**121. In an active shooter situation, the three things that staff members should be taught to do in order to survive are:**

a. run, hide, or fight.
b. barricade, hide, or fight.
c. confront, attack, or hide.
d. yell, run, or hide.

**122. The nurse executive plans to increase the focus on consumer education to improve patient outcomes and satisfaction. The "three Ps" of effective consumer education are:**

a. philosophy, priority, and performance.
b. physician, practitioner, and patient.
c. performance, permission, and persistence.
d. population, preparation, and provision.

**123. The key element in helping clinical staff institute evidence-based practice is:**

a. a mentor.
b. a reward system.
c. data/information.
d. coercion.

**124. According to Peplau's Interpersonal Relations Model of nursing, the nurse-patient relationship goes through overlapping phases that include orientation, problem identification, explanation of potential solutions, and:**

    a. problem evaluation.
    b. patient recovery.
    c. nurse-patient collaboration.
    d. problem resolution.

**125. The hospital is switching to a new integrated CPOE, CDSS and EHR, necessitating major changes in procedure and requiring much additional training of all staff. The initial method of implementation that is likely to be the least disruptive is:**

    a. small tests of change.
    b. pilot study.
    c. phased implementation.
    d. big bang implementation.

**126. A train derailment has resulted in an influx of patients who have been exposed to toxic chemicals; however the type of toxin has not yet been identified. According to OSHA, the minimum PPE that the receiving personnel should utilize includes:**

    a. gloves, gown, and a mask.
    b. chemical resistant suit, double-layer gloves, and an N95 mask.
    c. gloves, chemical resistant suit and boots, and an N95 mask.
    d. double-layered gloves, chemical resistant suit and boots, and a PAPR.

**127. The leader of a patient-centered medical home (PCMH) is generally a:**

    a. personal physician.
    b. nurse practitioner.
    c. case manager.
    d. therapist.

**128. When conferring with a unit supervisor, the nurse executive notes that the supervisor frequently licks her lips and constantly rubs her hands together. Based on this body language, the nurse executive may assume that the supervisor is:**

    a. angry.
    b. nervous.
    c. depressed.
    d. distracted.

**129. If developing a chart to display data about the age distribution of patients admitted to the oncology department over a one-month period, a useful type of graphic display is:**

    a. pie chart.
    b. digital dashboard.
    c. scattergram.
    d. balanced scorecard.

**130. When considering improvements to workflow processes, the first issue to address is whether steps in a process:**

    a. can be combined.

    b. should be increased.

    c. require alternate paths.

    d. can be eliminated.

**131. If a priest comes to a hospital and asks for information about Catholic patients, what information can be provided?**

    a. General condition, room number, and religious affiliation

    b. Name, diagnosis, and age

    c. Name, diagnosis, and religious affiliation

    d. Name, age, and general condition

**132. If a unit supervisor meets with the nurse executive and states, "I see, as usual, you have determined the best solution to the problem," the communication style the supervisor is using is:**

    a. aggressive.

    b. persuasive.

    c. assertive.

    d. passive-aggressive.

**133. Patients assigned to an accountable care organization (ACO) through Medicare:**

    a. must see specific physicians as directed rather than physicians of choice.

    b. will have some health information shared among different ACO providers.

    c. may have Medicare benefits changed after assignment to the ACO.

    d. can also be part of an HMO while participating in the ACO.

**134. A socioeconomic indicator that suggests a red flag for further screening for case management includes:**

    a. admission from sheltered living facility.

    b. residence in low-income urban area.

    c. divorced woman with adult children.

    d. inability to drive.

**135. A nurse executive who is able to understand the feelings of others and to understand why they have specific needs or desires is exhibiting which element of emotional intelligence?**

    a. Self-awareness.

    b. Motivation.

    c. Empathy.

    d. Social skills.

**136. The nurse executive listens to a staff member saying that he is concerned that a number of other staff members were laid off when a unit closed and responds, "You're worried about losing your job." The nurse executive is practicing:**

    a. paraphrasing.
    b. exploring.
    c. summarizing.
    d. reflecting.

**137. If the Board of Directors has asked the nurse executive to include subordinate evaluations as part of the annual performance review, the nurse executive should:**

    a. suggest that evaluations be anonymous.
    b. advise the Board that subordinate evaluations may be biased.
    c. request that subordinates sign the reviews.
    d. personally select subordinate evaluators.

**138. Actively listening to a subordinate's suggestions by making eye contact, nodding the head, and asking questions implies that the nurse executive:**

    a. will follow speaker's suggestions.
    b. agrees with the speaker's suggestions.
    c. shows respect for the speaker's suggestions.
    d. is simply placating the speaker.

**139. Which of the following is an example of using a normative re-educative strategy to facilitate and manage change?**

    a. The nurse executive provides facts and figures gleaned from research to support change.
    b. The nurse executive encourages the team to identify problems and solutions.
    c. The nurse executive uses authority to demand that staff make changes.
    d. The nurse executive utilizes a method of rewards and punishment to promote change.

**140. The nurse executive is utilizing the STAR model to facilitate systems change. According to this model, a change in one area usually:**

    a. is unsuccessful.
    b. results in unsuspected outcomes.
    c. promotes acceptance of change.
    d. necessitates change in another.

**141. When the nurse executive plans to initiate a change in processes or procedures, which is the most important factor to communicate to staff?**

    a. Reason.
    b. Cost effectiveness.
    c. Timeframe.
    d. Learning curve.

**142. The nurse executive is considering a suggestion to institute a telehealth program for a patient population primarily covered by original Medicare. The first issue to consider is:**

    a. cost of the program.
    b. need for staff and training.
    c. geographic location of target population.
    d. impact on inpatient services.

**143. Nurse-led clinics are generally part of:**

   a. accountable care organization.
   b. outpatient services.
   c. inpatient services.
   d. a patient-centered medical home.

**144. The nurse executive notes an increase in falls in an extended care facility. Which of the following interventions is likely to have the most positive impact on fall reduction?**

   a. Staff penalties
   b. Motion detector alarms
   c. Siderail use
   d. Hourly rounding

**145. Which of the following services are covered for eligible patients by Medicare and may be provided by home health agencies?**

   a. Speech language pathology services.
   b. 24-hour-a-day in-home care.
   c. Homemaker services.
   d. Meal services (preparation/delivered).

**146. Predictive analytics have identified a number of patients who are at risk for readmission because of previous failures to follow discharge treatment plans. The most effective intervention is to:**

   a. advise patients of risks.
   b. assign a case manager to patients.
   c. increase the length of stay.
   d. engage family members in patients' care.

**147. As part of an emergency response plan, continuity planning is necessary to ensure that:**

   a. incoming staff are able to take over for current staff without interruptions in care.
   b. critical functions (patient care, support services) are maintained during an emergent situation.
   c. patients in need of transport or more advanced care are managed appropriately.
   d. receiving facilities that can accept patients are identified when necessary.

**148. A reporter from the local newspaper has made an appointment to interview the nurse executive about the hospital's quality initiatives. In preparation, the first action the nurse executive should undertake is to:**

   a. prepare notes.
   b. write a formal statement.
   c. consult the public relations person.
   d. consult the Board of Directors.

**149. The purpose of an implantable loop recorder (IRL) is to:**

   a. monitor blood glucose levels.
   b. facilitate hearing.
   c. monitor heart rate and rhythm.
   d. pace the heartbeat.

**150. A patient with cancer experienced a sudden deterioration of health and is near the end of life, but she is unable to express wishes about care. The doctor advises stopping all curative treatment, and family members are in disagreement. The decision should be based on:**

    a.   the opinion of the next of kin.

    b.   family consensus.

    c.   physician's advice.,

    d.   patient's advance directive.

# Answer Key and Explanations for Test #1

**1. A**: Communication skills are required to develop professional relationships. Assertive communication incorporates sincerity, timing, gestures, and content. Fogging is a communication technique that allows a manager to remain sincere by agreeing in principle without becoming defensive. This passive skill allows the manager to maintain control over the direction of the conversation and discourages the critic from becoming more assertive. As with all communication skills, to be successful, this technique must be selected for the appropriate situation and would not be indicated with aggressive criticism.

**2. C**: The Cybernetic Model may be used by nurse executives who wish to implement programs that require evaluation. The Cybernetic Model includes three phases: Needs Assessment, Program Implementation, and Results Assessment. In phase 3, program objectives, cost, and impact are evaluated. The Collegial Model involves the collaboration and consensus of a group of peers and is often used in educational settings where professions share similar values and benefit from individual expertise. The Collegial Model approach to decision-making is suited for small-size groups. The Bureaucratic Model is used within a hierarchical organization, such as health care organizations, where operational policies and procedures are used to make decisions. While efficient implementation is gained with this model, creativity and process improvement may be diminished as a result of adherence to governing operations. The Garbage Can Model is based on accidental decision-making where changes may be implemented without a clear plan or actual problem identification.

**3. D**: Although the interviewer should be in control during the interview process, certain questions are not acceptable. To ask if an interviewee has children or is planning to have children may result in legal proceedings. If the rationale is to assess availability, inquiring about the number of hours the interviewee is available each week is prudent. Questions directly relating to nationality, native language, age, gender, race, disability, place of birth, and marital or family status are discriminatory. The interviewer's goal should be to choose the best candidate for the position in the presence of nondiscriminatory policies. Questions should relate to the position being offered and not to personal information.

**4. B**: Defamation of character is a type of intentional tort and refers to the communication of ideas that result in a negative image. The two types of defamation of character are slander and libel. Slander refers to spoken words as compared to libel, which refers to written words. Importantly, it is not always necessary that slander or libel be false information. In the scenario described in the question, even if the patient had a diagnosis of borderline personality disorder, when staff documented that the patient was "a borderline," it was not intended to benefit the patient and may, in fact, have reduced the patient's chances of receiving adequate treatment. Nurses must remember to identify correctly the purpose of documentation. Nursing documentation must not hinder treatment or cause damage to the patient.

**5. B**: All 50 states allow minors to consent to sexually transmitted disease testing and treatment except for HIV. Currently 27 states and the District of Columbia have passed laws allowing minors to consent to contraceptive services. State laws vary widely regarding the ability of a minor to provide informed consent for HIV testing and treatment. Very few states (currently only 2 and the District of Columbia) allow minors to consent to abortion. It is particularly important to remember that informed consent for a procedure or treatment for any minor or adult may not be provided by

169

a registered nurse. Only the primary provider, such as a physician or nurse practitioner, may provide the information required for informed consent.

**6. D**: Paternalistic actions and attitudes diminish the patient's autonomy. Paternalism relates to using one's own judgment to make decisions for another without considering their ideas. In this context, the principles of autonomy and beneficence are in conflict and create an ethical challenge. While respect for the autonomy of the patient should be observed, nurses and other health care providers must implement sound judgment under the principle of beneficence. To meet this challenge, nurses must recognize the importance of personal choice and equality in a professional nurse–patient relationship.

**7. D**: The framework of how nursing care is delivered in an organization is called a nursing care delivery model. There are four classic models; total patient care, functional nursing, team nursing, and primary nursing. In the total patient care model, a patient receives complete care by one nurse for an entire shift. In a functional nursing model, tasks are divided for groups of patients. The registered nurse (RN) performs advanced nursing functions for a group of patients, and other tasks, such as personal care and vital signs, may be assigned to ancillary staff members. In team nursing, an RN team leader manages care for a small group of patients by planning and delegating tasks to team members. Primary nursing is different from the total patient care model in that the RN holds 24-hour responsibility for the communication and direction of each patient's care, although some patient care may be delegated to support staff.

**8. B**: Nurse executives play a key role in the development of effective patient classification systems (PCS). A PCS is used to measure the level and amount of care or the acuity level for specific populations of patients. Examples include medical, pediatric, ambulatory, and psychiatric classification systems. One of the main goals in the development of a PCS is ensuring the delivery of safe care by providing appropriate staffing levels with competent personnel to care for patients from a specific population. Other goals include maintaining customer and staff satisfaction while adhering to financial resources.

**9. A**: In 1983, the Social Security Act was amended to include a prospective payment system for Medicare beneficiaries. Diagnosis-related groups (DRGs) were originally designed as part of a classification system used by Medicare to determine reimbursement at a fixed-fee. DRGs are based on several factors, including the International Classification of Disease (ICD-10) diagnoses, procedures, age, and the presence of comorbidities. Since the amendment, health care has evolved, leading to specialized types of DRGs, such as All Patient DRGs and Refined DRGs.

**10. C**: Medical waste is primarily regulated by state environmental and health departments. While the Environmental Protection Agency (EPA) used to have the authority to regulate medical waste, that authority was relinquished in 1991 when the Medical Waste Tracking Act of 1988 expired. Because medical waste disposal programs are regulated at the state level, laws vary depending on the state.

**11. A**: The Patient Self-Determination Act (PSDA), a federal statute, was an amendment to the Omnibus Budget Reconciliation Act of 1990. The PSDA requires federally funded health care facilities, such as hospitals, hospice providers, and nursing homes, to provide information in writing regarding advanced health care directives on admission. The purpose of the PSDA is to ensure that patients are aware of their right to make treatment decisions and that these decisions are communicated to their health care provider. On admission, patients must be asked if they have a living will or a durable power of attorney, and responses should be documented in the patient's medical record.

**12. B**: A SWOT analysis would most likely be used in strategic planning. SWOT analyses focus on the objective assessment of four main attributes: strengths, weaknesses, opportunities, and threats; these analyses are useful in developing strategic responses to opportunities and challenges. A VPEC-T analysis is often used to analyze expectations of involved parties without losing information in the transition from business needs to information technology development. The MoSCow analysis is also a business technique used in software development. The PC analysis, or principal component analysis, is a statistical tool used for multivariate analyses.

**13. D**: The zero-based budgeting method requires that all expenditures be justified for each new period (starting at a zero base). This budget method is time-consuming but provides more accurate and current results. Incremental budgeting is based on the previous budget and incorporates adjustments for additional planned increases, such as inflation and salary raises. Priority-based budgeting involves the development of a prioritization plan when determining the allocation of resources. The activity-based budgeting method focuses on creating a budget based on costs of key activities and their relationship to strategic goals.

**14. A**: A capital budget is developed to purchase long-term assets, such as equipment, computer hardware, and building facilities. It may require several years to pay off these assets. Multiyear assets such as the ones above are called capital assets. The operational budget represents the total value of all resources and expenses of a department or organization. Additional budgets, such as a labor budget, are subcategories of the operational budget.

**15. D**: There are several types of benchmarking, including generic, global, performance, and functional benchmarking. Additionally, benchmarking may occur at different levels, such as the best in an industry, internal or competitive. For example, internal benchmarking may occur in a hospital where each department's check out services are compared and evaluated to determine the best internal practices. These best practices are then implemented across all hospital departments.

**16. C**: When registered nurses (RNs) delegate tasks, they remain accountable for the overall care of the patient. Therefore, RNs must be aware of the qualifications of assistive personnel to delegate tasks appropriately. The American Nurses Association (ANA) provides guidelines and principles on delegation in the document "ANA Principles for Delegation." In addition to the ANA guidelines, delegation is addressed specifically by each state nursing practice act. Interventions may be delegated unless they require professional nursing judgment, knowledge, and skill to be completed. For example, the administration of oral medication for a stable patient may be delegated, but an initial nursing assessment may not be delegated.

**17. A**: Federal standards of the Occupational Safety and Health Administration (OSHA) require that new employees with the potential to be exposed to blood-borne pathogens be offered the hepatitis B three-injection series vaccination within 10 days of employment. New employees have the right to decline the vaccination, which should be documented in the employee's health file. A Hepatitis B Vaccine Declination is mandatory per OSHA standard 1910.1030 App A. OSHA does not require employees working in a health care environment to have an annual tuberculosis (TB) test; the Centers for Disease Control provides guidelines regarding TB testing, which have been adapted by many state regulations. Regarding post-exposure evaluation and treatment of a needle stick, OSHA standards require that the employer offer evaluation at no cost; however, an employee may decline. All post-exposure treatment, accepted or declined, should be documented in the employee's health file. OSHA standards do not require employees to have a titer following hepatitis B three-injection series vaccination. OSHA reports that the annual amount of hepatitis B infections in healthcare providers is anywhere from 12,000 to 18,000, and of those infected, approximately 200 to 300 will die from that hepatitis B infection.

**18. D**: The Nurse Reinvestment Act was passed in 2002 with the support of the American Nurses Association. The Act addresses the nursing shortage by authorizing several provisions, including loan repayment programs, long-term care training grants, and public service announcements to encourage people to enter the nursing profession. The Model Nursing Practice Act, developed by the National Council of State Boards of Nursing, was designed to provide guidelines for State Nurse Practice Acts. America's Partnership for Nursing Education Act of 2009 is currently a bill requesting an amendment to the Public Health Service Act. This amendment would make grants available to states with increasing population growth and a projected nursing shortage. The grants would be used to increase nursing faculty in those states. The National Nurse Act is another bill that was introduced in the House of Representatives on February 4, 2010. The bill is an amendment to establish the Office of the National Nurse with the same rank and grade as the Deputy Surgeon General of the Public Health Services. Duties of the National Nurse would include, but are not limited to, guidance and leadership in encouraging nurses to become nurse educators and increasing public safety and emergency preparedness.

**19. A**: Health care providers may share protected information to prevent or decrease an imminent threat to the public. The Health Insurance Portability and Accountability Act (HIPAA) privacy rules permit covered entities to impose reasonable fees for copying and mailing requested medical records. However, the fee may not include costs for searching or retrieving the requested information. HIPAA privacy rules do not require covered entities to retain tape-recorded information, following transcription of medical information. HIPAA rules permit temporary restrictions on individual access to medical information if involved in a clinical trial, providing the participant agreed during initial consent. However, the researcher must inform the participant that access will be reinstated following the clinical trial.

**20. A**: Meta-analysis is a statistical procedure to integrate the results of several studies on a particular topic. Advantages of meta-analysis include the ability to identify patterns across studies, detecting relationships that may not be identifiable in a single study and greater statistical power. Survey research involves the use of questionnaires or interviews to gather information. Market research, opinion polls, and the census are types of surveys. Surveys are generally less expensive than other types of research, and data collection through the internet has increased access to larger groups of specific populations. Needs assessment research focuses on collecting information to determine the needs for a specific group or organization.

**21. D**: Institutional Review Boards (IRBs) are regulated by the Food and Drug Administration and the Department of Health and Human Services. IRBs are required for all institutions performing research that receive federal funding. The main purpose of an IRB is to protect the rights of research participants. The Code of Federal Regulations contains specific laws regarding IRB membership. No IRB may consist entirely of members of one profession, and each IRB should contain at least one member not affiliated with the institution. Additionally, IRBs should contain at least one member whose primary concerns are in scientific areas and one member whose primary concerns are in nonscientific areas. While an IRB may invite special experts to assist in the review of complex issues, those individuals may not vote with the IRB.

**22. C**: Federal and state laws regarding the archiving of clinical data may vary, and both may apply. The HIPAA Privacy Rule requires securely maintaining clinical records for:

- Living adults: 6 years
- Post-mortem: 2 years
- Infants born in the facility: until child is 18
- Mammography records: 10 years or until a subsequent mammography taken

172

If no regulations exist for other types of clinical records, then 7 years of storage is usually sufficient. The method of record destruction must be recorded.

**23. D**: An effective change agent will recognize the importance of sharing goals with staff. Effective change strategies include encouraging involvement by all individuals who will be affected by change and supporting open communication. Additional change strategies include providing education or training if needed to reduce fear and prepare staff to move forward.

**24. D**: Effectively managed conflict can be beneficial for an organization. Conflict behavior styles include avoidance, accommodation, force, compromise, and collaboration. An awareness of these styles during periods of conflict is useful in determining communication techniques to manage conflict effectively. The avoidance style is nonconfrontational but does not often lead to conflict resolution or goal achievement. When the force style is used, it is considered a win/lose situation, with the opposing goals or values being disregarded. Persons using the accommodating style are nonassertive and cooperative at the expense of their own goals to satisfy others. The collaboration style includes an element of mutual respect where both conflict parties attempt to reach solutions that will retain the goals of both parties. Giving up some aspects of goals through assertive and cooperative behavior is a compromising style. A compromising style results in the partial satisfaction of both parties.

**25. C**: The Fair Labor Standards Act (FLSA) is a federal law administered by the Department of Labor. The FLSA establishes laws, such as child labor standards, overtime pay, and minimum wage. Employees are classified by the duties and responsibilities associated with their position. Although there are grey areas, nonexempt employees generally hold routine work, are paid hourly, and are entitled to receiving overtime. Exempt employees are exempt from receiving overtime pay and are known as salaried employees. The FLSA does not require payment for time not worked, including vacations or sick time. Additionally, the FLSA does not require breaks or meal periods to be provided to employees. However, employers must also adhere to additional state labor laws, which may be more detailed regarding breaks and vary from state to state. Some states such as Kentucky, Colorado, and Nevada require a 10-minute break for every 4 hours worked. Florida has no state law regulating rest periods for adult workers.

**26. A**: The Sentinel Event Policy has four main goals; to improve patient care, reduce the number of sentinel events, increase knowledge regarding sentinel events, and to uphold public confidence in accredited organizations. Although accredited hospitals must define sentinel events within their organization, hospitals are not required to report sentinel events to the Joint Commission. However, if the Joint Commission becomes aware of a reviewable sentinel event through voluntary self-reporting or otherwise, the organization is expected to conduct a root-cause analysis and action plan within 45 days of becoming aware of the sentinel event.

**27. D**: The Joint Commission Sentinel Event Policy defines both reviewable and non-reviewable sentinel events. Reviewable sentinel events are events that have resulted in unanticipated death or permanent loss of function to patients or residents. Reviewable sentinel events are subject to review by the Joint Commission. Non-reviewable sentinel events include "near miss" incidents, events that have not affected a recipient of care, and deaths or loss of function following an "against medical advice" discharge. For more information on the Joint Commission and the Sentinel Event Policy visit www.jointcommission.org.

**28. A**: The Joint Commission's official "Do Not Use" List identifies the documentation of trailing zeros (1.0) or lack of a leading zero (.1 mg) to be a potential problem. A missed decimal point may lead to an incorrect interpretation. For example, 1.0 mg may appear as 10 mg if the decimal point was not identified in a physician's order. Similarly, .1 mg may appear as 1 mg since it is lacking a leading zero. There is an exception for trailing zeros when reporting necessary increased levels of precision. Laboratory values, imaging studies, and lesion measurements may require trailing zeros for increased precision reporting. Trailing zeros may not be used in medication orders.

**29. D**: The Joint Commission defines malpractice as improper or unethical conduct or unreasonable lack of skill by a holder of a professional or official position and defines negligence as the failure to use such care as a reasonably prudent and careful person would use under similar circumstances. Several elements must be proven to hold a nurse liable for malpractice. Proof of a causal relationship must be established between the patient's injury and the nurse's failure to adhere to standards of care. However, the relationship must only demonstrate substantial cause, rather than a direct cause.

**30. D**: The Privacy Rule was issued in 2003 by the U.S. Department of Health and Human Services (DHHS) following the Health Insurance Portability and Accountability Act of 1996. The privacy rule has several effects on clinical research. Personal Health Information (PHI) must be protected during the disclosure of research. A Privacy Rule Authorization must adhere to section 164.508 as outlined in the privacy rule. Core elements of the Privacy Rule Authorization include a description of the protected health information (PHI) to be disclosed, the purpose of the disclosure, an expiration date or notice of no expiration, and a dated signature. In contrast, a signed informed consent is not used for the authorization for the disclosure of PHI. An informed consent is required by the DHHS and the Food and Drug Administration Protection of Human Subjects Regulations to consent to participate in the research. De-identification of PHI and waivers through an Institutional Review Board or Privacy Board are other possible methods of disclosing certain PHI.

**31. B**: The de-identifying of information is one method that allows the disclosure of protected health information (PHI) under the Health Insurance Portability and Accountability Act privacy rule for research purposes. There are 18 descriptive elements that must be removed before disclosure to prevent the identification of an individual. Names, geographic subdivisions smaller than a state, element of dates, and any unique identifying numbers, including an electronic mail address and internet protocol address number are a few of the 18 elements that must be removed during the de-identification of PHI.

**32. A**: To assist team leaders in accomplishing goals, it is important to understand group dynamics in organizational development. Tuckman's stages initially comprised a four-stage model and later expanded to include a final adjourning stage. In the first stage, called the forming stage, the group forms and initial communication begins. The group leader focuses on communicating the goals of the group. During the second stage, storming, team members may challenge authority and compete for roles. The group leader should facilitate open professional communication, support all members and continue to communicate goals. In the norming stage, hierarchy has been established, and the team begins to focus on the goals. The group leader promotes a cohesive team atmosphere. In the performing stage, members are working collaboratively toward goals. The final adjourning stage concludes a decision-making group.

**33. B**: Legitimate power is based upon the leader's position of authority in the organization. Referent power is created when the follower identifies positively with characteristics and qualities of the leader. Expert power is created when followers believe the leader has expert knowledge and competence. Coercive power is based on threat of punishment. Both expert and referent types of power indicate positive attitudes of followers toward their leaders, which enhances respect and commitment rather than simple compliance.

**34. D**: Lateral violence or horizontal violence between nurses is not uncommon and is often directed toward new nurses. Forms of lateral violence include sabotage, withholding information (as noted in the scenario described in the question), and nonverbal gestures, such as face-making. Managing lateral violence in the health care setting is challenging as this type of violence is frequently covert and met with denial during confrontation. Proactive education and policies regarding zero-tolerance to violence in the workplace can reduce unprofessional behavior. The Joint Commission issued a Sentinel Event Alert in 2008 on behaviors that undermine a culture of safety. The alert includes recommendations for reducing intimidating and disruptive behavior.

**35. B**: State and local laws require health care providers and laboratories to report specific infectious diseases to the state or public health authority. The state health department then compiles the data and reports nationally notifiable infectious diseases to the Centers for Disease Control (CDC) through the National Notifiable Diseases Surveillance System (NNDSS). The list of nationally notifiable infectious diseases is revised as necessary and is available for review on the CDC website. Morbidity and mortality weekly reports are generated from the data. Listeriosis is an infection caused by the bacteria *Listeria monocytogenes* and has been nationally reportable since 2000. In addition to national reporting, all persons with listeriosis should be interviewed by a health care provider, using the standard CDC *Listeria* case form. Although relatively rare, cases of listeriosis have risen since 2002. There are several methods of transmission, the most common of which is through ingestion of contaminated food, such as undercooked meat or contaminated vegetables, seafood, and dairy products. Direct contact may cause skin lesions. Flu-like symptoms, such as fever and muscle aches, are common with listeriosis infections. However, *Listeria* can infect the brain or spinal cord and may be transferred to a fetus in utero or during birth.

**36. C**: The mission of the Office of Inspector General (OIG) as mandated by public law includes protecting programs of the Department of Health and Human Services. The OIG, the Federal Bureau of Investigation, and the Department of Justice are federal agencies that collaborate with state agencies to detect and prevent fraud. Medicare and Medicaid fraud may be reported directly to the OIG for investigation. Examples of Medicare fraud include submitting false claims, door-to-door solicitation of beneficiaries, payment for referrals by Medicare providers, and misrepresentation of Medicare private plans.

**37. A**: In 1998, the American Nurses Association (ANA) developed the Utilization Guide to the Principles on Safe Staffing. Nine principles for safe staffing are identified within three categories; patient care unit–related staffing, staff-related staffing, and institution/organization–related staffing. Patient care unit–related staffing principles identify critical factors for consideration when determining a staffing plan, which include the number of patients, the level of experience and education of staff, and contextual issues, such as available technology. The guide questions the use of nursing hours per patient days (NHPPDs) in the development of staffing plans. NHPPDs do not reflect the variability of factors necessary to predict the requirements for every possible type of patient care setting. Averaging hours of care for each patient as opposed to measuring the intensity of care required is not appropriate in nursing practice.

**38. B**: Centralized decision-making occurs when the span of authority and the control of key business elements are retained by top-level management, for instance, the nurse manager approves all new hires through the nurse executive. Decision-making is not disbursed. Two advantages of centralization are the ability to make rapid decisions and consistency in communication. Obvious disadvantages are the possibilities of being managed by a dictator and the loss of employee creativity and knowledge.

**39. D**: During verbal communication, it is important to actively listen and understand possible cognitive distortions to identify pertinent facts and avoid misunderstandings and conflict. In the scenario described in the question, the nurse executive should recognize that the nurse manager is using all-or-nothing thinking. All-or-nothing, or black and white thinking, is often noted in perfectionists who are unable to meet unreasonable demands. The nurse manager sees herself as a failure because of her inability to complete the task. It would be prudent for the nurse executive to investigate the staff budgeting rather than focus on the manager's competence.

**40. D**: Published in 1978, the Ethical Principles and Guidelines for the Protection of Human Subjects of Research became known as the Belmont Report. The guidelines identify three ethical principles regarding the use of human subjects in research; respect, beneficence, and justice. These ethical principles are applied directly to research and pertain to informed, voluntary participation and protection of human subjects. Although the Belmont Report does not make specific recommendations or define regulations for human subjects of research, federal regulations under the HHS are based on these guidelines.

**41. C**: The Equal Employment Opportunity commission (EEOC) enforces federal laws against discrimination as a result of race, color, religion, sex, national origin, age, disability, and genetics. It is illegal to base wages or benefits on the discriminatory factors listed. Reducing benefits for older workers (if the reduction is equal to the cost of benefits for younger workers), may be legal in certain situations. It is important to note that discrimination based on sex also includes pregnant women, and discrimination based on age mainly focuses on persons over 40 years of age.

**42. A**: Healthy People 2030 (HP2030) is a health promotion and disease prevention program initiated in 2010 by the United States Department of Health and Human Services. HP2030 consists of 62 categories and hundreds of health objectives. National data from 190 data sources have been gathered over the last 10 years to measure the outcomes for the objectives. Collected data are based on a list of leading health indicators, which include physical activity, obesity, tobacco use, and access to health care, among others. Progress reviews analyze the data based on the 62 focus areas.

**43. B**: Employers' Liability Insurance protects employers against lawsuits of negligence or failure to provide safe working conditions. Many Workers' Compensation policies include a separate section for Employer's Liability coverage. Most states have laws requiring both types of insurance. Employers' Liability coverage does not protect against litigation related to discrimination. Public Liability Insurance provides insurance against third-party injuries.

**44. B**: Generally, PHI shared during a telephone call is not subject to the HIPAA Security rule unless it is already stored in electronic form. Once it is stored, it then becomes subject to the rule. The Privacy Rule, however, applies to all sharing of information, so PHI can only be shared for allowed communications, such as for communications regarding healthcare operations and treatment. Smart phones or other devices that contain confidential patient information should contain locking and tracking software. This ensures the device can be located and that data cannot be accessed if the device is misplaced.

**45. D**: Under section 5001(c) of the Deficit Reduction Act, the Centers for Medicare and Medicaid no longer cover certain illnesses acquired during hospitalization. The list of illnesses no longer covered includes pressure ulcers stages III and IV, certain infections following surgery, vascular and urinary catheter infections, air emboli, administration of incompatible blood, and foreign objects unintentionally retained after surgery.

**46. D**: An Exposure Control Plan (ECP) should include several elements: determination of employee exposure, implementation of methods of exposure control, hepatitis B vaccination documentation, post-exposure evaluation, employee training, recordkeeping, and procedures to evaluate exposure events. Lists of hazardous chemicals and safety data sheets are also requirements of the Occupational Safety and Health Administration within the Hazardous Communication Program. Templates for an ECP and a Hazardous Communication Program are available for review at: https://www.osha.gov/Publications/osha3186.pdf

**47. D**: A failure mode and effects analysis (FMEA) is a method used to identify potential failure modes or processes. Possible effects of those failures are analyzed and action recommendations are formulated. Benefits of regularly performing a FMEA include identifying change requirements, preventing negative occurrences, and improving patient care through prevention planning. A root-cause analysis is reactive to adverse occurrences and is performed following an event to investigate root causes.

**48. A**: The Pareto principle, also known as the 80/20 rule was initially created by Italian economist Vilfredo Pareto. The principle was based on a mathematical formula that was developed to analyze the unequal distribution of wealth in early 1900 Italy. In 1941, Dr. J. Juran, a quality-management consultant identified that Pareto's formula could be applied to other areas beyond economics, namely quality. The Pareto principal quickly became a useful analysis tool in many disciplines. Because of the 80/20 rule, the Pareto chart is useful in focusing and prioritizing significant factors or causes.

**49. D**: Gantt charts are linear bar charts used to display a project schedule. They are effective for small projects with up to 30 activities. While Gantt charts focus on schedule management and time, PERT flow charts focus on the relationship between activities and are often used for large complex projects because they can display connecting dependent networks of activities better than Gantt charts.

**50. D**: The National Committee for Quality Assurance (NCQA) is a non-profit organization that promotes quality in health care. NCQA offers several accrediting programs for health plans, managed behavioral health care organizations, medical groups, and physicians. A multicultural health care distinction is available through NCQA. The distinction is available for organizations that meet evidence-based criteria for cultural competency.

**51. B**: Tobacco use is a leading health indicator for Healthy People 2030 (HP2030). HP2030 reports that cigarette smoking is the most preventable cause of disease and death in the United States, and that more than 16 million adults have disease secondary to smoking. HP2030 objectives regarding tobacco use include reducing cigarette smoking by adults and adolescents and increasing resources to help individuals quit smoking. The Centers for Disease Control report that cigarette smoking causes 1 of every 5 deaths in the United States each year.

**52. A**: With the professional practice model of differentiated nursing practice, responsibilities for patient care differentiate according to level of education and/or clinical expertise. In this model, the hierarchy of responsibility begins with the APN, then to the BSN, to the AS RN, the LPN/LVN, and the UAP. Differentiated nursing practice is in common use, although a shortage of advanced practiced and BSN nurses means that in, some cases, nurses with less education, such as AS RNs, are in positions of authority. Differentiated nursing practice takes advantages of differences in training among nursing personnel.

**53. C**: Under the HIPAA Privacy Rule, a person's right to privacy extends 50 years following death. The HIPAA Privacy Rule allows a covered entity to make disclosures regarding a decedent's PHI without authorization in 2 circumstances:

- The disclosure is to a healthcare provider who is treating a surviving family member, and the information is necessary for treatment purposes.
- The disclosure is to a decedent's legal representative, executor, or a person legally authorized to act on behalf of the estate, and the PHI is relevant.

**54. B**: Corporate compliance requires adherence to state and federal regulations and legal and ethical standards. Corporate compliance guidance is provided by the Officer of Inspector General of HHS. A compliance officer should review all compliance issues and ensure that the organization is in compliance and meets all regulatory requirements for reporting. Compliance issues may include privacy and security concerns, accountability standards, regulatory requirements, record retention, employer screening/employment standards, risk assessment, communication of requirements, and third-party due diligence.

**55. D**: HIPAA has a list of reasons for which a covered entity is allowed to call a patient, and the assessment of a patient regarding new health issues is not on that list. The acceptable reasons are limited to administrative issues, such as appointments and reminders, lab test results, and post-discharge follow-up. It is generally accepted that if a patient provides a covered entity with a telephone number, the patient consents to be contacted at that number. Messages should only be left with family members or on voicemail with the consent of the patient.

**56. A**: The Consumer Credit Protect Act (Title III) prohibits employers from discharging employees because of wage garnishment and also, in most instances, caps garnishment at 25% of the employee's salary or the amount the wages exceed 30 times the Federal minimum hourly wage. The purpose of the law is to allow those with debts to continue to work while paying off the debts rather than to be punished and left with no means to repay the amounts owed.

**57. C**: If an evidence-based intervention has been implemented but outcome measures show that the results are not on par with those experienced by other organizations, the most likely reasons is lack of treatment fidelity. That is, staff members are inconsistent in applying the intervention exactly as required. This may be because staff members lack sufficient training on the intervention or they are resistive and purposely modify the intervention or use previous methods.

**58. B**: If a unit supervisor comes to the nurse executive and discusses a problem the supervisor is trying to solve, the nurse executive should listen without offering advice unless the supervisor specifically asks for the advice. The nurse executive may, if appropriate, ask clarification questions but should avoid asking "why" questions, such as "Why did you do that?" In many cases, people only want to vent about problems or to get a response regarding potential solutions.

**59. A**: If a full-time employee who has met eligibility requirements requests unpaid medical leave under the Family Medical Leave Act, the employer may request a medical certificate to prove that the leave is medically necessary. Employees in eligible companies (companies with more than 50 employees) can take unpaid, job-protected leave for up to 12 weeks in a one-year period for:

- Childbirth/Adoption.
- Child bonding.
- Care for spouse, child, or parent with severe illness.
- Personal health condition.
- Qualifying circumstances for military spouse.

**60. D**: The key to leveraging diversity in the workplace is communication. The more diversity present, the more communication is needed. Communication must be both horizontal and vertical and should include open and frank discussions about ideas and values as well as approaches to care. It's important to provide sensitivity training to help staff members learn to communicate better and to understand that each individual offers different strengths and abilities that are essential to the organization.

**61. B**: If an organizational goal is to decrease the rate of postoperative infections, the method of communication of results that is likely the most effective in encouraging ongoing efforts is dashboard updates. The dashboard is an easy to read and access computer program that provides a number of different performance measures, such as rates of infection, usually in a visual presentation with graphs or charts. The dashboard should be updated on a regular basis, such as weekly or monthly.

**62. C**: Increasing costs are likely to be most disruptive of healthcare quality because of the costs involved in making significant changes or remaining current (such as through purchase of new equipment) and the trend toward decreased reimbursement and value-based reimbursement. For example, an increased nurse-to-patient ratio directly correlates with better patient outcomes but is one of the most expensive approaches to patient care. Hospitals are increasingly contracting for services, and this can negatively impact continuity of care and commitment to quality.

**63. D**: Before facilitating change in a healthcare organization, it's especially important to have an understanding of the organizational culture, which comprises attitudes, beliefs, behaviors, and shared assumptions. Different basic types of organizational cultures include:

- Stable learning cultures where people exercise skills and advance over time.
- Independent cultures in which people have valued skills that are easily transferable to other organizations.
- Group cultures in which there is strong identification and emphasis on seniority.
- Insecure cultures with frequent staff layoffs and reorganization.

**64. B**: The most effective method of establishing a professional network is to become active in professional organizations, including those at the local, state, and national levels. Becoming active involves not only attending conferences, but also actively participating, such as by giving conference presentations and serving on committees. The nurse should maintain contact with other professionals though social media or other means and should focus on areas of particular interest, making an effort to keep up-to-date and knowledgeable.

**65. D:** Patient authentication procedures are necessary to prevent unauthorized disclosure/access to PHI. Identification should be verified at first contact with a photo ID or photograph taken during the visit, and copies of the ID/photo should be securely stored for future reference. It's important to ask for information without inadvertently supplying the information. Questions that require only a response of "yes" or "no" are also inadvisable. For example, "Do you still live at the same address?" and "Do you still live at 24 Burch Street, Camelot, California?" provide no authentication, while "What is your address?" requires the person to provide information.

**66. C**: The skill mix of nursing staff is a nursing sensitive quality indicator. The skill mix refers to the percentage of each type of nursing personnel (advanced practice registered nurses, registered nurses, LVNs/LPNs, and nurse aids). Because registered nurses cost more per hour than other staff, the skill mix is often one area of nursing that is reviewed when cost-cutting efforts must be made despite evidence that shows that patients have better outcomes with a skill mix weighted toward registered nurses.

**67. C**: Close-call events are errors that could have resulted in patient injury but were detected in time to prevent injury. Close-call events frequently occur in healthcare--much more frequently than actual adverse events--and many are not reported; however, analysis of close calls may help to identify safety concerns. For example, if an EHR does not display critical information, such as the patient's name, or information is not easily accessible, then this can increase the risk of errors.

**68. D**: Change theory (Lewin/Schein):

- Motivation to change (unfreezing): Dissatisfaction occurs and beliefs questioned, and survival anxiety may occur. Learning anxiety about having to learn different strategies causes resistance that can lead to denial, blame, and trying to maneuver or bargain without real change.
- Desire to change (unfrozen): Dissatisfaction is strong enough to override defensive actions. Desire to change is strong, but needed changes must be identified.
- Development of permanent change (refreezing): The new behavior becomes habitual, often requiring a change in perceptions of self and establishment of new relationships.

**69. A**: Emergency planning should begin with hazard vulnerability analysis, which assesses any potential hazards or threats that may impact the provision of care that must be maintained during an emergency situation. The primary vulnerabilities (flood, fire, terrorist attack, airline crash, chemical spill, nuclear reactor accident) should be identified and plans formulated. A hazard vulnerability analysis should be done on an annual basis and emergency preparedness plans updated according to the results of the analysis.

**70. A**: If the organization's overall staff turnover rate exceeds the benchmark (<6%) set by the organization, the next step should be to analyze the rate by job class. If, for example, the data is 9% staff turnover in nursing and 4% to 6% in other job classes, then strategies for retention need to be focused on nursing rather than on the other job classes. At this point, surveys and interviews should be carried out to obtain more data about nursing and focus groups formed.

**71. C**: If censuses in the oncology unit and medical-surgical unit fluctuate widely, often resulting in overstaffing or understaffing, the best solution is to cross train staff members so that at least some of the staff members are able to float between the two units, depending on the census and workload. Nurses should train together as much as possible so they can build relationships and should be familiar with common medications, equipment, and treatments used on both units.

**72. D**: If the nurse executive wants to increase patient engagement, according to the Patient Activation Measure (Hibbard et.al., 2004), the stages are:

1. Believing in the importance of the patient's role.
2. Having the ability (resources) to take action.
3. Taking action to improve health.
4. Persisting even in the face of stress.

Patients must progress through all four stages to be considered activated or engaged.

**73. A**: If, in order to improve relations between physicians and nurses, the nurse executive stresses support for the "platinum rule" associated with interdisciplinary collaboration, this means that a person should treat others as they want to be treated. This also means that showing respect for other persons is of paramount importance as is taking the time to determine people's needs and to consider their responses. The platinum rule looks outward instead of inward to guide interactions.

**74. B**: If a union is organizing employees, 30% of employees must sign union authorization cards before the union requests that the organization voluntarily recognize the union as the bargaining agent for the employees. However, the employer is not required to recognize the union at this point. If the employer refuses, the union can petition the National Labor Relations Board to verify the signatures and set a date for an election, which is often after a prolonged period of many months.

**75. D**: According to force field analysis (Lewin), the two forces that must be considered for change include:

- Driving forces: These are forces responsible for instigating and promoting change, such as leaders, incentives, and competition.
- Restraining forces: These are forces that resist change, such as poor attitudes, hostility, inadequate equipment, or insufficient funds.

Both forces must be considered when promoting change and a plan developed to diminish or eliminate restraining forces. A balance between forces represents the *status quo* or equilibrium.

**76. C**: Strategies for change include:

- Normative-reeducative approach: Focusing on the need to get along with others, this approach tries to convince people to be cooperative and to go along with the majority.
- Power-coercive approach: Using power to coerce others, this approach imposes change based on the authority to do so.
- Rational-empirical approach: Using data to influence others, this approach depends on providing information and evidence to support change.

**77. A:** Carrying out drills is an important element of an emergency operations plan. Drills addressing various emergency situations, such as pandemics, floods, hurricanes, or heatwaves, should be carried out depending on the risks around the health care organization. Drills are necessary to identify deficits in the plan or elements that are ineffective or unworkable. Feedback derived from the drills should be used to revise or modify the emergency operations plan as needed.

**78. A:** Training output estimating is used primarily to estimate the supply of health practitioners based on the number of people enrolled in and completing training programs. For example, if projecting the need for nurses and the available supply, the nurse executive would survey nurse training programs and trends in enrollment, especially programs in the local area and state from which a hospital is likely to draw employees. If the need is greater than the supply, then recruitment is likely to pose a problem.

**79. D**: To ensure that new hires are correctly licensed and credentialed, it is necessary to carry out a primary source verification. That means that sealed transcripts must be obtained for academic credits and certifying agencies must be contacted directly. It's also important to obtain copies of current license and credentials and to contact previous employers, although privacy constraints limit the information employers can provide. A credential verification organization may be contracted to carry out verifications.

**80. C**: The four core criteria for credentialing and privileging include:

- Licensure: Must be current through the appropriate state board, such as state medical board.
- Education: Includes training and experience appropriate for the credential and may include technical training, professional education, residencies, internships, fellowships, doctoral and post-doctoral programs, and board and clinical certifications.
- Competence: Evaluations and recommendations by peers regarding clinical competence and judgment.
- Performance ability: Demonstrated ability to perform the duties to which the credentialing/privileging applies.

**81. B**: As with any changes in procedures or policies, the staff should be provided detailed guidelines and training of each element of SBAR as well as worksheets they can use to organize information. Elements include:

- Situation: Name, age, physician, diagnosis.
- Background: Brief medical history, co-morbidities, review of lab tests, current therapy, IV's, VS, pain, special needs, educational needs, discharge plans.
- Assessment: Review of systems, lines, tubes, and drains, completed tasks, needed tasks, future procedures.
- Recommendations: Review plan of care, medications, precautions (restraints, falls), treatments, wound care.

**82. C**: Pay-for-performance programs are usually based on four types of quality measures:

- Performance: Based on carrying out practices demonstrated to improve health outcomes.
- Outcomes: Based on achieving positive outcomes (but does not always consider social or other variables that the healthcare provider cannot control).
- Patient experience (satisfaction): Based on patient's perceptions of care received and their satisfaction.
- Structures/Technology: Based on facilities and equipment used for care, and may reward some types of upgrades, such as an upgrade to an electronic health record.

**83. A**: According to the general systems theory, changed behavior would be classified as an output. The general systems theory involves a cycle that includes 4 elements:

- Input: This is what goes into a system in terms of energy or materials, such as knowledge and facts.
- Throughput/Processes: These are the actions that take place in order to transform input, such as lived experience.
- Output: This is the result of the interrelationship between input and processes, such as changed behavior.
- Feedback: This is information that results and can be used for evaluation of the system, such as praise and support.

**84. D**: If the nurse executive appears to have staff support for proposed changes as no one voices opposition, but anonymous surveys indicate widespread opposition, the type of power that the nurse is likely utilizing is coercive. When faced with coercive power, staff members often feel that their opinions are not respected and that they may have repercussions if they voice them. This may effectively silence staff members but result in widespread discontent and lack of cooperation.

**85. B**: After selecting a number of possible vendors for a complex upgrade of equipment and services, the next step is to develop a request for proposal. With the request for proposal, there may be considerable differences among the different vendors related to the types of equipment and the costs or services. A request for quotation, on the other hand, is usually submitted for products or services that are essentially the same or very similar with cost being one of the deciding factors.

**86. D**: Communication is a critical element of emergency response, and it is the first of six critical areas to be addressed. This is because effective communication is necessary to initiate response not only among staff members of the health care organizations, but also among federal, state, and local agencies that will have a role in the emergency response. The six critical areas are (1) communication, (2) resources and assets, (3) safety and security, (4) staff responsibilities, (5) utilities, and (6) clinical and support activities.

**87. D**: In a just culture, if a nurse who misread a medication order and administered an incorrect dosage to a patient should be consoled and supported as this is a human error. The just culture differentiates among:

- Human error: Inadvertent actions, mistakes, or lapses in proper procedure—Consider processes, procedures, training, and/or design to determine the cause of the error, console and support.
- At-risk behavior: Unjustified risk, choice—Provide incentives for correct behavior and disincentives for incorrect, provide coaching.
- Reckless behavior: Conscious disregard for proper procedures—Take remedial action and/or punitive action.

**88. A**: Once an evidence-based change has been implemented, the next critical element is to measure outcomes to determine how the change has impacted care, especially those elements that are important for reimbursement and reporting: rates of complications and sentinel events, length of stay, rates of rehospitalization, and costs of care. After measures are evaluated and data collected, the outcomes should be widely disseminated throughout the organization.

**89. B**: If the hospital has a high turnover rate and difficulty recruiting staff, the strategy that is most likely to increase retention is providing career ladders that outline opportunities for advancement in people's careers. Studies show that some strategies, surprisingly, increase staff morale but do not affect retention. These strategies include such things as providing educational benefits and on-site childcare. Providing amenities such as employee lounges have little effect on either morale or retention.

**90. D**: If the hospital has begun developing a transitional care model for at-risk patients, the patients' care is generally coordinated by an advanced practice nurse. The APRN coordinates care with the patient's physician and other healthcare providers, such as therapists, while the patient is in the hospital and then takes on the role of case manager when the patient is discharged, ensuring that the patient's home care is adequate and needs are being met.

**91. C**: When estimating employment costs (salary plus benefits), benefits account for approximately 30% of the total costs, according to the Bureau of Labor Statistics, so they must be figured in to each hiring cost. Benefits include the costs of medical insurance, dental insurance, vision insurance, Workers' Compensation, malpractice insurance, disability insurance, and paid sick time, vacation time, and holiday time. The benefit package may also include retirement programs and payment for the costs of training, hiring bonuses, and tuition coverage.

**92. B**: Mass casualty events result in large numbers of patients in need of care, such as with a pandemic. During mass casualty events, infrastructure remains generally intact, at least in the early stages. Mass effect events, however--which include most types of natural disasters, such as hurricanes, earthquakes, floods, and tornados--often result in disruption of infrastructure. For example, power may be out, communication may be severed, and roads may be impassable. Emergency preparedness plans must take into account the possible results of mass effect events and mass casualty events.

**93. A**: The four leadership styles (Hersey, 2008) associated with situational leadership are:

- Telling: The leader gives clear orders with specific instructions as to how, when, and where. The follower has limited ability and motivation.
- Selling: The leader explains the reasons for an action and answers questions. The follower has some ability but limited motivation
- Participating: The leader discusses needs and shares decision-making. The follower has good ability and some motivation.
- Delegating: The leader delegates decision-making to others. The follower has good ability and good motivation.

**94. D**: If the hospital is considering hiring additional fulltime staff in order to reduce overtime costs, cost-benefit analysis would use the average cost of overtime and the cost of hiring fulltime staff to demonstrate savings. A cost-effective analysis measures the effectiveness of an intervention rather than the monetary savings. Efficacy studies may compare a series of cost-benefit analyses to determine the intervention with the best cost-benefit. Cost-utility analysis (a subtype of cost-effective analysis) measures benefit to society in general, so it is hard to quantify.

**95. B**: The first step in planning continuing education opportunities for staff members is to conduct a needs assessment to determine what content is most applicable. This needs assessment may include a staff survey but that should be only one of multiple measures. Next, the coordinator should define objectives and determine the method of delivery, develop lesson plans, select pilot group (if appropriate), schedule classes/training, and carry out evaluations.

**96. C**: The patient assessment instrument (PAI) that inpatient rehabilitation facilities (IRFs) must submit in order to receive reimbursement from Medicare and Medicaid is <u>IRF-PAI</u>. The patient's condition and need for rehabilitative care must be carefully documented. Minimum Data Set (<u>MDS</u> version 3.0) is used by long-term care facilities and is part of the resident assessment instrument (RAI). Outcome and Assessment Information Set (<u>OASIS</u>) is the assessment instrument used by home health agencies.

**97. A**: If a nurse executive avoids hiring nurses in their mid-20s because of the belief that they will require family leave have and/or care for children, the type of discrimination this represents is statistical discrimination. In this case, the nurse executive is basing hiring decisions on the fact that, statistically, the mid-20s (average currently about age 26) are the most common child-bearing years. The nurse executive is using information about a large group to make decisions about an individual.

**98. D**: If the nurse executive wants to reassure staff members that internal whistleblowing will be dealt with anonymously and without repercussions, the best method for reporting is multiple methods because this allows the whistleblower to use the method with which the person feels most comfortable and also signals that whistleblowing is encouraged and taken seriously.

**99. C**: SAMHSA has developed a number of different resources to utilize in planning for disaster preparedness and dealing with behavioral health problems of those affected. SAMHSA maintains the Disaster Technical Assistance Center (DTAC), which carries out research and provides consultation, training, technical assistance, and expertise. SAMHSA also offers numerous fact sheets and toolkits aimed at different populations, including *Helping Survivors Cope with Grief After a Disaster or Traumatic Event*.

**100. C**: If the hospital has a limited marketing budget but needs to attract more patients to services, the most effective approach is probably targeted marketing. The hospital can utilize available demographic and consumer data to target the groups that may most benefit from and utilize the services. Once a population is selected, then the marketing campaign is aimed specifically at that group, effecting the types and sites of advertising.

**101. A**: According to Kotter and Cohen's theory of change (2002), the first step in bringing about change is creating a sense of urgency through encouraging others and stressing the need to change the *status quo*. This is followed by building a team to guide change, determining the right vision and strategy, communicating the value of the change, empowering people and removing barriers, creating short term achievements ("wins"), continuing, and taking steps to ensure that the changes persist.

**102. B**: For performance appraisal, the method that is likely to provide the most equitable measure is the behavioral anchored rating scale (BARS). The BARS provides a rating scale with specific descriptions for each point on the scale. For example, leadership qualities may be assessed on a scale of 1 to 4 with 1 described as "lacks appropriate interpersonal skills and has poor working relationships with staff" with 4 described as "exhibits excellent interpersonal skills, is supportive of staff members, and promotes quality nursing care."

**103. C**: For staffing purposes, a staff nurse who works 20 hours a week throughout the year would be considered 0.5 FTE. FTE (full-time equivalent) is based on working 40 hours a week for 52 weeks a year (including paid sick time and vacation time). Those who work three 12-hour shifts (total 36 hours) are classified as 0.9 FTE even though they may be paid the full-time rate because the missing 4 hours must be covered by other personnel.

**104. A**: The affirmative action plan for the organization must provide equal hiring opportunities for qualified individuals but should not establish a quota system for hiring as quotas are illegal. The affirmative action plan may describe training programs as well as outreach efforts to increase the diversity of applicants. Affirmative action covers qualified minorities, women, covered veterans, and persons with disabilities who can work with or without reasonable accommodations.

**105. C**: There are three types of bargaining that can be used in the negotiation process. Those types include:

- Distributive: A competitive process in which one side wins and the other loses [zero-sum, win-lose], and may lead to compromise or stalemate.
- Integrative: A collaborative process [win-win] where the parties involved bargain jointly, trying to solve problems).
- Mixed: Combines some aspects of distributive and integrative.

Collaborative bargaining is not a formal type of bargain, though collaboration is generally involved in the process.

**106. C**: While all elements of a Disaster Preparedness Plan (DPP) are important, in the event of possible or impending flooding, the evacuation plans are the most critical. The hospital should already have Memoranda of Understanding (MOUs) in place with receiving facilities outside of the flood zone and transportation plans to facilitate transfers. Protocols regarding medical records, equipment, medications, and supplies needed for the evacuation should be outlined in the Disaster Preparedness Plan.

**107. C**: Under hospital 501(r) requirements for not-for-profit hospitals, hospitals must perform a community health needs assessment (CHNA) at least every 3 years. Additionally, the hospital must publish the results on a website and take steps to meet the needs that were identified. The hospital must also limit the costs of care for those eligible for financial assistance and must inform patients of programs for financial assistance before collection activities.

**108. B**: HealthGrades is a website that provides information and star ratings about the quality of hospitals, dentists, and doctors in the area for consumers and allows an "experience match" so that profiles can match the criteria used for searching. HealthGrades receives almost 20 million queries each month, and customers can post reviews of hospitals, doctors, and dentists. However, the ratings can be based on as few as one review, so monitoring the site is important.

**109. A**: The most important element of a disaster/emergency preparedness plan is being readily available and having practice drills. Because disaster/emergency situations are generally rare, staff members may not recall how to activate the plan and carry out procedures unless they have had frequent opportunities to review the plan and practice. Disaster/emergency preparedness drills should be carried out at least annually and the plan updated, especially the chain of command and "phone tree" (including text or email) to reflect current staffing.

**110. A**: When collecting clinical outcomes data, primary consideration should be given to the needs of the patient population and to the mandated reporting requirements because compliance is essential for not only reimbursement but also hospital ratings and accreditation. If possible, outcomes selected for data collection should be directly associated with the organization's mission. The team selecting outcomes measures should be interdisciplinary and should include advance practice nurses that are familiar with data analysis and the use of benchmarks.

**111. C**: Utilizing the worst-case scenario method of decision-making is most indicated for decisions that pose risks. This method includes asking, "What is the worst that could happen," and "How could we manage X if it happened?" It's important to review each step-in process as well as possible system failures. For example, if implementing a new EHR, the worst-case scenario might include what could happen if data was entered incorrectly as well as what might happen during a disaster that included power failure.

**112. B**: According to Provision 1 of the ANA Code of ethics, the nurse must respect the right of the patient, but when patient's choices are risky or self-destructive, the nurse's best approach is to address the behavior in a nonjudgmental but factual manner and offer resources, such as information about 12-step groups or smoking cessation. Provision 1 recognizes the patient's right to self-determination while also indicating that the nurse has a responsibility to the patient's welfare.

**113. D**: If a physician at hospital A is able to access patient information from hospital B and another physician, the system that allows this exchange of information is a health information exchange. HIEs allow three types of exchanges:

- Directed: Allows secure transmission of information among healthcare providers.
- Query-based: Allows healthcare providers to search for or request patient information.
- Consumer-mediated: Provides some control to patients to decide what information can be shared with healthcare providers.

**114. A**: The primary protection included in the Patient's Bill of Rights under the Affordable Care Act is the right to insurance coverage for those with pre-existing conditions. The person cannot be denied insurance or dropped from insurance because of the pre-existing condition. Additionally, the Patient's Bill of Rights extends the age to which parents can cover dependents on their insurance to age 26 and also includes the right to some preventive care, such as physical examination and mammograms, at no additional cost to the insured.

**115. C**: To meet ORYX® quarterly reporting requirements for hospitals with a daily census greater than 10, the hospital must report on 9 chart-extracted electronic clinical quality measures (eCQMs):

- 5 required: ED-1, ED-2, PC-01, VTE-6 and IMM-2. If the hospital has greater than 300 live births, then four additional perinatal care (PC) measures are required.
- 4 of choice: The hospital chooses at least 4 out of 13 possible measures, selecting those that are most applicable to the patient population and the services the hospital provides.

**116. D**: The four criteria used to classify accountability measures (formerly core measures) are:

- Research: Evidence should support interventions.
- Proximity: Process and outcome being measured are closely associated.
- Accuracy: Measure accurately assesses the effectiveness of the intervention.
- Adverse effects: Measure avoids unintended adverse effects.

These 4 criteria are important factors in achieving positive patient outcomes. The accountability measures align with CMS measures.

**117. B**: A nurse executive who promotes pervasive leadership will encourage decision making by others, recognizing that leadership potential exists at all levels of an organization and should be encouraged and celebrated. With pervasive leadership, the nurse executive demonstrates respect and trust in others in the organization and encourages innovative and proactive solutions to problems at the local level. Pervasive leadership is based on the idea of "we" make decisions rather than the traditional leader-follower model.

**118. B:** When evacuating a facility, the first step is to reduce the number of patients that require assisted transportation. This can be done by identifying patients who can safely be discharged early and can be transported by family or friends. Protocols should be in place to immediately discharge these patients, who are generally ambulatory and in need of minimal assistance. Attending physicians must be notified, and medical record summaries must be prepared for all patients who will be transferred to other facilities.

**119. A:** If a group of nurses on the staff have expressed interest in researching evidence-based practice but admit to having limited time to do so and ask the nurse executive for advice, the best suggestion is to advise them to form a journal club. Each member can then read and report on one or two articles to the group, and the group can discuss the information and how it might apply to clinical services. In this way, they all benefit from the research but only have to expend a small amount of time.

**120. C:** Appreciative inquiry veers away from problem solving to promote change and looks to the power of inquiry. Principles of appreciative inquiry include:

- Constructionist: People's actions are associated with what they believe.
- Simultaneity: Questions affect the organization about which they are inquiring.
- Poetic: Words have an impact and constantly effect and change an organization.
- Anticipatory: Ideas about the future affect current actions.
- Positive: Positive thoughts and actions are needed to sustain change.

**121. A:** In an active shooter situation, staff members have little time to decide on a course of action. The normal response to a fearful situation is the three Fs (freeze, flight, fight), but staff need to be retrained to run if they are in imminent danger, hide if they possibly can to avoid the shooter, and fight if they have to protect themselves or others. Fighting most often means throwing whatever is available at the shooter or tackling the shooter. Whenever possible, the staff should call 911 or yell warnings.

**122. A:** If the nurse executive plans to increase the focus on consumer education to improve patient outcomes and satisfaction, the "three Ps" of consumer education are:

- Philosophy: Patient education is viewed as a positive investment.
- Priority: Patient education is important to both quality nursing and to patients, who want information and involvement.
- Performance: Nurses must have the necessary skills and knowledge of various techniques to effectively provide consumer education.

**123. A:** The key element in helping clinical staff institute evidence-based practice is a mentor. The mentor, often an advanced practice nurse or other nurse trained in evidence-based research and practice, can serve as a guide and resource person for other staff members as well as a model of evidence-based practice. It is the role of the mentor to ensure that point-of-care healthcare practitioners understand the evidence-based process.

**124. D:** According to Peplau's Interpersonal Relations Model of nursing, the nurse-patient relationship goes through overlapping phases that include orientation, problem identification, explanation of potential solutions, and problem resolution. Peplau believed that collaboration

# M⊘metrix

between the nurse and patient was especially important and that the nurse acts as a "maturing force" to help the patient. Peplau also stressed the importance of the patient being treated with dignity and respect and believed that a positive or negative environment could affect a patient accordingly.

**125. A:** If the hospital is switching to a new integrated CPOE, CDSS and EHR, necessitating major changes in procedure and requiring much additional training of all staff, the initial method of implementation that is likely to be the least disruptive is small tests of change. This allows testing of small parts of the whole in order to identify any problems that may require modification. Small tests of change can also help to identify areas that require additional training.

**126. D:** According to OSHA guidelines, the following PPE will adequately protect receiving personnel from toxic chemicals:

- Double layer protective gloves.
- Chemical resistant suit (openings sealed with tape).
- Head and eye coverings.
- PAPR (protective factor of 1000) (99.97% HEPA /organic vapor/aid gas respirator cartridges).
- Chemical protective boots.

**127. A:** The leader of a patient-centered medical home (PCMH) is generally a personal physician, who establishes ongoing relationships with patients. The team may comprise various members, such as nurses, various therapists, and a case manager. The goal of PCMH is to provide quality care and to reduce complications and the need for hospitalization, thus reducing costs of care. The PCMH team provides all levels of care (acute, chronic, end-of-life, hospice) and ensure that patients are able to obtain the medical care they need.

**128. B:** If, when conferring with a unit supervisor, the nurse executive notes that the supervisor frequently licks her lips and constantly rubs her hands together, based on this body language, the nurse executive may assume that the supervisor is nervous. Being nervous may make the mouth and lips dry, and rubbing the hands together is a self-comforting action. The person may also avoid direct eye contact, staring at the desk, for example, instead of looking at the nurse executive. Some may fidget or move about restlessly.

**129. C:** If developing a chart to display data about the age distribution of patients admitted to the oncology department, a useful type of graphic display is a scattergram, which has an X (age) axis and a Y (admissions) axis in order to show the relationship between two variables (in this case admissions to the unit by date and age). A data point is applied for each admission, corresponding to the patient's age. Once the data are charted, then the data are reviewed to determine if a pattern has emerged.

**130. D:** When considering improvements to workflow processes, the first issue to address is whether steps in a process can be eliminated because the goal is to simplify while still maintaining the integrity of the process. Eliminating steps may result from purchasing of new equipment, altering product design, or changing the environment (such as carrying out a process at point of care rather than in another area). In some cases, steps may be simplified by combining some steps with others or changing the order of steps.

**131. A:** Priests and other clergy may have access to limited information about patients; however, hospitals are not obligated to provide this information, and such disclosure should be outlined in the privacy notice. While visitors and families must provide the name of the person they wish to visit, clergy members, like priests, for example, may ask for a list of Catholic patients so that they can provide spiritual services. The information they receive can only include the names, general conditions (critical, poor, fair, good), locations (room number, unit) and religious affiliations.

**132. D**: If a unit supervisor meets with the nurse executive and states, "I see, as usual, you have determined the best solution to the problem," the communication style the supervisor is using is passive-aggressive. Passive-aggressive communication often includes an element of sarcasm, such as "as usual," but may be delivered with a smile. The passive-aggressive individual may appear on the surface to be in agreement but often works behind the other person's back to undermine decisions and authority.

**133. B**: Patients who are assigned to an accountable care organization (ACO) through Medicare will have some health information shared among different ACO healthcare providers in able to ensure coordination of care and to prevent duplication of services, such as laboratory testing. However, patients have the right to request that specific information not be shared. Patients who are participating in an ACO cannot also participate in a Medicare Advantage Plan, such as an HMO or PPO.

**134. A**: While all of these issues may be considered, the red flag is admission from a sheltered living facility. Other red flag concerns include homelessness, poor living conditions, limited financial and insurance resources, and dependency on others for care. While reportable events (child/elder abuse, violent crime, domestic violence) automatically require full case management services, other situations must be considered individually. For example, the inability to drive for someone with a spouse or with availability of public transportation may not be a problem while it may prevent others from accessing care.

**135. C**: A nurse executive who is able to understand the feelings of others and to understand why they have specific needs or desires is exhibiting the empathy element of emotional intelligence. The 5 basic elements of emotional intelligence include:

- Self-awareness: Recognizing own feelings and self-worth.
- Self-regulation: Being able to exhibit self-control in expressing emotions and managing negative emotions, being flexible and innovative.
- Motivation: Having initiative, optimism, and drive to succeed.
- Empathy: Being able to sense feelings of others.
- Social skills: Having the ability to influence others, communicate effectively, and work well with others.

**136. D**: If the nurse executive listens to a staff member saying that he is concerned that a number of other staff members were laid off when a unit closed and responds, "You're worried about losing your job," the nurse executive is practicing reflecting. The nurse executive is stating the intent of the staff member's words to help the person better understand his feelings and concerns. Reflecting is a way to show that one is paying attention and to encourage the other person to share concerns.

**137. A**: If the Board of Directors has asked the nurse executive to include subordinate evaluations as part of the annual performance review, the nurse executive should suggest that evaluations be anonymous. While evaluations are more likely to focus on the positive if they are signed, this is because evaluators may fear repercussions. Anonymous evaluations are usually more honest and, therefore, helpful to use to improve performance. However, disgruntled employers may give excessively negative evaluations.

**138. C**: Actively listening to a subordinate's suggestions by making eye contact, nodding the head, and asking questions implies that the nurse executive shows respect for the speaker's suggestions. It does not, however, obligate the nurse executive to follow the suggestions or commit to any action. If the nurse executive does not agree, it's appropriate to give the reasons without passing negative judgments about the suggestion. Active listening is an important skill to encourage others to participate.

**139. B**: An example of a normative-re-educative strategy to facilitate and manage change is to encourage the team to identify problems and solutions because this causes them to become active participants in the process of change. While this method of facilitating change may take longer than the empirical-rational model, which relies on facts and figures to bring about rational decisions, or the power-coercive strategy, which enforces change with power, it is often the most successful.

**140. D**: According to the STAR model, a change in one area usually necessitates a change in another area because of the interrelatedness of systems. The STAR model is based on a diagram with the points of the STAR representing strategy, structure, human resources, incentives, and information/decision making. Values that are core to this model include the idea that a systemic problem is rarely related to laziness or incompetence, there are multiple optimal systems, many points are equally important, and cultural values may be ingrained, impeding progress, and cannot be changed directly.

**141. A**: The most important factor for the nurse executive to communicate to staff when proposing changes in processes and procedures is the reason why changes are needed. Staff members are more likely to be cooperative if they understand why they are asked to make changes. The nurse executive should be prepared to present evidence-based rationale for changes and to discuss anticipated outcomes so that the staff fully understands that the changes are not arbitrary and that they should result in positive results.

**142. C**: If the nurse executive is considering a suggestion to institute a telehealth program for a patient population primarily covered by original Medicare, the first issue to consider is the geographic location of the target population. Medicare limits coverage for telehealth services primarily to rural areas, so designated as a Health Professional Shortage Area (HPSA) according to the US Census Bureau. Some chronic care management may also include remote monitoring, and some special Medicare programs, such as Medicare Advantage, may include telehealth services (at higher cost to patient).

**143. B**: Nurse-led clinics are generally part of outpatient services provided by an organization, managed by a nurse practitioner or other advanced practice nurse. However, they may also be private practices. Most nurse-led clinics focus on population-based care and/or care of patients with chronic disease and preventive medicine. Nurse-led clinics are often placed in the community where patients have easy access and may be open in the evening or weekends to better accommodate employed patients.

**144. D**: Hourly rounding is often effective in reducing falls, especially in extended care facilities where patients are often elderly and have difficulty communicating or using call bells. Patients often fall when climbing out of bed to go to the bathroom or get a drink of water. During rounds, patients should each be spoken to briefly, checked to confirm that they are comfortable and dry (if incontinent), offered a drink of water, and asked if they need to use the bathroom or have pain.

**145. A**: Speech language pathology services are covered for eligible patients by Medicare and may be provide by home health agencies. Patients must be essentially homebound and require such other services as intermittent skilled nursing care (such as dressing changes), physical therapy, or occupational therapy. The patient must be under a physician's care, and the physician must certify the patient's homebound status. Patients may attend adult daycare programs and still be considered homebound.

**146. B:** Predictive analytics uses historical data to make predictions about present or future health needs. As is the case in this question, if a patient has a history of readmissions and failures to follow treatment plans, then the most effective intervention is likely to assign a case manager to the patient so that he or she can have monitored follow-up care. This may include home health care, referrals to community resources, and reminders regarding medical appointments and treatments.

**147. B:** Continuity planning is an essential component of any emergency response plan. Continuity planning ensures that critical functions, such as patient care and support services, are maintained during various types of emergent situations, such as mass casualty events or hurricanes. Continuity planning should consider the minimum needs to maintain patient care and typically includes the use of additional staff to manage patient loads, stockpiled water and supplies (including drugs and dressings), as well as generators to maintain electrical output, critical equipment, and lighting.

**148. C:** If a reporter from the local newspaper has made an appointment to interview the nurse executive about the hospital's quality initiatives, in preparation, the first action the nurse executive should undertake is to meet with the public relations person. It's important that publicity about the hospital be cohesive and follows a plan to ensure that all hospital representatives are providing complementary rather than contradictory information. PR may, for example, want to focus on patient advantages rather than cost-savings.

**149. C:** Cardiac implantable loop recorders (ILRs) are miniaturized, implantable devices that are inserted by injection into the left chest in order to monitor heart rate and rhythm, such as tachycardia and atrial fibrillation. They monitor continuously and send reports to the physician. Examples of these devices include Reveal LINQ and Reveal XT, Confirm Rx ICM, and BioMonitor 2. These devices typically do not interfere with MRIs, but radiology should be notified because some precautions may be indicated. The devices are palpable and patients should be advised to avoid applying pressure directly over the device.

**150. D:** Under the *Patient Self Determination Act*, patients have a right to express their wishes for end-of-life care with an advance directive. The presence of an advance directive should be documented in the patient's healthcare record. When a patient is incapacitated, the advance directive should supersede the wishes of the next of kin and other family members. In practice, however, this does not always occur. Healthcare providers can also, under the law, refuse to comply with an advance directive based on a conscious objection.

# Nurse Executive Practice Test #2

**1. If a job applicant has a history of trying to unionize at a previous job and the healthcare organization declines to hire the applicant for that reason, this is a(n):**

a. Unfair labor practice
b. Violation of civil rights
c. Abuse of power
d. Legal action

**2. One of the eligibility criteria for the American Nurses Credentialing Center's Magnet Recognition Program is that all nurse leaders must have, at a minimum, a(n):**

a. Registered nurse (RN) certificate
b. Associate of science in nursing (ASN) degree
c. Bachelor of science in nursing (BSN) degree
d. Master of science in nursing (MSN) degree

**3. If a mass-casualty incident occurs and triggers the need for critical incident stress management, the first step to critical incident stress debriefing is:**

a. Debriefing sessions
b. Education sessions
c. Retreat sessions
d. Defusing sessions

**4. To reduce the use of the emergency department for routine healthcare, the hospital has opened a free clinic in an area with a large population of undocumented immigrants, but few people come to the clinic. The best method of outreach is likely to:**

a. Gain the support of community leaders.
b. Advertise in the language of the community.
c. Post signs encouraging participation.
d. Record radio commercials about the clinic.

**5. If an employee feels that the healthcare organization has not provided a safe working environment, the employee may file a complaint with:**

a. CDC
b. OSHA
c. FDA
d. DOL

**6. Which of the following facilities is required by the Centers for Medicare & Medicaid Services (CMS) to conduct an annual review of the emergency preparedness plan/program?**

a. Critical access hospitals
b. Hospitals
c. Long-term-care facilities
d. Transplant centers

**7. If the turnover rate of staff has been >40% and a new leader works with the staff to improve the working environment, resulting in a reduction of turnover to 10%, the strength that the leader is exhibiting is:**

    a. Executing
    b. Influencing
    c. Strategic thinking
    d. Relationship building

**8. The nurse executive's ability to impact the patient experience is likely most affected by the nurse executive's role in:**

    a. recruitment and retention of staff.
    b. orientation and in-service.
    c. budgeting.
    d. the nursing model.

**9. If an employee has not met performance expectations, the initial intervention should be to:**

    a. Require the employee work under direct supervision.
    b. Begin disciplinary procedures that may end in termination.
    c. Monitor for improvement until the annual performance evaluation.
    d. Immediately counsel the employee regarding expectations.

**10. According to The Joint Commission, healthcare organizations must carry out competency validation for new hires and staff members:**

    a. On hiring and on an ongoing basis
    b. On hiring—one time only
    c. Annually
    d. As needed only

**11. If a job applicant has an obvious disability, under provisions of the Americans with Disabilities Act (1990), the nurse executive may ask:**

    a. About the extent of the disability
    b. If the disability will interfere with job functions
    c. If the applicant can carry out job functions with or without accommodations
    d. How many sick days the applicant has used in the past year

**12. The nurse executive is planning to distribute surveys regarding patient satisfaction with care and treatment during hospitalization. Which of the following is likely to have the greatest effect on patient satisfaction?**

    a. Cost of care
    b. Environment (room, lab facilities, rehab center)
    c. Interaction with healthcare providers
    d. Amenities (meals on demand, televisions, wifi)

**13.** A nurse leaves a clinical unit without notifying anyone, leaving patients unattended to take care of personal business, and fails to provide pain medication to a patient who has requested it. Subsequently, the patient gets out of bed to look for the nurse, falls, and breaks a hip. How many elements of negligence does this represent?

    a.  1
    b.  2
    c.  3
    d.  4

**14.** Nurses report that patients are often self-monitoring their activity, steps, and heartrates with their smart watches. This is an example of:

    a.  telemedicine.
    b.  telehealth.
    c.  eHealth.
    d.  mHealth.

**15.** CMS record retention requirements for healthcare providers include:

    a.  10 years for regular Medicare and 5 years for Medicare managed care programs
    b.  10 years for regular Medicare and Medicare managed care programs
    c.  5 years for regular Medicare and 10 years for Medicare managed care programs
    d.  5 years for regular Medicare and Medicare managed care programs

**16.** The factor evaluation system of patient classification:

    a.  Classifies patients into broad categories
    b.  Predicts patient needs based on patient category
    c.  Is primarily subjective and descriptive
    d.  Uses patient care activities to determine direct hours of care

**17.** The nurse executive asks staff members and community members who are ethnic minorities to share healthcare experiences, negative and positive, as part of staff training. This is an example of:

    a.  Leveraging diversity
    b.  Outreach
    c.  Strategic planning
    d.  Relationship building

**18.** If inexperienced nurses complain of lateral violence (e.g., bullying, insults, gossiping) from more experienced nurses in a healthcare organization, the nurse executive should:

    a.  Encourage the inexperienced nurses to be less sensitive to criticism.
    b.  Explain that this is a pervasive problem in healthcare.
    c.  Establish a zero-tolerance policy that outlines expectations and consequences.
    d.  Reprimand nurses and others engaging in lateral violence.

**19. The nurse executive notes that a large part of the budget goes to inventory, but outdated products have resulted in unnecessary waste. Which approach is likely the most cost effective?**

    a. Ordering when item numbers drop to a preestablished count
    b. Using just-in-time ordering
    c. Looking for less expensive supplies
    d. Educating staff members about avoiding waste

**20. The Fair Labor Standards Act (FLSA, 1938) requires that employers provide:**

    a. A basic minimum wage and overtime payment
    b. Holiday and sick pay
    c. Premium payment for working holidays
    d. Immediate severance pay

**21. In order to function as an effective team, a group of people must:**

    a. Work together
    b. Work collectively
    c. Have different skill sets
    d. Establish a hierarchy

**22. The first element of a business plan for a proposed new clinic should be the:**

    a. Market survey
    b. Marketing strategies
    c. Timeline
    d. Executive summary

**23. The nurse executive believes that a hospital needs to make improvements in the provision of patient-centered care. Which of the following elements is likely to be the most important in transforming care?**

    a. Leadership
    b. Staff support
    c. Organizational structure
    d. Physician support

**24. The core measure sets developed by the Core Quality Measures Collaborative for Primary Care are intended for use in:**

    a. Value-based payment programs
    b. CMS programs
    c. Fee-for-service
    d. Managed care programs

**25. When considering hours per patient day (HPPD) as part of staffing and budget planning, the clinical unit type that typically requires the greatest number of HPPD is:**

    a. Adult surgical
    b. Adult critical care
    c. Pediatric critical care
    d. Level II neonatal continuing care

**26. The rights of employees to organize and engage in collective bargaining is provided by the:**

    a. Equal Pay Act (1963)
    b. Fair Labor Standards Act (1938)
    c. Labor-Management Reporting and Disclosure Act (1959)
    d. National Labor Relations Act (1935)

**27. Skill-mix staffing is often used as a method of:**

    a. Improving patient care
    b. Reducing staffing costs
    c. Filling staffing positions
    d. Meeting legislative requirements

**28. Which of the following methods of rendering unsecured protected health information (PHI) unusable, unreadable, or indecipherable is specifically excluded under Health Insurance Portability and Accountability Act of 1996 (HIPAA) provisions?**

    a. Redaction
    b. Encryption
    c. Shredding
    d. Destruction

**29. The acuity model of staffing is based on:**

    a. Providing cost-effective care
    b. The hours of care needed
    c. The type of equipment used with the patient
    d. Patient diagnoses

**30. If a staff member exerts power over others by exploiting a personal relationship that the individual has with a board member, this is an example of:**

    a. Legitimate power
    b. Coercive power
    c. Connection power
    d. Referent power

**31. The nurse executive takes care in practice to avoid conflicts of interest or boundary violations. What provision of the American Nurses Association (ANA) Code of Ethics does this support?**

    a. Provision 1: practices with compassion and respect
    b. Provision 2: primary commitment is to the patient
    c. Provision 3: protects rights, health, and safety
    d. Provision 8: collaborates with other health professionals and the public

**32. Although mandated nurse-to-patient ratios are still not common, the average nurse-to-patient ratio for medical-surgical patients in acute care is:**

    a. 1:4
    b. 1:5
    c. 1:6
    d. 1:7

**33. A team's members have developed positive feelings toward each other, work well together, and identify with and feel attached to the team. According to Tuckman's group development stages, this represents the stage of:**
- a. Forming
- b. Storming
- c. Norming
- d. Performing

**34. In the communication component of the emergency preparedness plan for the healthcare organization, succession planning refers to identifying:**
- a. Staff who can assume the role of someone else who is absent during an emergency
- b. Off-duty staff who can replace on-duty staff during an emergency
- c. Sites to move patients to if an emergency renders the facility unsafe/unusable
- d. The chain of command and an alternate chain of command

**35. The type of budget that comprises general expenses, such as salaries, education, insurance, maintenance, depreciation, and debts as well as profits is a(n):**
- a. Master budget
- b. Operating budget
- c. Capital budget
- d. Cash balance budget

**36. If the healthcare organization carries out periodic updates (revenue, costs, volume) to the operational budget prior to the next budget cycle, this type of budget approach is:**
- a. Zero-based
- b. Flexible
- c. Fixed/forecast
- d. Continuous/rolling

**37. As the last step CMS requires for compliance regarding emergency preparedness, healthcare organizations with inpatient providers must test their emergency preparedness plan:**
- a. Annually with one full-scale exercise
- b. Every 6 months with one full-scale exercise
- c. Annually with one full-scale exercise and one additional exercise (full-scale or less)
- d. One time with one full-scale exercise and annually with less than a full-scale exercise

**38. Which of the following will be included when calculating nonproductive full-time equivalent (FTE) hours?**
- a. Staff break times
- b. Education/training time
- c. Night shift hours
- d. Time spent for handoffs

**39. A primary goal of transformational leadership is to:**
- a. Empower staff members
- b. Exercise control over staff members
- c. Advocate for nursing
- d. Consult with staff members

**40. If the nurse executive ensures that goals are met through a system of sanctions and rewards, this type of leadership is categorized as:**

a. Transformational
b. Situational
c. Transactional
d. Laissez-faire

**41. According to the Agency for Healthcare Research and Quality (AHRQ) TeamSTEPPS program, the three phases needed to develop a team approach to a culture of safety are (1) assessment of the need, (2) planning, training, and implementation, and (3):**

a. Sustainment
b. Evaluation
c. Replication
d. Dissemination

**42. A nurse executive adapts leadership styles to accommodate staff members' levels of competence, varying from a task-oriented approach to a relationship-oriented approach. This type of leadership is:**

a. Laissez-faire
b. Transformational
c. Reactive
d. Situational

**43. In an extended care facility, a patient whom staff members have described as angry and demanding approaches the nurse executive and complains loudly about the care he is receiving. He criticizes the meals, treatments, and response to call bells. The most appropriate response is:**

a. "I'll discuss your concerns with your nurses."
b. "The nurses are trying their best to care for you."
c. "What would you like me to do to resolve this problem?"
d. "I'm sorry you're so upset. How can we work together to improve things?"

**44. Which of the following federal acts requires that healthcare providers who are enrolled in Medicare, Medicaid, or the Children's Health Insurance Program adopt compliance programs?**

a. Deficit Reduction Act
b. Health Insurance Portability and Accountability Act
c. Affordable Care Act
d. Healthcare Quality Improvement Act

**45. The three aspects of care that nursing-sensitive indicators reflect are structural indicators, process indicators, and:**

a. Outcomes indicators
b. Compliance indicators
c. Research indicators
d. Staffing indicators

**46. Remote patient monitoring is especially beneficial for patients:**

    a. Who lack transportation resources
    b. Who live a far distance from healthcare providers
    c. With adequate insurance coverage
    d. With chronic health problems

**47. Predictive analytics helps to predict outcomes based on:**

    a. Observations
    b. Algorithms
    c. Statistical analysis
    d. Laboratory and imaging

**48. If a breach of unsecured PHI of 20 patients occurred and the covered entity is unable to contact 12 individuals to make notification, the next step is to:**

    a. Take no further action.
    b. Hire a private detective.
    c. Post a notice on the website for 90 days.
    d. Provide a substitute form of notice.

**49. A hospital has experienced a breach of unsecured PHI for 580 patients. What type of notice is required?**

    a. Individual and major media outlet notification
    b. Individual notification only
    c. Major media outlet notification only
    d. Website notification only

**50. Which of the following is outside of the scope of practice for the nurse executive/administrator?**

    a. Managing and supervising nursing staff
    b. Developing and managing budgets
    c. Ensuring compliance with regulations
    d. Managing and supervising physicians

**51. The first step in facilitating a patient experience program is to:**

    a. Define goals
    b. Gain the participation of key stakeholders
    c. Develop a plan/strategy
    d. Assess the current status

**52. When using Lean Six Sigma as a method for process improvement, the focus is on:**

    a. Individual projects
    b. Long-term goals and strategies
    c. Short-term goals
    d. Increasing profits

**53. Which method of problem solving is better suited to solving specific problems than organizational problems?**

a. PDCA
b. FOCUS
c. IMPROVE
d. FADE

**54. If a problem such as increased rate of surgical site infections has occurred, the first step in developing process improvement plans should be to:**

a. Identify key stakeholders
b. Conduct a cost–benefit analysis
c. Conduct surveys
d. Conduct a root cause analysis (RCA)

**55. As part of quality improvement, new processes have been developed. What type of study is indicated before full implementation?**

a. Quality inspection plan
b. Five whys
c. Failure mode and effects analysis
d. Feasibility study

**56. Which of the following payor methods rewards healthcare providers for the quantity of patients seen rather than the quality of healthcare given or positive outcomes and disincentivizes cost-saving efforts?**

a. Bundling
b. Capitation
c. Fee for service
d. Value based, gain share

**57. When conducting a literature review, the first issue to consider is the:**

a. Source of the material
b. Date of the material
c. Author(s)
d. Research format

**58. The payor system with which the healthcare provider receives incentive payments if the costs of care are lower than predicted but also has to bear additional costs if costs are higher than predicted is:**

a. Capitation
b. Bundling
c. Value based, gain share
d. Value based, risk share

**59. A research question should:**

a. Require further knowledge to find the answer
b. Be answered by using problem solving
c. Be answered by knowledge that already exists
d. Apply to only one population or problem

**60. Population health focuses on:**
- a. Disease treatment
- b. Chronic illness
- c. Prevention
- d. Aging

**61. If a research project has been completed and the nurse executive wants to disseminate the findings, the first step is to:**
- a. Assess stakeholders
- b. Develop a dissemination plan
- c. Determine the audience
- d. Do a cost analysis

**62. A hospital has seen a recent increase in falls among patients. When responding, the nurse executive should seek input from:**
- a. The risk management department
- b. Legal counsel
- c. The board of directors
- d. The patient advisory board

**63. A staff member states, "You're doing a good job, considering how little experience you've had." What type of communication does this represent?**
- a. Assertive
- b. Passive
- c. Passive-aggressive
- d. Aggressive

**64. According to Kurt Lewin's change management theory, an example of refreezing is:**
- a. Staff members are unhappy that goals are not being met.
- b. The new team-focused nursing model is accepted and successful.
- c. Staff members recognize the need for change but are unsure how.
- d. Staff members are resistant to change out of fear.

**65. According to Havelock's six-stage model for planned change, an integral part of the change process is:**
- a. Resistance
- b. Compliance
- c. Cooperation
- d. Resources

**66. According to force field analysis (Lewin), the two subgroups for proposed changes are:**
- a. Positive attitudes and negative attitudes
- b. Compliance and resistance
- c. Restraining forces and driving forces
- d. Leaders and followers

**67. In a conflict between a supervisor and a nurse on a unit, the nurse cedes to the supervisor, who is in a position of power. This approach to conflict resolution is categorized as:**

a. Avoiding
b. Compromising
c. Accommodating
d. Forcing

**68. If the nurse executive wants to resolve a conflict between two staff members, the first step is to:**

a. Encourage cooperation
b. Allow both parties to present their sides of the conflict
c. Use humor and empathy
d. Summarize the issues

**69. The model for change of health behavior that focuses on changes in behavior based on an individual's decisions is:**

a. 7S framework
b. Kotter's change management
c. Accelerated rapid-cycle change
d. The transtheoretical model

**70. If proactive strategies, such as compromise, have been unable to resolve a conflict, which of the following is defensive a measure that provides an indirect solution?**

a. Making an organizational change that eliminates the basis for the conflict
b. Separating the parties to the conflict by changing assignments
c. Advising the parties to avoid discussing the conflict
d. Parties agreeing to disagree and dealing with other issues

**71. According to the ANA, a healthy work environment has the following elements: safety, empowerment, and:**

a. Security
b. Sanctity
c. Support
d. Satisfaction

**72. If an organization supports the concept of pervasive leadership, this means that:**

a. Everyone is believed to have leadership potential.
b. The leader is expected to actively supervise all staff members.
c. The goals of the organization should be clearly outlined by leadership.
d. Leadership lies with a central authority rather than being shared.

**73. A nursing supervisor has filed a complaint with the human resources department and the nurse executive regarding the performance of a staff member. If the supervisor subsequently asks about the type of disciplinary action that has been taken, the most appropriate response is to:**

a. Tell the supervisor that steps are being taken to resolve the problem.
b. Outline the disciplinary actions that have been taken in detail.
c. Ask the supervisor what disciplinary actions he or she would advise.
d. Remind the supervisor that all disciplinary actions are confidential.

**74. According to the Model for Ethical Decision Making (Chally and Loriz, 1998), when faced with an ethical dilemma, the first step is to:**

a. obtain more data about the issue.
b. clarify the issue and determine responsibility for decision.
c. obtain legal advice regarding the issue.
d. consider alternative solutions.

**75. If the organization has determined the need for reengineering, the focus is likely to be on:**

a. Improving outcomes
b. Educating staff
c. Reducing costs
d. Clarifying roles

**76. The four behavior types associated with situational leadership include (S1) telling, (S2) selling, (S3) participating, and (S4):**

a. Sharing
b. Collaborating
c. Delegating
d. Empowering

**77. With appreciative inquiry, which focuses on the positive in all individuals and organizations, the constructionist principle refers to the idea that:**

a. Questions themselves promote change.
b. People's words create the life of the organization and cause emotions.
c. People act currently in accordance with their beliefs about the future.
d. Belief creates reality, and interaction creates situations and organizations.

**78. With Bridges' transition model of change, the bridge stage during which people may feel anxious and resentful is referred to as:**

a. Ending, losing
b. Letting go
c. Neutral zone
d. New beginning

**79. If conducting a strengths, weaknesses, opportunities, and threats (SWOT) analysis of the organization, increasing costs of equipment and supplies would be placed in the category of:**

a. Internal environment, strengths
b. Internal environment, weaknesses
c. External environment, strengths
d. External environment, weaknesses

**80. If using the six-step ethical decision-making model developed by Chally and Loriz to deal with ethical dilemmas, the first step is to:**

a. Consider alternative solutions.
b. Obtain more data, including information about legal issues.
c. Clarify the extent/type of dilemma and the person ultimately responsible for making the decision.
d. Assess the outcomes of the decision to determine if the action was effective.

**81. The federal government establishes annual corporate compliance programs for healthcare through the:**

a. Office of Inspector General (OIG)
b. Agency for Healthcare Research and Quality (AHRQ)
c. Bureau of Industry and Security (BIS)
d. Chief compliance officer

**82. A walk-in clinic has two RNs who each work 80 hours (total 160) in a 2-week period and four RNs who each work 40 hours (total 160) in the 2-week period. How many full-time equivalent (FTE) positions are staffed in the clinic?**

a. 2
b. 4
c. 6
d. 8

**83. In a group in which the members participate in decision making but the final decision rests with the leader, the type of decision making used is:**

a. Autocratic
b. Delegated
c. Joint
d. Consultative

**84. Considering the security of information systems in the healthcare organization, survivability refers to:**

a. Ability to maintain security despite threats, system failure, and accidents
b. Life expectancy of hardware and software
c. Ability of hardware to survive electric surges
d. The duration that software can survive before replacement is needed

**85. The nurse executive, in reviewing the use of resources (supplies), notes that one unit has at least double the resource usage of all the other units. The most appropriate response is to:**

    a. Decrease the resource allocation to that unit.

    b. Carry out a utilization study, including necessity and waste.

    c. Demand an accounting by the unit leader.

    d. Assume that the unit has greater needs than other units.

**86. Six critical elements of an emergency operations plan, according to The Joint Commission's Emergency Management Standards, include (1) communications plans, (2) resources and assets, (3) staff roles and responsibilities, (4) safety and security, (5) power/utilities, and (6):**

    a. Transfer protocols

    b. Clinical support activities

    c. Chain of command

    d. Facility damage assessment

**87. The nurse executive is interested in including a patient experience coordinator as part of the staff to improve the patient experience. The primary role of a patient experience coordinator is:**

    a. developing strategies to improve patient satisfaction and outcomes.

    b. communicating with patients and families regarding patients' needs.

    c. reviewing current trends in patient care and advising staff.

    d. gathering data to determine better means of improving patient satisfaction.

**88. The HIPAA Security Rule states that:**

    a. Protected information includes anything in the medical record.

    b. Protected information includes conversations between the doctor and other healthcare providers.

    c. Procedures must be in place to limit access to PHI and disclosures.

    d. Access controls to electronic health information must include encryption/decryption.

**89. Under the Medicare Inpatient Prospective Payment System for acute hospitals, if a hospital-acquired condition (HAC) is present at discharge and the present-on-admission (POA) indicator on the claim is U, this means that Medicare:**

    a. Pays for the condition if the HAC was present and accounted for on admission

    b. Will not pay for the condition if the HAC is present on discharge but not on admission

    c. Will not pay for the condition if the HAC is present and documentation is not adequate to determine if the condition was POA

    d. Will pay for condition if the HAC is present and the healthcare provider cannot determine if the condition was POA

**90. An Advance Beneficiary Notice of Noncoverage (ABN) must be provided for noncovered services to patients with:**

    a. Original Medicare

    b. Medicare managed care programs

    c. Private fee-for-service reimbursement

    d. Medicare Advantage plans

**91.** If a covered entity has a breach of unsecured PHI for 475 patients, the covered entity must notify the secretary of the Department of Health and Human Services (HHS):

    a. Within 60 days
    b. Within 90 days
    c. Annually
    d. No notification is necessary

**92.** Which of the following is an appropriate form of communication to use for telehealth?

    a. SMS text messaging
    b. Skype
    c. Email
    d. Secure messaging

**93.** If a state has a right-to-work law in place, this means that:

    a. No employee is forced to join a union or pay union dues as a requirement of employment.
    b. No employee can be fired if they are part of a union.
    c. Employees have no right to carry out unionization efforts.
    d. Unionization requires 100% support of all employees.

**94.** According to CMS regarding emergency preparedness, each organization must create an emergency plan and conduct a(n):

    a. Audit of supplies
    b. All-hazards risk assessment
    c. Staffing assessment
    d. Feasibility study

**95.** A bedridden patient with end-stage kidney disease has elected not to receive dialysis treatments to prolong life because the quality of life is so poor. Besides the ethical principle of autonomy, which other principle applies to this situation?

    a. Nonmaleficence
    b. Beneficence
    c. Justice
    d. Veracity

**96.** If the hospital has promoted a just culture, and a nurse misreads an order and gives the wrong dosage of a medication, the response should be to:

    a. Identify the cause and console the nurse.
    b. Provide coaching for the nurse.
    c. Take remedial action toward the nurse.
    d. Take punitive/disciplinary action the nurse.

**97.** If employee union organizers want to address fellow employees and ask them to sign authorization cards to show support for the union, they must:

    a. Do so off of company premises
    b. Do so off of company premises and only during off-duty hours
    c. Do so only during off-duty hours
    d. Use only outside organizers on the company's premises

**98. If nurses are assigned to work four 12-hour shifts weekly (totaling 48 hours), how many hours of overtime must the nurses be paid for each week?**

  a. 16
  b. 12
  c. 8
  d. 4

**99. When considering cost allocation for a healthcare facility, which of the following is a direct cost?**

  a. Custodial services
  b. Human resources
  c. Utilities
  d. Nursing staff

**100. When utilizing an ethical framework to facilitate healthcare decision making, *values clarification* refers to:**

  a. objective descriptions of ethical issues.
  b. consideration of medical issues and possible barriers.
  c. determination if personal values impact decisions.
  d. utilization of ethical principles.

**101. The primary advantage of participating in a group purchasing organization (GPO) is to:**

  a. Simplifying ordering
  b. Reducing costs
  c. Establishing relationships
  d. Managing inventory

**102. The CMS Core measure regarding Delivery and Newborn Care, Baby Electively Delivered Early, measures the percentage of infants electively delivered (vaginally or per Caesarean) prior to:**

  a. 36 weeks.
  b. 37 weeks.
  c. 38 weeks.
  d. 39 weeks.

**103. A pro forma is a financial statement that:**

  a. Reviews expenses/revenues that were associated with a new program
  b. Outlines projected expenses/revenues associated with a new program
  c. Outlines expenses associated with planning for a new program
  d. Separates direct and indirect costs associated with a new program

**104. To effectively measure current performance, it's necessary to first:**

  a. Communicate needs
  b. Establish benchmarks
  c. Establish an assessment team
  d. Review past performance

**105. The type of display that is used to manage schedules and estimate times needed to complete tasks when developing improvement projects is the:**

a. Gantt chart
b. PICK chart
c. SIPOC diagram
d. Ishikawa (fishbone) diagram

**106. According to the Patient's and Resident's Bill of Rights, patients and residents of healthcare facilities have the right to expect:**

a. Any requested treatment
b. Freedom from all pain
c. Protection of confidentiality and privacy
d. Legal advice regarding healthcare

**107. According to the Safe Medical Practices Act, manufacturers and medical device user facilities must report problems (e.g., death, serious injuries) with medical devices to MedWatch within:**

a. The annual report
b. 90 working days
c. 30 working days
d. 10 working days

**108. Which of the following is a tool used to determine causes and effects?**

a. Flowchart
b. Ishikawa fishbone diagram
c. Pareto chart
d. Control chart

**109. Electronic clinical quality measures (eCQM) are those that are:**

a. submitted electronically.
b. extracted electronically from certified electronic health records technology (CEHRT)
c. calculated manually.
d. based on direct observations.

**110. When developing a staffing schedule for a unit, which of the following is likely the most useful?**

a. Average daily census
b. Percentage of occupancy
c. Average length of stay
d. Nursing productivity

**111. When carrying out performance appraisal using a rating scale (0 to 5), the nurse executive should be aware of the risk of the "halo" effect, which means that:**

a. Everyone is rated high.
b. Experienced staff are rated higher than inexperienced.
c. Favored staff are rated higher than unfavored.
d. Favored staff are rated lower than unfavored.

**112. If increased numbers of nursing staff report burnout, this usually reflects:**

   a. Individual problems
   b. Nursing problems
   c. Administrative problems
   d. Systemic problems

**113. Characteristics of a high-reliability organization include:**

   a. Eagerness to simplify
   b. Preoccupation with failure
   c. Lack of sensitivity to operations
   d. Downplaying expertise

**114. For a nurse wanting to review a procedure that has not been performed recently, a technique that is especially valuable for preventing error is:**

   a. STAR
   b. SBAR
   c. ARCC
   d. Stop and resolve

**115. One of the five components of the Magnet model is:**

   a. Positive patient outcomes
   b. Job satisfaction
   c. Systemic collaboration
   d. Empirical-quality results

**116. Appreciative inquiry refers to:**

   a. Showing appreciation for staff's contributions
   b. Basing assessment on positive qualities
   c. Looking for the best in people and organizations
   d. Considering positive aspects of research

**117. The major elements of organizational culture are values, vision, and:**

   a. Attitudes
   b. Assumptions and beliefs
   c. Personal relationships
   d. Shared concerns

**118. An individual who has a particular passion or interest in performance improvement and has formed a team to promote performance improvement may be best classified as a:**

   a. Team player
   b. Stakeholder
   c. Leader
   d. Champion

**119. If a hospital does not meet CMS requirements regarding the Hospital Inpatient Quality Reporting (IQR) program, Medicare reimbursement rates may be reduced by:**

    a. 25%.
    b. 20%.
    c. 15%.
    d. 10%.

**120. When hiring travel workers, such as RNs and therapists, it's important to remember that they:**

    a. Are employed by the agency and not the healthcare organization
    b. May leave at any time they choose
    c. Will need a license waiver to work in the state
    d. Are less expensive than other types of employees

**121. In order to calculate FTEs for the entire nursing staff for tax credits, the nurse executive totals all of the employee hours (not counting overtime) and divides by:**

    a. 2,040
    b. 2,400
    c. 2,080
    d. 2,800

**122. Phase one of the strategic planning process is:**

    a. Review of the mission statement, including goals and objectives
    b. Identification of strategies
    c. Assessment of outcomes
    d. Assessment of external and internal environments

**123. A hospital is located in a socioeconomically depressed area in which major employers have closed plants and left, the population has decreased, and three elementary schools have closed. Which proposed program is likely to be most used?**

    a. Family planning
    b. Well-baby
    c. Cardiovascular/stroke rehabilitation
    d. Genetic counseling

**124. When considering nursing hours per patient day, approximately what percentage of a staff member's total hours is typically considered productive hours?**

    a. 90%
    b. 80%
    c. 70%
    d. 60%

**125. Because Medicare does not reimburse adequately for the cost of some laboratory and imaging testing, the hospital has billed twice for procedures that were actually only done one time. This is an example of:**

    a. Embezzlement
    b. Fraud
    c. Abuse
    d. Misrepresentation

126. Conversations between a physician and other healthcare providers about a patient are considered protected information under the:
   a. HIPAA Privacy Rule
   b. HIPAA Security Rule
   c. Stark Law
   d. HITECH Act

127. SMART objectives are specific, measurable, agreed on, realistic, and:
   a. Transferable
   b. Thoughtful
   c. Teachable
   d. Time bound

128. The nursing staff is transitioning to utilization of a warm handoff. Warm handoff refers to transitions between caregivers conducted:
   a. through video conferencing.
   b. after brief rounding.
   c. in front of the patient.
   d. through written format.

129. Which of the following characteristics may be counterproductive for a good team player?
   a. Collaborative
   b. Competitive
   c. Competent
   d. Self-improving

130. Essential to the success of an employee assistance program (EAP) to help with personal or family problems is:
   a. Low or no cost
   b. Paid time off to participate
   c. Confidentiality
   d. Referral

131. The nurse executive has established an employee suggestion program but has had little participation. Which of the following is most likely to encourage participation?
   a. Recognition and rewards
   b. Personal appeals
   c. Confidentiality
   d. Standardized forms

132. When conflicts arise among team members, the approach that is likely to be the most successful at bringing about resolution is:
   a. Researching
   b. Bargaining
   c. Voting
   d. Problem solving

**133. To meet HIPAA requirements, records of HIPAA training must be retained for:**

   a. clinical staff.

   b. support staff.

   c. clinical and administrative staff.

   d. all staff.

**134. According to the National Institute for Occupational Safety and Health (NIOSH) hierarchy of control for exposure to workplace hazards, which of the following is the least effective?**

   a. Administrative controls

   b. Engineering controls

   c. Substitution

   d. Personal protective equipment

**135. An employee absenteeism program should include:**

   a. Posting of daily absences

   b. Attendance policy for employees

   c. Telephone contact for employees using sick time

   d. Timeline for decreased absenteeism

**136. An employee who fell and tore a rotator cuff while on the job is returning to work, but the physician has indicated that she has work restrictions because of the injury. The first step is to:**

   a. Assess the job to determine if the employee can carry out job functions.

   b. Reassign the employee to a less strenuous job until cleared for full work.

   c. Provide the employee with paid time off.

   d. Ask the employee if she would prefer to work or stay home.

**137. Which of the following is especially valuable for compliance efforts to ensure that the healthcare organization is meeting industry standards?**

   a. Clinical observations

   b. Record review

   c. Internal benchmark data

   d. External benchmark data

**138. The nurse executive promotes the use of the CRAF method of recording minutes of meetings for consistency. The C stands for:**

   a. Considerations for the next meeting

   b. Central issues

   c. Conclusions of group discussion

   d. Communication

**139. A patient with Alzheimer's disease has run out of insurance benefits and is being discharged from a skilled nursing facility because the patient does not qualify for Medicaid and cannot afford to pay for care. The ethical principle that is threatened is:**

   a. Autonomy

   b. Justice

   c. Nonmaleficence

   d. Beneficence

**140. When developing a website to promote the hospital and the nursing department, layout considerations include:**

    a. The colors red and green should be avoided.
    b. Complex designs are more effective than simple designs.
    c. Borders should be used around text and photos.
    d. Images and text should be scattered around the page.

**141. Which of the following outlines the four elements needed to create and sustain a patient safety culture?**

    a. The National Academy of Medicine (formerly the Institute of Medicine)
    b. The National Quality Forum
    c. The Agency for Healthcare Research's Quality Indicators
    d. The Leapfrog Group

**142. Under HIPAA compliance regulations regarding workforce security, workforce clearance procedures refer to:**

    a. supervising individuals who have access to electronic PHI.
    b. establishing safeguards to prevent access to electronic PHI.
    c. terminating access to electronic PHI when individuals are no longer employed.
    d. determining whether individual's access to electronic PHI is appropriate.

**143. When conducting research, which type of study provides the best evidence?**

    a. Systematic review of randomized trials
    b. Systematic review of observational studies
    c. Single observational study
    d. Physiologic studies

**144. The primary cause of nursing turnover in hospitals is:**

    a. Job opportunities elsewhere
    b. Job dissatisfaction
    c. Aging of the nursing workforce
    d. Pay-related

**145. If members of the nursing staff work a fluctuating workweek at a fixed salary that doesn't vary, the overtime rate the staff members must receive for each overtime hour greater than 40 hours per week is at least:**

    a. 0.5
    b. 1.0
    c. 1.5
    d. 2.0

**146. Oncology staff are interested in beginning a volunteer peer mentoring program for breast cancer patients to help them navigate treatment. Which of the following is the most important element to ensure the program is successful in the long-term?**

    a. Evidence-based metrics
    b. Staff engagement
    c. Financial aid
    d. Volunteer training

**147. Which of the following is the most appropriate example of assertive communication?**

a. "I'm very unhappy with the way you are shouting at me."
b. "You need to calm down, show respect, and stop shouting at me."
c. "I can see that you are upset, but I need you to stop shouting so we can find a solution."
d. "This is the way you always respond when you are upset!"

**148. According to the ADKAR (Hiatt) method for facilitating change, during the first step (awareness), the role of the leader is to:**

a. Provide training to prepare staff for change.
b. Communicate the need for change.
c. Recommend specific changes.
d. Seek input about the need for change.

**149. With servant leadership, the focus is on:**

a. Following orders and supporting leadership
b. Collaboration and participation at all levels
c. Development of leadership potential in staff
d. Meeting goals and positive outcomes

**150. According to FEMA, the four phases of an Emergency Management Program include (1) mitigation, (2) preparedness:**

a. (3) impact assessment, and (4) participation.
b. (3) participation, and (4) response.
c. (3) response, and (4) recovery.
d. (3) risk assessment, and (4) participation.

# Answer Key and Explanations for Test #2

**1. A:** If a job applicant has a history of trying to unionize at a previous job and the healthcare organization declines to hire the applicant for that reason, this is an unfair labor practice because, under the Labor Management Relations Act of 1947 (aka the Taft-Hartley Act), discrimination in employment because of union activities is not allowed. Other unfair labor practices include interference with employees in their right to organize, interference with a labor organization, discrimination against employees who have filed charges or provided testimony related to the act, refusal to engage in good-faith bargaining, or engagement in "hot cargo" agreements.

**2. C:** One of the eligibility criteria for the Magnet Recognition Program is that all nurse leaders must have, at a minimum, a BSN in nursing. This also applies to nurse managers and the top nurse educator. Nurses in specialty roles, such as wound ostomy nurses, must also have a minimum of a BSN. The chief nursing officer (CNO) must have, at a minimum, an MSN. If the master's degree is outside of nursing (such as in administration), then the CNO must have a BSN or a doctorate in nursing.

**3. D:** If a mass-casualty incident occurs and triggers the need for critical incident stress management, the first step to critical incident stress debriefing is defusing sessions. Steps in defusing include the following:

1. Defusing sessions begin during or immediately after the stressful event; they are used to educate actively involved personnel about what to expect over the next few days and to provide guidance in handling feelings and stress.
2. Debriefing sessions are held in 1 to 3 days and repeated periodically. These may include those directly and indirectly involved. The six phases of debriefing are introduction, fact sharing, discussing feelings, describing symptoms, teaching, and reentry.
3. Follow-up happens usually after approximately 1 week.

**4. A:** To encourage a community with a large population of undocumented immigrants to attend a free clinic, the best method of outreach is to gain the support of community leaders (not necessarily elected officials). Community leaders may include priests, ministers, business owners, and others that the community members respect and trust. Undocumented immigrants are often afraid to seek help and need assurance from someone they trust that they will not be reported to immigration officials.

**5. B:** If an employee feels that the healthcare organization has not provided a safe working environment, the employee may file a complaint with the Occupational Safety and Health Administration (OSHA). The employee can also request that OSHA conduct an inspection of the workplace. Complaints can be submitted through an online complaint form; by fax, mail, or email; in person; and by telephone. If the employee experiences retaliation, the employee can also file a whistleblower complaint.

**6. C:** Although long-term-care facilities must carry out the same testing exercises as other inpatient facilities, such as critical access hospitals, hospitals, and transplant centers, only long-term-care facilities must conduct an annual review of the emergency preparedness plan/program and must also conduct annual training in the plan/program to ensure that staff members know their roles during an emergency. Other inpatient facilities must only conduct review and training of their plans/programs biennially (every 2 years).

216

**7. D:** If the turnover rate of staff has been >40% and a new leader works with the staff to improve the working environment, resulting in a reduction of turnover to 10%, the strength that the leader is exhibiting is relationship building. Executing is the ability to make decisions and act. Influencing is the ability to convince others, and strategic thinking is the ability to plan ahead and make necessary changes.

**8. A:** The nurse executive's role in the recruitment and retention of staff who are skilled, compassionate, and motivated is a critical factor in improving patient experience. Patient satisfaction is tied closely to the quality of interactions patients have with healthcare providers. The nurse executive's role in budgeting is also important, as answer C suggests, because staffing is dependent on the budget. The nurse executive may have a role in determining budgeting priorities and must be a strong advocate for hiring staff members.

**9. D:** If an employee has not met performance expectations, the initial intervention should be to immediately counsel the employee regarding expectations and areas in which the employee has failed to meet performance expectations to allow the employee time to rectify the situation. All actions taken must be carefully documented. If counseling does not resolve the situation, the next step is to begin disciplinary procedures that may end in termination in some cases.

**10. A:** According to The Joint Commission, healthcare organizations must carry out competency validation for new hires and staff members on hiring and on an ongoing basis for all staff members. A competency validation plan should be developed that lists skills and the necessary frequency of competency validation. Advanced skills that are done infrequently may need more frequent competency validation than skills that are carried out daily. Competency validation should also be done as needs arise.

**11. C:** If a job applicant has an obvious disability, under provisions of the Americans with Disabilities Act, the nurse executive may ask if the applicant can carry out job functions with or without accommodations. The nurse executive may not ask about the extent of the disability, whether it will interfere with job duties, or how many sick days the applicant has used in the past year. Questions should remain focused on the person's ability to carry out the functions needed for the job and not on the disability.

**12. C:** Patient surveys provide a valuable resource in evaluation of healthcare quality. Studies have consistently shown that the interactions between the patient and/or family with healthcare providers is likely to have the greatest effect—either negative or positive—on patient satisfaction. For example, patients are more likely to be satisfied with treatment if the healthcare provider takes the time to explain the treatment in terms the patient can understand and treats the patient's concerns and opinions with respect.

**13. D:** If a nurse leaves a clinical unit without notifying anyone, leaving patients unattended, this violates (1) the duty owed to the client. Then the nurse failed to provide pain medication that a patient had requested, so this constitutes (2) a breach of duty. The subsequent fall (3) can be traced to the nurse's lack of response to the pain medication request, and the broken hip (4) is the damage caused by the accident. If four elements of negligence are present, then this meets the requirement for malpractice.

**14. D:** When individuals utilize mobile technology, such as a smart watch, to monitor health activities, this is referred to as mHealth. While initially mHealth was used almost exclusively to monitor fitness (activity, steps), the capability of the devices has improved. Some devices now monitor heartrate and rhythm, can detect abnormalities, and transmit an electrocardiogram in real time when abnormalities occur. The line between fitness devices and medical devices is becoming more blurred over time as individuals opt to utilize health monitoring by their devices without medical guidance.

**15. C:** CMS record retention requirements for healthcare providers include 5 years for regular Medicare and 10 years for Medicare managed care programs. However, retention issues can become complicated. State laws govern retention of health records and in some cases may extend these time periods. Although HIPAA does not contain retention provisions, it does require that covered entities (such as those billing Medicare) retain the required documentation for 6 years.

**16. D:** The factor evaluation system of patient classification uses patient care activities to determine direct hours of care needed for the patient. Each intervention is given a rating or time expectation, and these are added to determine overall needs. This system is primarily objective as opposed to the prototype evaluation system, which is subjective and narrative and classifies patients into broad categories based on their diagnoses and then predicts needs based on those categories.

**17. A:** Asking staff and community members who are ethnic minorities to share healthcare experiences, both negative and positive, as part of staff training is leveraging diversity. The nurse executive is including ethnic minorities to participate in an open dialogue in order to promote a diverse perspective and acceptance and awareness of cultural diversity.

**18. C:** If inexperienced nurses complain of lateral violence (e.g., bullying, insults, gossiping) from more experienced nurses in a healthcare organization, the nurse executive should establish a zero-tolerance policy that outlines expectations and consequences. Although lateral violence is a pervasive problem in healthcare, that is not an excuse. All staff should be educated about the policy and staff members assured that they can report any incidence of lateral violence (directed toward them or others) without retribution.

**19. B:** If the nurse executive notes that a large part of the budget goes to inventory but outdated products have resulted in unnecessary waste, the approach that is likely the most cost effective is just-in-time ordering. With just-in-time ordering, new supplies are ordered when the stock is almost depleted so that less money is tied up in inventory, but this is most effective with automatic reordering, which is more efficient with computerized inventories.

**20. A:** The FLSA requires that employers provide a basic minimum wage and overtime payment, although some states may impose additional requirements. The FLSA does not address holiday and sick pay, premium payment for working holidays, or immediate severance pay. The basic minimum wage is periodically increased. FLSA provisions apply toward businesses with annual gross sales of at least $500,000, healthcare organizations, public agencies, and schools.

**21. B:** In order to function as an effective team, a group of people must work collectively to achieve the same goals. A team is a consistent group of people and is different from a work group, whose members may refer to themselves as part of a team but whose membership changes depending on who is scheduled to work. Team members are typically assigned specific roles, although the role of leader may rotate among the team members.

**22. D:** The first element of a business plan for a proposed new clinic should be the executive summary, which outlines all of the key elements of the business proposal, including customers, product/services, goals, risks, opportunities, costs, management, and timelines. Complete elements include the summary as well as a description of the product/service, management organization, market survey, marketing strategies, organizational structure, timeline, risk factors, and appendices (e.g., samples of forms and any other necessary additional information).

**23. A:** Patient-centered care involves engaging the patient and family in all aspects of care in order to achieve desired outcomes. Traditional care has often been disease-driven or provider-driven, with the focus on diagnosis and treatment rather than individual patient needs. In order to make improvements in the provision of patient-centered care, leadership is the critical element. The leader must actively endorse patient-centered care, lead by example, provide evidence-based data in support of change, and establish expectations.

**24. A:** Core measure sets developed by the Core Quality Measures Collaborative for Primary Care are intended for use in value-based payment programs. Measures are included for cardiovascular care (controlling high blood pressure), diabetes (hemoglobin A1C testing), care coordination/patient safety (medication reconciliation), prevention and wellness (cervical cancer screening), use and cost/overuse (imaging for low back pain), patient experience (surveys), behavioral health (12-month depression response), pulmonary (asthma medication ratio), and readmissions (plan all-cause readmission).

**25. C:** When considering HPPD as part of staffing and budget planning, the unit type that typically requires the greatest number of HPPD is pediatric critical care (approximately 19 hours) followed by adult critical care (approximately 16 hours). Neonatal care (approximately 12 hours) also has a high HPPD requirement, but adult surgical (approximately 6 hours) requires a lower HPPD. Staffing needs can be projected based on the unit type and the average patient census.

**26. D:** The rights of employees to organize and engage in collective bargaining is provided by the National Labor Relations Act (1935). The act provides private-sector employees the right to unionize and carry out not only collective bargaining but also collective actions, including strikes. The act also banned unfair labor practices, such as union busting, and established the National Labor Relations Board.

**27. B:** Skill-mix staffing, in which various levels of nursing (e.g., registered nurse [RN], licensed vocational nurse [LVN]/licensed practical nurse [LPN], and unlicensed assistive personnel [UAP]) are engaged in patient care rather than only RNs or licensed personnel, is often used as a method of reducing staffing costs because it allows for higher nurse-to-patient ratios. A team-nursing approach with good communication among the different levels of nursing is essential in order to maintain the quality of care.

**28. A:** Redaction is a method of rendering unsecured PHI unusable, unreadable, or indecipherable that is specifically excluded under HIPAA provisions. Acceptable methods include encryption (consistent with NIST Sp. Pub. 800-111 or complies with NIST Sp. Pub. 800-52 or 800-77). The media on which data are stored may be destroyed, shredded, or (for electronic storage) purged (consistent with NIST Sp. Pub. 800-88). Whichever method is used, the PHI should not be retrievable.

**29. B:** The acuity model of staffing is based on the hours of care needed. The acuity rating may be calculated using different parameters, such as diagnoses and interventions needed. In some cases, the nurses caring for the patients assign an acuity rating for the oncoming staff members. In other cases, a software program calculates acuity ratings based on specific types of input (e.g., ages, treatments, diagnoses). Using an acuity tool provides more consistency than depending on subjective assessment.

**30. D:** If a staff member exerts power over others by exploiting a personal relationship that the individual has with a board member, this is an example of referent power—power that is gained by affiliating with those in power. Legitimate power is that received through licensure, education, and credentialing. Coercive power comes from the ability to apply punishment or discipline. Connection power comes from relationships that enhance one's resources.

**31. B:** If the nurse executive takes care in practice to avoid conflicts of interest or boundary violations, this supports provision 2 of the ANA Code of Ethics: "The nurse's primary commitment is to the patient, whether an individual, family, group, community, or population. The elements of this provision include (2.1) the primacy of the patient's interests, (2.2) conflict of interest for nurses, (2.3) collaboration, and (2.4) professional boundaries."

**32. B:** Although mandated nurse-to-patient ratios are still not common, the average nurse-to-patient ratio for medical-surgical patients in acute care is 1:5. This is also the ratio that is mandated by California, the only state with mandated nurse-to-patient ratios for units other than the intensive care unit. (Note that California raised the ratios during the coronavirus pandemic because of nursing shortages.) Healthcare facilities in many states can set their own staffing standards, and some states require only that the facilities have plans to manage staffing ratios.

**33. C:** According to Tuckman's group development model, the norming stage is characterized by team members developing positive feelings toward each other, working well together, and identifying with and feeling attached to their team. The stages are as follows:

- Forming: the leader provides direction, and members are unsure of their roles.
- Storming: conflicts may arise and leadership may be challenged.
- Norming: the team is expressing positive feelings toward each other and feeling attached.
- Performing: the team is working effectively and achieving goals.
- Adjourning/Mourning: some of the team members may find it difficult to leave the team.

**34. A:** In the communication component of the emergency preparedness plan for the healthcare organization, succession planning refers to identifying staff who can assume the role of someone else who is absent during an emergency. For example, the plan may include all those trained to manage patients on ventilators or to work in surgery. It may be the case that the absence is caused by death or injury related to the emergency as well. The communication plan should include a system to locate all on-duty staff and patients and to contact off-duty staff.

**35. B:** The operating budget includes general expenses, such as salaries, education, insurance, maintenance, depreciation, and debts, as well as profits. The capital budget includes allocations for remodeling, repairing, building, and equipment. The cash balance budget project cash balances for a specific period of time (including operating and capital budget items). The master budget combines all of the various budgets of an organization.

**36. D:** A continuous/rolling budget approach involves carrying out periodic updates to the operational budget prior to the next budget cycle. With a zero-based approach, all cost centers are evaluated each budget period to determine if they should be funded or eliminated. With a fixed/forecast approach, revenue and expenses are forecast for the entire budget period and budget items are fixed. With a flexible approach, estimates are made regarding anticipated changes in revenue and expenses and both fixed and variable costs are included.

**37. C:** As the last step CMS requires for compliance regarding emergency preparedness, healthcare organizations with inpatient providers must test their emergency preparedness plan annually with one full-scale exercise and one additional exercise (full-scale or less). Outpatient providers are required to carry out one exercise annually. The other five steps required include performing a risk analysis, establishing a plan, developing policies and procedures against risks, developing a communication plan, and training staff to readily be able to implement the plan.

**38. B:** Nonproductive FTEs are those hours for which staff members are paid but are not working. Nonproductive FTEs include paid holiday time, vacation time, sick time, and education and training time. Other nonproductive FTEs can include jury time, military leave, and personal leave (such as to attend a funeral). Nonproductive FTEs must be calculated in order to determine the costs for replacement FTEs. Nonproductive FTEs usually average 10% or more of the total hours.

**39. A:** A primary goal of transformational leadership is to empower staff members without relinquishing total control. The transformational leader leads by example, looks for leadership qualities in others, and encourages and supports collaboration rather than competition. Transformational leadership generally includes some form of shared governance (such as staff-led councils) so that staff members feel like they have a voice in decision making and are motivated to provide better care.

**40. C:** Transactional leaders ensure that goals are met through a system of sanctions and rewards. This type of leader focuses on supervision and performance and is very task oriented, but criticism may be used more than reward in order to achieve goals. Transactional leadership may work well in emergent situations, but it is less successful over the long term because staff members are more encouraged to follow rules than to think innovatively.

**41. A:** According to the AHRQ TeamSTEPPS program, the three phases needed to develop a team approach to a culture of safety are:

- Assessment of the need: Determine readiness.
- Planning, training, and implementation: Design a plan to train staff regarding team-building skills and the use of specific tools, such as SBAR, to facilitate communication.
- Sustainment: Continue team-building improvements and the use of strategies that were taught.

**42. D:** If a nurse executive adapts leadership styles to accommodate staff members' levels of competence, varying from a task-oriented approach (directive) to a relationship-oriented approach (collaborative), this type of leadership is situational. This is the most flexible leadership style because the leader is able to assess each situation and task, establish goals, and use a leadership approach based on each staff member's abilities and need for guidance. Most leaders tend to use the same leadership style in all situations, but the needs of inexperienced and experienced staff members may be widely divergent.

**43. D:** Some patients are very complacent and complain little, while others may complain about almost everything. The latter are often labeled as "difficult" or "demanding," and this can affect not only their perception of care, but the provision of care as well. Patients who appear angry and demanding are often responding to their own fear and loss of autonomy. The most appropriate response is to empathize with how the patient is feeling, saying something like, "I'm sorry you are so upset," and then suggesting collaboration by asking something like, "How can we work together to improve things?" This will make the patient feel a sense of control.

**44. C:** The Affordable Care Act (2010) requires that healthcare providers who are enrolled in Medicare, Medicaid, or the Children's Health Insurance Program adopt compliance programs. Earlier, the Deficit Reduction Act (2005) required that healthcare organizations that received revenues from Medicaid of greater than $5 million have a compliance program in place. This act included provisions that employees and business partners be informed about the False Claims Act.

**45. A:** The three aspects of care that nursing-sensitive indicators reflect are structural indicators, process indicators, and outcome indicators:

- Structural: hours of direct care, skill mix, turnover, and education/certification.
- Process: pain assessment, risk assessment, no-shows/cancellations, median encounter time, emergency department encounters involving hospital admission, and a patient leaving without receiving care or against medical advice.
- Outcomes: unplanned hospital transfers, falls/falls with injury, number of visits with any errors, and number of visits with burns.

**46. D:** Although patient monitoring is helpful for those who lack transportation resources or live a far distance from healthcare providers, it is especially beneficial for patients with chronic health problems because of the large number of these patients and the costs of care. Studies have shown that those with remote patient monitoring have fewer hospitalizations, a shorter length of stay, and greater patient satisfaction. Because the response is almost immediate when problems arise, morbidity and mortality are decreased.

**47. B:** Predictive analytics helps to predict outcomes based on algorithms. Based on the patient's diagnosis, historical and current data are input into a software program that uses the data to make predictions about patient risk, such as the risk of rehospitalization or deep venous thrombosis. Armed with this information, healthcare providers can take preventive steps and make decisions about clinical care. Predictive analytics may guide care for inpatients and at-home patients for follow-up care.

**48. C:** If a breach of unsecured PHI of 20 patients occurred and the covered entity is unable to contact more than 10 individuals, the next step is to post a notice on the entity's website for at least 90 days. As an alternative, the covered entity may provide notice in major print or broadcast outlets. If unable to reach fewer than 10 individuals, then the covered entity may provide a substitute form of notice, such as by telephone.

**49. A:** If a hospital has experienced a breach of unsecured PHI for more than 500 patients, the notices that are required are individual notices (a written letter or email if the patient previously agreed to this method of contact) for each patient and notices to major media outlets, typically through a press release that will be disseminated to print and broadcast media in the area where the breach occurred.

**50. D:** Managing and supervising physicians is outside of the scope of practice for the nurse executive/administrator. The nurse administrator is responsible for managing and supervising nursing staff, assistant administrators, and other workers. The nurse administrator also has a number of business and administrative duties, including developing and managing budgets, reporting to the board of directors, handling human resources issues, and ensuring compliance with regulations.

**51. D:** The first step in facilitating a patient experience program is to assess the current status, usually through patient satisfaction surveys, interviews, or focus groups. The next step is to define the goals of the program and to gain the participation of key stakeholders. The final steps are to develop a plan or strategy to achieve the goals that have been outlined; speak directly to patients, families, and caregivers about their experiences; develop an advisory committee; make engagement a priority; and educate the staff.

**52. B:** When using Lean Six Sigma as a method of process improvement, the focus is on long-term and strategies. The basis of this program is to reduce error and waste within the organization through continuous learning and rapid change. Characteristics of Lean Six Sigma include the following:

- Long-term goals with strategies in place for 1- to 3-year periods
- Performance improvement as the underlying belief system
- Cost reduction through quality increases, supported by statistics evaluating the cost of inefficiency
- Incorporation of an improvement methodology, such as DMAIC, PDCA, or other methods

**53. A:** Plan-do-check-act (PDCA) is a method of problem solving that is better suited to solving specific problems than organizational problems. Steps of PDCA include the following:

- Plan: Identifying, analyzing, and defining the problem and goals and establishing a process through brainstorming, data collection, and analysis
- Do: Generating solutions, selecting one or more of them, and then implementing each solution on a trial basis
- Check: Gathering and analyzing data to determine the effectiveness of the solution
- Act: Identifying changes needed to fully implement a solution, adopting the solution, and continuing to monitor the results

**54. D:** If a problem such as an increased rate of surgical site infections has occurred, the first step in developing process improvement plans should be to conduct an RCA, which is a retrospective attempt to determine the cause of an event. RCA involves interviews, observations, questionnaires, and reviews of medical records. Every step in the hospitalization and care experience, including every treatment, medication, and contact, is traced. The focus of the RCA is on systems and processes rather than on individuals.

**55. C:** Failure mode and effects analysis is indicated before full implementation of new processes developed as part of quality improvement. This team-based prospective analysis aims to identify and correct failures in a process before implementation. Steps include:

1. Defining: Outlining the process in detail
2. Creating a team: Ad hoc team of those involved in the process or those with expertise
3. Describing: A numbered flowchart describes each step and substep
4. Brainstorming: Each step/substep is analyzed for potential failures

**56. C:** Fee for service is the payor method that rewards healthcare providers for the quantity of patients seen rather than the quality of healthcare given or positive outcomes and disincentivizes cost-saving efforts. A set payment for service is established, and the healthcare provider receives the payment regardless of outcome. There is little motivation with this type of payment structure for the healthcare provider to innovate or to avoid unnecessary testing.

**57. A:** When conducting a literature review, the first issue to consider is the source of the material. Juried journals are the most reliable (although not infallible), whereas articles in the popular press cannot be relied upon for evidence-based research. The next step is to review the date and the author(s) as well as the credentials of the author(s). For current practice, the date should be within 5 years, but it may be older if reviewing historical information.

**58. D:** The payor system with which the healthcare provider receives incentive payments if the costs of care are lower than predicted but also has to bear additional costs if costs are higher than predicted is value based, risk share. The majority of current value-based plans are value based, gain share in which the healthcare provider receives a percentage of the savings. The primary goal of value-based reimbursement plans is to increase the quality of healthcare while reducing costs.

**59. A:** A research question should require further knowledge to find the answer. If a question can be answered by using problem solving or through literature research to find already existing knowledge, then the question relates to the need for information but not to new research. The answer to the research question should have the potential to provide information and create or refine knowledge about a subject.

**60. C:** Population health focuses on prevention—keeping people healthy and avoiding unnecessary and costly procedures. Preventive measures are especially aimed at chronic illness because this has such an impact on patient care and the costs of care. Population health depends on the leadership of primary care physicians to identify those at risk, the active participation of patients in their own healthcare, and increased collaboration and coordination of care.

**61. B:** If a research project has been completed and the nurse executive wants to disseminate the findings, the first step is to develop a dissemination plan. Elements of the plan should include the overall purpose of dissemination (inform, increase awareness, obtain feedback), the target audience (general public, nursing, other healthcare professionals), the key information that should be shared (conclusions), the method of delivery (print, video, audio, in person), and the timing for dissemination.

**62. A:** If a hospital has seen a recent increase in falls among patients, when responding, the nurse executive should seek input from the risk management department. The task of risk management is to reduce risk factors that may cause a negative effect, such as through loss of income, loss of reputation, or liability costs. Steps to risk management include identifying, assessing, mitigating risk, monitoring, and reporting risk.

**63. C:** If a staff member states, "You're doing a good job, considering how little experience you've had," this type of communication is passive-aggressive. The person is making what appears to be a compliment, but it is followed by an indirect insult. People who are passive-aggressive often deny anger and resentment but express it indirectly, delay or fail to carry out duties, suggest they didn't understand directions, fail to share important information, try to make others look bad, and pretend to joke when insulting someone.

**64. B:** According to Kurt Lewin's change management theory, an example of refreezing is when the new team-focused nursing model is accepted and successful. The three stages:

- Motivation (unfreezing): Dissatisfaction occurs but also fear of change or anxiety, leading to resistance.
- Desire to change (unfrozen): The desire for change is evident, but needed changes must be identified.
- Development of permanent change (refreezing): The new behavior becomes habitual.

**65. A:** According to Havelock's six-stage model for planned change, an integral part of the change process is resistance. Havelock proposes that change can be planned and carried out in a series of

224

sequential phases. Change agents should build relationships with the system through understanding the dynamics and culture, diagnosing problems, obtaining necessary resources, selecting a solution, garnering acceptance, stabilizing the change, and facilitating self-renewal.

**66. C:** According to force field analysis (Lewin), the two subgroups for proposed changes are:

- Restraining forces: These are forces that resist change, such as poor attitudes, hostility, inadequate equipment, or insufficient funds.
- Driving forces: These are forces responsible for instigating and promoting change, such as leaders, incentives, and competition.

Steps to force field analysis include listing proposed changes and dividing them into two subgroups (i.e., driving forces and restraining forces), brainstorming, discussing the value of the proposed changes, and developing a plan.

**67. C:** If, in a conflict between a supervisor and a nurse on a unit, the nurse cedes to the supervisor, who is in a position of power, this approach to conflict resolution is categorized as accommodating. Conflict resolution approaches are as follows:

| | |
|---|---|
| **Accommodating** | One party ceding to the other |
| **Avoiding** | Avoiding the conflict |
| **Collaborating or negotiating** | Trying to please both parties |
| **Competing** | One party trying to win at all costs |
| **Compromising** | Each party ceding something in return for harmony |
| **Confronting** | Using "I" messages and assertive problem solving |
| **Forcing** | One party issuing orders to force a solution |
| **Reassuring** | Attempting to make everyone happy |
| **Problem solving** | Trying to find a solution that works for everyone using a step-by-step approach |
| **Withdrawing** | One party withdraws, so the conflict is unresolved |

**68. B:** Steps to conflict resolution include:

1. Allow both parties to present their side of the conflict without bias, maintaining a focus on opinions rather than on individuals.
2. Encourage cooperation through negotiation and compromise.
3. Maintain the focus, providing guidance to keep the discussions on track and avoid arguments.
4. Evaluate the need for renegotiation, a formal resolution process, or a third party.
5. Use humor and empathy to defuse escalating tensions.
6. Summarize the issues, outlining key arguments.
7. Avoid forcing a resolution, if possible.

**69. D:** The model for change of health behavior that focuses on changes in behavior based on an individual's decision is the transtheoretical model. Stages of the transtheoretical model include:

- Precontemplation: The person has no intention of changing a behavior in the next 6 months.
- Contemplation: The person intends to change in the next 6 months but is not ready yet.
- Preparation: The person intends to initiate change in the near future (≤1 month) and is ready.

- Action: The person is modifying a behavior according to a set criterion.
- Maintenance: The person works to maintain changes and gains confidence that he or she will not relapse.

**70. A:** If proactive strategies such as compromise have been unable to resolve a conflict, making an organizational change that eliminates the basis for the conflict is an indirect solution. Other defensive measures may provide direct solutions, including the following:

- Separating the parties to the conflict: This can mean assigning them to different teams or to different shifts or work schedules with different days off in order to avoid contact between those in conflict.
- Avoiding/suppressing conflict: The parties in conflict may choose to avoid discussing the issue or problems or may be advised to do so by supervisory personnel.
- Ignoring the conflict: The parties in conflict may agree to disagree and to set the conflict aside and deal with other issues.

**71. D:** According to the ANA, a healthy work environment has the following elements:

- Safety: Workers are entitled to environmental safety (e.g., fire escapes and good air quality, lighting, and heating) and physical and emotional safety (e.g., freedom from bullying and violence).
- Empowerment: Healthcare workers should have autonomy commensurate with their position and training and should participate in decision making through some type of shared governance.
- Satisfaction: Contributing factors include adequate wages, reasonable workload, good scheduling of work hours, flexible working schedules, and a supportive, nonpunitive environment.

**72. A:** If an organization supports the concept of pervasive leadership, this means that everyone is believed to have leadership potential and can influence others. Pervasive leadership uses mentoring, training, and role modeling to help staff members become better leaders, and power and data are shared. Pervasive leadership recognizes the power found in groups and allows group members a greater degree of autonomy in making decisions and solving problems rather than having to wait for a central authority to make decisions.

**73. D:** If a nursing supervisor asks about the disciplinary action taken toward a particular staff member, the most appropriate response is to remind the supervisor that all disciplinary actions are confidential. Any discussion of performance or discipline should always take place in private, and steps to the disciplinary process should be followed consistently.

**74. B:** Chally, a professor of nursing, and Loriz, a professor and director of a school of nursing, developed the Model for Ethical Decision Making in 1998 to assist nurses in dealing with ethical dilemmas. Steps to ethical decision-making include:

1. Clarifying the extent/type of dilemma and who is ultimately responsible for making the decision.
2. Obtaining more data, including information about legal issues, such as the obligation to report.
3. Considering alternative solutions.
4. Arriving at a decision after considering risk/benefits and discussing it with the individual.

5. Acting on the decision and utilizing collaboration as needed.
6. Assessing the outcomes of the decision to determine if the chosen action was effective.

**75. A:** If the organization has determined the need for reengineering, the focus is likely to be on improving outcomes. Rather than simply reviewing processes and trying to find ways to improve them, reengineering starts from scratch and tries to identify new processes that will result in improved outcomes as well as be cost-effective. Priorities may be changed, and resources may be reallocated in order to improve efficiency. Reengineering is dependent on input from consumers, such as through patient satisfaction surveys, and the support and engagement of staff.

**76. C:** The four behavior types associated with situational leadership include:

- (S1) Telling: The leader is in charge with one-way communication.
- (S2) Selling: The leader is in charge with two-way communication and provision of social and emotional support.
- (S3) Participating: The leader uses shared decision making for aspects of tasks.
- (S4) Delegating: The leader is involved but is no longer responsible for tasks.

This leadership style is flexible and changes according the situation and the skills and needs of the workers. Situational leaders need the ability to diagnose, adapt, and communicate.

**77. D:** With appreciative inquiry, which focuses on the positive in all individuals and organizations, major principles include:

- Constructionist: Belief creates reality and interaction creates situations and organizations.
- Simultaneity: Questions themselves promote change.
- Poetic: People's words create the life of the organization and cause emotions.
- Anticipatory: People act currently in accordance with their beliefs about the future.
- Positive: Change necessitates social cohesion and positive sentiments.

**78. C:** With Bridges' transition model of change, the stages of transitions that people experience are:

- Ending, losing, letting go: People are often resistive and experience various emotions, such as fear and denial, when they have to face the end of something with which they are familiar and comfortable.
- Neutral zone: This is the bridge stage during which people may feel anxious and resentful, especially as caseloads may increase or change; however, this is also a time of creative energy.
- New beginning: People have begun to accept and feel positive about change and can benefit from rewards and celebration.

**79. B:** If conducting a SWOT analysis of the organization, increasing costs of equipment and supplies would be placed in the category "internal environment, weaknesses." Examples of internal and external environment analyses include:

| Internal environment | | External environment | |
|---|---|---|---|
| Strengths | Weaknesses | Opportunities | Threats |
| Financial stability | Increasing costs | Increased population | Low reimbursement |
| Programs, | Outdated | New programs | Regulations |
| services | equipment | New markets | Competition |
| Staff persons | Ineffective | Stakeholders | Political changes |
| Client/Staff | programs | | |
| satisfaction | Marketing | | |

**80. C:** If using the six-step ethical decision-making model developed by Chally and Loriz to deal with ethical dilemmas, the steps are:

1. Clarifying the extent/type of dilemma and who is ultimately responsible for making the decision
2. Obtaining more data, including information about legal issues, such as the obligation to report
3. Considering alternative solutions
4. Arriving at a decision after considering risks/benefits and discussing them with the individual
5. Acting on the decision and using collaboration as needed
6. Assessing the outcomes of the decision to determine if the chosen action was effective

**81. A:** The federal government establishes annual corporate compliance programs for healthcare through the OIG. Each organization must develop an individual compliance plan, which should establish internal controls so that the organization does not violate state or federal rules, laws, or regulations, such as by carrying out fraudulent billing practices. Corporate compliance includes developing written standards of conduct and policies and procedures to ensure adherence. A chief compliance officer must be responsible for monitoring compliance, and staff must be educated about compliance issues.

**82. B:** If a walk-in clinic has two RNs who each work 80 hours (total 160) in a 2-week period and four RNs who each work 40 hours (total 160) in the 2-week period, four FTE positions are staffed in the clinic. One FTE is equal to a combination of one or more than one staff member who works 80 hours in 14 days. In this case, two nurses work full time (80 hours per 14 days) for two FTEs and four work half time (40 hours in 14 days) for two FTEs.

**83. D:** In a group in which the members participate in decision making but the final decision rests with the leader, the type of decision making used is consultative. With autocratic decision making, the leader makes decisions and, although the leader may receive input, there is no vote. In joint decision making, the final decision is made by the members of the group rather than the leader, who has the same vote as other members. In delegated decision making, the leader may have input, but the members make the decision and the leader does not have a vote.

**84. A:** Considering the security of information systems in the healthcare organization, survivability refers to the ability of a system to maintain security despite threats, system failures, and accidents. Planning should be in place to assess risks in these areas and to prevent problems. Risks to survivability can include attacks or threats (e.g., insiders, hackers), vulnerability (e.g., inherent weakness), malicious software, phishing (e.g., fake emails or websites that try to get information such as passwords), and spam (which may introduce malware or viruses).

**85. B:** If the nurse executive, in reviewing the use of resources (supplies), notes that one unit has at least double the resource usage of all other units, the most appropriate response is to carry out a utilization study, including necessity and waste. The study may be aimed at only the high-use unit or all units because there may be underutilization on some units and the acuity level and needs of patients may differ considerably, so having a greater use of resources may indicate a greater necessity.

**86. B:** An emergency operations plan, according to The Joint Commission's Emergency Management Standards, is intended to provide guidance for response to an emergency situation in which a hospital cannot rely on the community or others for support and for recovery. The six critical elements are (1) communications plans, (2) resources and assets, (3) staff roles and responsibilities, (4) safety and security, (5) power/utilities, and (6) clinical support activities.

**87. A:** A patient experience coordinator has many roles in an organization, but the primary role is the development of strategies to improve patient satisfaction and outcomes. In order to achieve this, the patient experience coordinator collaborates with the executive team and clinical staff, reviews survey data, provides feedback, and meets with patients and families. Additionally, the patient experience coordinator observes the interactions between staff members, patients, and their families to determine if the patient is receiving necessary physical and emotional support.

**88. D:** The HIPAA Security Rule states that access controls to electronic health information must include encryption/decryption as well as a unique identifier, a procedure to access the system in emergencies, and automatic logoff. Any electronic health information must be secure and protected against threats, hazards, or nonpermitted disclosures. Security requirements include limiting access to authorized personnel, use of unique identifiers for each user, automatic logoff, encryption and decryption of PHI, authentication that healthcare data have not been altered/destroyed, the monitoring of logins, authentication, and security of transmissions.

**89. C:** Under the Medicare Inpatient Prospective Payment System for acute hospitals, if an HAC is present at discharge and the POA indicator on the claim is U, this means that Medicare will not pay for the condition if the HAC is present and documentation is not adequate to determine if the condition was POA. Other POA indicators:

- Y: Medicare pays for the condition if the HAC was present and accounted for on admission.
- N: Medicare will not pay for the condition if the HAC is present on discharge but not on admission.
- W: Medicare will pay for the condition if the HAC is present and the healthcare provider cannot determine if the condition was POA.

**90. A:** An ABN is provided for noncovered services to patients with original Medicare in addition to patients with Medicare fee-for-service. Patients must indicate whether they choose to have or forego the noncovered service and sign the document. Patients with Medicare managed care or private fee-for-service reimbursement do not receive the ABN. Medicare does not require that patients with Medicare Advantage plans receive an ABN, but one may be provided voluntarily for information only, although the patient should not sign the document or indicate a choice.

**91. C:** If a covered entity has a breach of unsecured PHI for fewer than 500 patients, the secretary of HHS need be notified only on an annual basis but no later than 60 days after the end of the calendar year in which the breaches occurred. If, however, the breach occurred for 500 or more patients, then the secretary should be notified of the breach as soon as possible and no later than 60 days after the breach occurred.

**92. D:** Secure messaging is an appropriate form of communication to use for telehealth because it is HIPAA compliant. Communication forms that can be hacked, including SMS text messaging, Skype, and email, should not be used, although during the COVID-19 pandemic, some of the rules regarding HIPAA compliance were relaxed. Secure messaging limits and provides a secure channel for communication. Secure messaging does not require special software or hardware. Users log in to a secure messaging service.

**93. A:** A right-to-work law means that no employee is forced to join a union or pay union dues as a requirement of employment. Thus, if some employees are unionized and others opt out, those who opt out still benefit from collective bargaining carried out by the union but do not contribute. Right-to-work laws prohibit "closed shops," businesses that hire only union members. State right-to-work laws may vary somewhat from one state to another.

**94. B:** According to CMS regarding emergency preparedness, each organization must create an emergency plan and conduct an all-hazards risk assessment. Hazards include epidemic/pandemic, biological, chemical, nuclear/radiological, explosive-incendiary, natural incidents, emerging infectious diseases, and cybersecurity incidents. The emergency plan should be adequate to respond to any of these types of emergency situations. The plan should focus on the capacities and capabilities of the healthcare organization. Plans should be specific to the area, considering the potential hazards.

**95. A:** Besides the ethical principle of autonomy, the other principle that applies to this situation is nonmaleficence, which means that one should not intentionally cause harm to a patient. In this case, dialysis may only prolong the person's suffering (causing harm) but not ultimately alter the outcome because the patient is dying.

**96. A:** The just response to a nurse misreading an order and giving the wrong dosage of a medication would be to identify the cause and console the nurse. Types of errors addressed by a just culture include the following:

- Human error: Inadvertent actions, mistakes, or lapses in proper procedure. Management includes considering processes, procedures, training, and/or design to determine the cause of the error and consoling the person.
- At-risk behavior: Unjustified risk, choice. Management includes providing incentives for correct behavior and disincentives for incorrect behavior and coaching the person.
- Reckless behavior: Conscious disregard for proper procedures. Management includes remedial action and/or punitive action.

**97. C:** If employee union organizers want to ask fellow employees to sign authorization cards to show support of the union, they must do so only during off-duty hours, but they may do so on company premises. If outside organizers are used, they may solicit on company premises only if the organization does not have a no-solicitation policy that is consistently enforced. Management may not interfere with union organizing efforts but can address employees on the premises regarding unionization.

**98. C:** If nurses are assigned to work four 12-hour shifts weekly for a total of 48 hours, they must be paid regular wages for the first 40 hours and overtime pay for 8 hours each week because overtime pay is required for hours greater than 40 a week. Overtime is paid at the rate of 1.5 times the regular hourly wage. State laws may vary somewhat. California, for example, requires 2 times the regular hourly wage for any hours more than 12 in a single shift.

**99. D:** When considering cost allocation, direct and indirect costs must be considered. Direct costs are directly incurred in the production of a product or performance of a service. They include labor costs, such as nursing staff costs, and costs of needed supplies. Indirect costs are costs not incurred in the performance of a service or the production of a product, such as the costs of custodial services, human resources, utilities, and administration. A percentage of the indirect cost is allocated, based upon the utilization. For example, if team leaders represent 5% of total employees, then 5% of indirect employee costs would be allocated to this line item.

**100. C:** Values clarification is an important consideration in ethical decision-making because the aim is to determine if decision-making is impacted by personal values or the values of others and whether a conflict exists. Values reflect a person's basic beliefs about what is important or has meaning. For example, individuals may differ widely in beliefs about the beginning of life and the sanctity of life. Individuals may carry both unconscious and conscious bias toward others based on other individuals' lifestyle choices, ethnicity, or religion.

**101. B:** The primary advantage of participating in a GPO is reducing costs. GPOs aggregate purchase orders in order to buy in large volumes that are lower in cost with savings to healthcare organizations usually ranging from 10% to 15%. GPOs do not directly purchase materials but negotiate the contracts under which the healthcare organizations purchase. Contracting with a GPO also reduces the number of staff and amount of time needed for purchasing, resulting in further cost savings.

**102. D:** CMS establishes core measures, which are national standards of treatment and care. For example, there are standards for the treatment **of** heart failure and acute myocardial infarction. The core measure Delivery and Newborn Care, Baby Electively Delivered Early is based on recommendations of the ACOG and AAP that elective deliveries should not be carried out prior to 39 weeks gestation because of increased risk to the neonate.

**103. B:** A pro forma is a financial statement that outlines projected expenses/revenues associated with a new program and is usually presented in a spreadsheet that covers projections for at least the first year. It should include net revenues (minus debts and discounts), expenses (all types), direct expenses (salary/nonsalary), indirect expenses (overhead), the contribution margin (the net revenue minus direct expenses), and the total cost margin (the contribution margin minus indirect expenses).

**104. B:** To effectively measure current performance, it's necessary to first establish benchmarks. A baseline may be established by measuring where an organization is at a point in time or a period of time, such as the number of readmissions averaged each month in the previous year. State or national data may also be used to establish benchmarks. Insurance companies may also provide data. A healthcare organization may also use local data, such as from similar hospitals in the same area, to set benchmarks.

**105. A:** Gantt charts are used to manage schedules and estimate times needed to complete tasks when developing improvement projects. It is a bar chart with a vertical list of tasks and a horizontal time scale that presents a visual representation of the beginning and end point of time when different steps in a process should be finished. The Gantt chart is typically created after brainstorming and creating a timeline and action plans.

**106. C:** According to the Patient's and Resident's Bill of Rights, patients and residents of healthcare facilities have the right to expect protection of confidentiality and privacy. Additionally, rights include respect, response to needs, ability to make informed decisions, clear procedures for registering complaints, freedom from abuse/neglect, protection during research, appraisal of outcomes, information about all aspects of the organization, appeal procedures, code of ethical behavior, and procedures for donating and procuring organs/tissues.

**107. D:** According to the Safe Medical Practices Act, manufacturers and medical device user facilities must report problems (e.g., death, serious injuries) with medical devices to MedWatch within 10 working days. User facilities must maintain records for 2 years and must develop written procedures for the identification, evaluation, and submission of medical device reports. MedWatch provides:

- Reporting forms (downloadable) for voluntary and mandatory reports
- Recalls and safety information about recalls, market withdrawals, and safety alerts, organized by month and year

**108. B:** The Ishikawa fishbone diagram is a tool used to determine cause and effect. The fish head is labeled with the problem (effect), and the bones are labeled with categories (causes), which are identified through brainstorming.

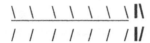

Traditional codes used for the categories include:

- M: Methods, materials, manpower, machines, measurement, and Mother Nature (environment)
- P: People, prices, promotion, places, policies, procedures, and product
- S: Surroundings, suppliers, systems, and skills

**109. B.** Electronic clinical quality measures (eCQM) are extracted electronically from certified electronic health records technology (CEHRT), including EHRs and HIT systems, and may be transmitted either manually or electronically. The data is captured in order to provide information about healthcare quality. In addition, CMS utilizes the data in incentive programs. CMS provides guidelines regarding eCQMs, including implementation guidelines, reporting, standards, references, and technical specifications.

**110. B:** When developing a staffing schedule for a unit, the percentage of occupancy is likely the most useful. To calculate the percentage of occupancy, the daily patient census is divided by the number of beds on a unit. For example, if there are 30 beds on a unit and the daily census is 28, then 28/30 equals 93% occupancy. The percentage of occupancy can be calculated for a period of time (such as a week or month) by using the average patient census.

**111. C:** When carrying out performance appraisal using a rating scale (0 to 5), the nurse executive should be aware of the risk of the halo effect, which means that favored staff are rated higher than unfavored staff. This is often done unconsciously because people tend to view those that they like as being more competent and efficient. Rating scales are easy to devise, but they lack specificity because they tend to focus on generalizations, such as "Is reliable" or "Works well with other staff."

**112. D:** If increased numbers of nursing staff report burnout (a state of mental and physical exhaustion exacerbated by stress), this usually reflects systemic problems. Burnout is often a result of an unhealthy working environment in which staffing is inadequate and nurses don't feel that their voices and concerns are heard or appreciated. Nurses may feel too much pressure to perform while lacking the time or energy to do so. Increased levels of burnout usually result in increased turnover.

**113. B:** A high-reliability organization is one that operates under constant challenges but manages to function well. Standardized care practices are used as part of a culture of safety. Characteristics of a high-reliability organization include:

- Preoccupation with failure (taking steps to avoid).
- Resistance to simplifying (because the work is complex).
- Sensitivity to operations (understanding different systems).
- Commitment to resilience (understanding challenges and failures).
- Deference to expertise (experts, evidence-based practice).

**114. A:** For error prevention training, a technique that is especially valuable for a nurse wanting to review a procedure that has not been performed recently is STAR (stop, think, act, and review). SBAR (situation, background, assessment, and recommendation) is used for handoff. ARCC (ask a question, request a change, voice a concern, and invoke the chain of command) provides steps to voice concerns about patient safety and move up the chain of command as needed. Stop and resolve provides a chance to reassess a situation before proceeding.

**115. D:** The Magnet model is a framework to improve the quality of nursing by providing excellence and serves as a guide to achieving Magnet recognition. The five components of the Magnet model are:

- Transformational leadership
- Structural empowerment
- Exemplary professional practice
- New knowledge, innovation, improvements
- Empirical-quality results

**116. C:** Appreciative inquiry refers to looking for the best in people and organizations and determining what forces result in an organization's effectiveness. Core characteristics include (1) constructionist (beliefs affect actions), (2) simultaneity (change begins with questioning), (3) poetic (the past, present, and future all provide opportunities for learning), (4) anticipatory (future expectations affect behavior), (5) positive (positive questions lead to positive changes). The model used to guide appreciative inquiry includes five Ds: define, discover, dream, design, and destiny.

**117. B:** The major elements of organizational culture are:

- Values: These are core ethics/principles that guide an organization.
- Vision: This is an organization's outlook for the future, including long- and short-term goals.
- Assumptions and beliefs: These include basic underlying assumptions and beliefs that influence behavior and outlook for change. Assumptions and beliefs may be conscious or unconscious.

**118. D:** An individual who has a particular passion or interest in performance improvement and has formed a team to promote performance improvement may be best classified as a champion. A champion is especially effective in combatting resistance, which is the common response to change. This process champion (also called a sponsor) is often a member of upper management with the authority to make decisions, but champions may exist at all levels within an organization.

**119. A:** The Hospital Inpatient Quality Reporting program started in 2003 to allow CMS to reward or penalize healthcare providers based on quality measures and data provided for the public to make comparisons. Hospitals that are unable to meet CMS's list of requirements (which are updated annually) face a 25% reduction in Medicare reimbursement. Mandatory annual requirements include four electronic clinical quality measures (eCQM).

**120. A:** When hiring travel workers, such as RNs and therapists, it's important to remember that they are employed by the agency and not the healthcare organization, so their salary is paid to the agency that then pays the employee. Costs are usually higher than when hiring locally. Typically, a traveling nurse works under contract for a limited period of time, such as 4 to 12 weeks, although some assignments may last up to 2 years. Nurses may have to relicense if moving to another state unless it is part of the Nurse Licensure Compact. Most agencies require 1 to 2 years of nursing experience for hire as an RN.

**121. C:** In order to calculate FTEs for the entire nursing staff for tax credits, the nurse executive totals all of the employee hours and divides by 2,080 (which is equal to 40 hours weekly times 52 weeks), excluding seasonal workers who work <120 days during the year (although this usually does not apply to healthcare). No more than 2,080 hours may be counted for any one employee, so hours exceeding this limit are eliminated. Decimal numbers are rounded down, not up, to the whole number. Full time at 36 hours per week is counted as 0.9 FTE.

**122. D:** Phase one of the strategic planning process is the assessment of external and internal environments. The external assessment looks at the sociopolitical, technological, demographic, and cultural aspects of the community and assesses competitors and their likely response to a strategic plan. The internal assessment looks at the organizational culture and the relationships among the different departments. Phase two reviews the mission statement including goals and objectives, phase three involves the identification of strategies, phase four is implementation, and phase five is evaluation.

**123. C:** If a hospital is located in a socioeconomically depressed area in which major employers have closed plants and left, the population has decreased, and three elementary schools have closed, the proposed program that is likely to be most used is the cardiovascular/stroke rehabilitation program. These facts about changes in the area all point to a change in demographics with younger families leaving the area in search of work. The remaining population is likely to skew toward older adults, who tend to have chronic illnesses and may benefit from cardiovascular/stroke rehabilitation.

**124. B:** When considering nursing hours per patient day, approximately 80% of a staff member's total hours are typically considered productive hours. So, if an FTE nurse is paid for 2,080 hours over the course of a year, but 20% is nonproductive (e.g., sick time, vacation time, and holiday time), the nurse is unavailable for 416 hours of those hours: 2080 – 416 = 1,664 hours.

**125. B:** Billing twice for procedures that were actually only done once is fraud. CMS considers fraud to include the theft of medical identity, billing for unauthorized or unnecessary materials or services, billing for materials or services not actually provided, upcoding, unbundling, and kickbacks. Abuse is conduct that is below acceptable standards and results in fraudulent reimbursement, such as for medically unnecessary services.

**126. A:** Conversations between a physician and other healthcare providers about a patient are considered protected information under the HIPAA Privacy Rule. HIPAA mandates privacy and security rules (CFR, Title 45, part 164) to ensure that health information and individual privacy are protected:

- Privacy Rule: Protected information includes any information included in the medical record (electronic or paper), conversations between the doctor and other healthcare providers, billing information, and any other form of health information.
- Security rule: Any electronic health information must be secure and protected against threats, hazards, or nonpermitted disclosures.

**127. D:** Objectives should be written clearly and should be easy to understand. SMART objectives are:

- **S**pecific: Outlines the expected result and target date
- **M**easurable: can be quantified
- **A**greed on: Based on mutual agreement/consensus
- **R**ealistic: Possible to achieve
- **T**ime bound: Includes a time frame

**128. C:** The AHRQ recommends warm handoff (i.e., bedside reporting) as a means to increase patient engagement. Warm handoff refers to transitions between caregivers (such as at a change of shift) conducted in front of the patient—as well as the patient's family, if the patient agrees—so that the patient hears the report and is free to ask any questions or to comment. Warm handoff is a patient-centered approach that includes the patient as an active member of the team. Warm handoffs can also be used for other transitions, such as when a lab technician comes to obtain blood samples.

**129. B:** A characteristic that may be counterproductive for a good team player is being competitive. The goal is to work together rather than to win, and power struggles with other team members can lead to a dysfunctional team, which often gets little accomplished. According to Maxwell (2002), positive characteristics of team players include being adaptable, collaborative, committed, communicative, competent, dependable, disciplined, enlarging, enthusiastic, intentional, mission conscious, prepared, relational, self-improving, selfless, solution oriented, and tenacious.

**130. C:** Confidentiality is essential to the success of an EAP to help with personal or family problems. Participants must be told in advance of any issues that must be disclosed, such as diversion of drugs. EAPs may provide counseling, referrals, wellness programs, support groups, financial advisors, and legal assistance. EAPs may be offered on-site or off-site. In some cases, all services are free, but in others, some fees may apply.

**131. A:** If the nurse executive has established an employee suggestion program but has little participation, recognition and rewards for suggestions are most likely to encourage participation. Employees like to feel appreciated and listened to, and being able to make suggestions may increase their job satisfaction. An employee suggestion program should not be confused with an employee complaint program (which requires confidentiality and serves a different purpose).

**132. D:** Although all of these approaches to resolving conflicts among team members have value, using a problem-solving approach is likely to be the most successful. Researching can be time-consuming and may delay resolution. Bargaining is only successful if conflict applies to two equally positive choices. Voting may devolve into a popularity contest rather than a true assessment. Problem solving means to discuss both sides of an issue and to consider the pros and cons of each.

**133. D:** HIPAA regulations include the requirement that records of HIPAA training must be retained for all staff for a period of at least 6 years. Support staff should be included in training because, even though they are not directly involved in patient care, they may inadvertently encounter PHI. For example, a member of the housekeeping staff may recognize a famous patient and share this information with family and friends, which constitutes a HIPAA violation.

**134. D:** According to NIOSH's hierarchy of control for exposure to workplace hazards, personal protective equipment is the least effective and often indicates the inability to carry out effective controls at a higher level. Eliminating hazards is the most effective, followed by substituting a different piece of equipment or substance. Engineering controls include the use of shields, barriers, guardrails, soundproofing, air-conditioning, and equipment guards. Administrative controls include signage, training, adjusted work schedules, and rest periods.

**135. B:** An employee absenteeism program should include:

- Attendance policy: Expectations regarding attendance and being on time should be outlined as well as the organization's definition of excessive absenteeism and tardiness and any disciplinary actions.
- Performance review: Attendance should be considered as part of performance, and workers should receive positive reinforcement for good attendance and adhering to the attendance policy.
- Wellness program: Focusing on improving health habits through smoking cessation, substance abuse treatment, emotional support, exercise, and diet may reduce absenteeism.
- Flexible work schedule: Allowing workers to work from home or to have flexible work hours may reduce absenteeism.

**136. A:** When an employee is returning to work with work restrictions due to an on-the-job injury, the first step is to assess the job to determine if the employee can carry out the job functions with or without accommodations. Employees with work restrictions should be carefully monitored to determine that they are, in fact, able to carry out the job functions without pain and undue effort and that any accommodations provided are adequate.

**137. D:** External benchmark data are especially valuable for compliance efforts to ensure that the healthcare organization is meeting industry standards. Benchmark data are available from many sources including internal data, state boards of health, CMS, the CMS Hospital Compare website, professional organizations (such as the Society for Thoracic Surgeons), the Institute for Healthcare Improvement, and accreditation agencies (such as The Joint Commission). Benchmarking data should be made widely available within an organization, such as on an organizational dashboard.

**138. C:** The nurse executive promotes the use of the CRAF method of recording minutes of meetings for consistency:

- **C**onclusions of the group discussion: Includes any decisions made regarding future actions.
- **R**ecommendations made by the group: Plan for decisions.
- **A**ctions that the group or individual members decided to take: List of tasks.
- **F**ollow-up activities: Determine if the actions are completed, assess.

**139. B:** If a patient with Alzheimer's disease has run out of insurance benefits and is being discharged from a skilled nursing facility because the patient does not qualify for Medicaid and cannot afford to pay for care, the ethical principle that is threatened is justice, which implies that all patients will be treated fairly and have equal access to needed care. Unfortunately, this is often not the case because those with better insurance or greater income typically have greater access to care.

**140. A:** When developing a website to promote the hospital and nursing department, layout considerations include avoiding red and green because some people are colorblind to these colors. Simple designs are more effective than complex ones, and unnecessary lines, such as borders around text and photos, should be avoided. Images and texts should be arranged so that the eyes move in a continuous line (usually top to bottom) rather than skipping around a page.

**141. B:** The National Quality Forum outlines the four elements needed to create and sustain a patient safety culture:

- Leadership must ensure that structures are in place for organization-wide awareness and compliance with safety measures, including adequate resources and direct accountability.
- Measurement, analysis, and feedback must track safety and allow for interventions.
- Team-based patient care with adequate training and performance improvement activities must be organization-wide.
- Safety risks must be continuously identified, and interventions must be taken to reduce patient risk.

**142. D:** HIPAA includes the Workforce Security standard and required implementations:

- Workforce clearance: determining whether an individual's access to electronic PHI is appropriate
- Authorization/Supervision: supervising individuals who have access to electronic PHI
- Termination procedures: terminating access to electronic PHI when individuals are no longer employed

**143. A:** When conducting research, the type of study that provides the best evidence is the systematic review of randomized trials. The hierarchy (weakest to best) for evidence sources is:

1. Unsystematic clinical observations
2. Physiologic studies (e.g., bone density, vital signs, and weights)
3. Single observational study (addressing important outcomes)
4. Systematic review of observational studies (addressing important outcomes)
5. Randomized trial
6. Systematic review of randomized trials

**144. B:** The primary cause of nursing turnover in hospitals is job dissatisfaction. Turnover rates vary from 7% to approximately 40% depending on the area and the circumstances of the individual hospitals. Understaffing and overwork are common causes of turnover as well as a lack of opportunity for advancement and a lack of power. The aging of the nursing workforce also has an impact on turnover with the average age of nurses now approximately 51, meaning that over the next decade many more nurses will likely be leaving the profession.

**145. C:** If members of the nursing staff work a fluctuating workweek at a fixed salary that doesn't vary, the overtime rate that the staff members must receive for each overtime hour greater than 40 hours per week is at least 1.5 times their base rate. In order to use the fluctuating workweek method to determine overtime, five criteria must be met: (1) work hours fluctuate from week to week, (2) the employee earns a fixed salary, (3) the hourly wage is above the federal minimum, (4) there is a "clear and mutual" understanding between the employee and employer, and (5) overtime pay is at least 1.5 times the regular hourly rate.

**146. A:** While all of these are important for a peer mentoring program, evidence-based metrics are especially important. Part of planning should include how to assess effectiveness and to modify the program to better meet needs. If the program does not meet the needs of the patients who are enrolled, then it will ultimately fail. Additionally, a program is more likely to be funded or to receive grants if there is evidence to show that the program results in positive outcomes.

**147. C:** The most appropriate example of assertive communication is "I can see that you are upset, but I need you to stop shouting so we can find a solution." The speaker is showing empathy ("I can see that you are upset") while still making a direct request regarding the action that the person needs to take ("I need you to stop shouting") and providing a rationale for that action ("so we can find a solution"). It's important to maintain a neutral tone of voice and facial expression and to avoid responding in kind to aggressive comments.

**148. B:** According to the ADKAR (Hiatt) method for facilitating change, during the first step (awareness), the role of the leader is to communicate the need for change. The steps of the ADKAR method are as follows:

1. **A**wareness: Leaders must communicate the need for change.
2. **D**esire: Individuals must overcome resistance and fear of change.
3. **K**nowledge: Individuals must receive education and hands-on training in order to understand the processes of change.
4. **A**bility: Individuals gain the skills necessary to effectively implement change.
5. **R**einforcement: Feedback, corrections, and recognition help to maintain change.

**149. B:** With servant leadership, the focus is on collaboration and participation at all levels. The leader's first priority is to be a servant in the sense of serving others and considering the needs of the organization and the individuals within it to determine how best to meet these needs and encourage growth and well-being. Servant leaders provide support and encouragement to workers and exhibit skills in listening, empathy, and persuasion. The servant leader helps to develop skills in others and shares decision making.

**150. C:** FEMA has outlined the four phases of emergency management:

- Mitigation: preventive actions (levees, fire insurance) or activities that reduce damages
- Preparedness: plans, rescue operations, stockpiling
- Response: actions during an emergency, such as turning off gas or seeking shelter
- Recovery: actions following an emergency, such as recovery activities, financial support, or shelters

# Nurse Executive Practice Test #3

To take this additional Nurse Executive practice test, visit our bonus page:
**mometrix.com/bonus948/nurseexec**

# How to Overcome Test Anxiety

Just the thought of taking a test is enough to make most people a little nervous. A test is an important event that can have a long-term impact on your future, so it's important to take it seriously and it's natural to feel anxious about performing well. But just because anxiety is normal, that doesn't mean that it's helpful in test taking, or that you should simply accept it as part of your life. Anxiety can have a variety of effects. These effects can be mild, like making you feel slightly nervous, or severe, like blocking your ability to focus or remember even a simple detail.

If you experience test anxiety—whether severe or mild—it's important to know how to beat it. To discover this, first you need to understand what causes test anxiety.

## Causes of Test Anxiety

While we often think of anxiety as an uncontrollable emotional state, it can actually be caused by simple, practical things. One of the most common causes of test anxiety is that a person does not feel adequately prepared for their test. This feeling can be the result of many different issues such as poor study habits or lack of organization, but the most common culprit is time management. Starting to study too late, failing to organize your study time to cover all of the material, or being distracted while you study will mean that you're not well prepared for the test. This may lead to cramming the night before, which will cause you to be physically and mentally exhausted for the test. Poor time management also contributes to feelings of stress, fear, and hopelessness as you realize you are not well prepared but don't know what to do about it.

Other times, test anxiety is not related to your preparation for the test but comes from unresolved fear. This may be a past failure on a test, or poor performance on tests in general. It may come from comparing yourself to others who seem to be performing better or from the stress of living up to expectations. Anxiety may be driven by fears of the future—how failure on this test would affect your educational and career goals. These fears are often completely irrational, but they can still negatively impact your test performance.

## Elements of Test Anxiety

As mentioned earlier, test anxiety is considered to be an emotional state, but it has physical and mental components as well. Sometimes you may not even realize that you are suffering from test anxiety until you notice the physical symptoms. These can include trembling hands, rapid heartbeat, sweating, nausea, and tense muscles. Extreme anxiety may lead to fainting or vomiting. Obviously, any of these symptoms can have a negative impact on testing. It is important to recognize them as soon as they begin to occur so that you can address the problem before it damages your performance.

The mental components of test anxiety include trouble focusing and inability to remember learned information. During a test, your mind is on high alert, which can help you recall information and stay focused for an extended period of time. However, anxiety interferes with your mind's natural processes, causing you to blank out, even on the questions you know well. The strain of testing during anxiety makes it difficult to stay focused, especially on a test that may take several hours. Extreme anxiety can take a huge mental toll, making it difficult not only to recall test information but even to understand the test questions or pull your thoughts together.

# Effects of Test Anxiety

Test anxiety is like a disease—if left untreated, it will get progressively worse. Anxiety leads to poor performance, and this reinforces the feelings of fear and failure, which in turn lead to poor performances on subsequent tests. It can grow from a mild nervousness to a crippling condition. If allowed to progress, test anxiety can have a big impact on your schooling, and consequently on your future.

Test anxiety can spread to other parts of your life. Anxiety on tests can become anxiety in any stressful situation, and blanking on a test can turn into panicking in a job situation. But fortunately, you don't have to let anxiety rule your testing and determine your grades. There are a number of relatively simple steps you can take to move past anxiety and function normally on a test and in the rest of life.

# Physical Steps for Beating Test Anxiety

While test anxiety is a serious problem, the good news is that it can be overcome. It doesn't have to control your ability to think and remember information. While it may take time, you can begin taking steps today to beat anxiety.

Just as your first hint that you may be struggling with anxiety comes from the physical symptoms, the first step to treating it is also physical. Rest is crucial for having a clear, strong mind. If you are tired, it is much easier to give in to anxiety. But if you establish good sleep habits, your body and mind will be ready to perform optimally, without the strain of exhaustion. Additionally, sleeping well helps you to retain information better, so you're more likely to recall the answers when you see the test questions.

Getting good sleep means more than going to bed on time. It's important to allow your brain time to relax. Take study breaks from time to time so it doesn't get overworked, and don't study right before bed. Take time to rest your mind before trying to rest your body, or you may find it difficult to fall asleep.

Along with sleep, other aspects of physical health are important in preparing for a test. Good nutrition is vital for good brain function. Sugary foods and drinks may give a burst of energy but this burst is followed by a crash, both physically and emotionally. Instead, fuel your body with protein and vitamin-rich foods.

Also, drink plenty of water. Dehydration can lead to headaches and exhaustion, especially if your brain is already under stress from the rigors of the test. Particularly if your test is a long one, drink water during the breaks. And if possible, take an energy-boosting snack to eat between sections.

Along with sleep and diet, a third important part of physical health is exercise. Maintaining a steady workout schedule is helpful, but even taking 5-minute study breaks to walk can help get your blood pumping faster and clear your head. Exercise also releases endorphins, which contribute to a positive feeling and can help combat test anxiety.

When you nurture your physical health, you are also contributing to your mental health. If your body is healthy, your mind is much more likely to be healthy as well. So take time to rest, nourish your body with healthy food and water, and get moving as much as possible. Taking these physical steps will make you stronger and more able to take the mental steps necessary to overcome test anxiety.

# Mental Steps for Beating Test Anxiety

Working on the mental side of test anxiety can be more challenging, but as with the physical side, there are clear steps you can take to overcome it. As mentioned earlier, test anxiety often stems from lack of preparation, so the obvious solution is to prepare for the test. Effective studying may be the most important weapon you have for beating test anxiety, but you can and should employ several other mental tools to combat fear.

First, boost your confidence by reminding yourself of past success—tests or projects that you aced. If you're putting as much effort into preparing for this test as you did for those, there's no reason you should expect to fail here. Work hard to prepare; then trust your preparation.

Second, surround yourself with encouraging people. It can be helpful to find a study group, but be sure that the people you're around will encourage a positive attitude. If you spend time with others who are anxious or cynical, this will only contribute to your own anxiety. Look for others who are motivated to study hard from a desire to succeed, not from a fear of failure.

Third, reward yourself. A test is physically and mentally tiring, even without anxiety, and it can be helpful to have something to look forward to. Plan an activity following the test, regardless of the outcome, such as going to a movie or getting ice cream.

When you are taking the test, if you find yourself beginning to feel anxious, remind yourself that you know the material. Visualize successfully completing the test. Then take a few deep, relaxing breaths and return to it. Work through the questions carefully but with confidence, knowing that you are capable of succeeding.

Developing a healthy mental approach to test taking will also aid in other areas of life. Test anxiety affects more than just the actual test—it can be damaging to your mental health and even contribute to depression. It's important to beat test anxiety before it becomes a problem for more than testing.

# Study Strategy

Being prepared for the test is necessary to combat anxiety, but what does being prepared look like? You may study for hours on end and still not feel prepared. What you need is a strategy for test prep. The next few pages outline our recommended steps to help you plan out and conquer the challenge of preparation.

### STEP 1: SCOPE OUT THE TEST

Learn everything you can about the format (multiple choice, essay, etc.) and what will be on the test. Gather any study materials, course outlines, or sample exams that may be available. Not only will this help you to prepare, but knowing what to expect can help to alleviate test anxiety.

### STEP 2: MAP OUT THE MATERIAL

Look through the textbook or study guide and make note of how many chapters or sections it has. Then divide these over the time you have. For example, if a book has 15 chapters and you have five days to study, you need to cover three chapters each day. Even better, if you have the time, leave an extra day at the end for overall review after you have gone through the material in depth.

If time is limited, you may need to prioritize the material. Look through it and make note of which sections you think you already have a good grasp on, and which need review. While you are studying, skim quickly through the familiar sections and take more time on the challenging parts.

Write out your plan so you don't get lost as you go. Having a written plan also helps you feel more in control of the study, so anxiety is less likely to arise from feeling overwhelmed at the amount to cover.

## STEP 3: GATHER YOUR TOOLS

Decide what study method works best for you. Do you prefer to highlight in the book as you study and then go back over the highlighted portions? Or do you type out notes of the important information? Or is it helpful to make flashcards that you can carry with you? Assemble the pens, index cards, highlighters, post-it notes, and any other materials you may need so you won't be distracted by getting up to find things while you study.

If you're having a hard time retaining the information or organizing your notes, experiment with different methods. For example, try color-coding by subject with colored pens, highlighters, or post-it notes. If you learn better by hearing, try recording yourself reading your notes so you can listen while in the car, working out, or simply sitting at your desk. Ask a friend to quiz you from your flashcards, or try teaching someone the material to solidify it in your mind.

## STEP 4: CREATE YOUR ENVIRONMENT

It's important to avoid distractions while you study. This includes both the obvious distractions like visitors and the subtle distractions like an uncomfortable chair (or a too-comfortable couch that makes you want to fall asleep). Set up the best study environment possible: good lighting and a comfortable work area. If background music helps you focus, you may want to turn it on, but otherwise keep the room quiet. If you are using a computer to take notes, be sure you don't have any other windows open, especially applications like social media, games, or anything else that could distract you. Silence your phone and turn off notifications. Be sure to keep water close by so you stay hydrated while you study (but avoid unhealthy drinks and snacks).

Also, take into account the best time of day to study. Are you freshest first thing in the morning? Try to set aside some time then to work through the material. Is your mind clearer in the afternoon or evening? Schedule your study session then. Another method is to study at the same time of day that you will take the test, so that your brain gets used to working on the material at that time and will be ready to focus at test time.

## STEP 5: STUDY!

Once you have done all the study preparation, it's time to settle into the actual studying. Sit down, take a few moments to settle your mind so you can focus, and begin to follow your study plan. Don't give in to distractions or let yourself procrastinate. This is your time to prepare so you'll be ready to fearlessly approach the test. Make the most of the time and stay focused.

Of course, you don't want to burn out. If you study too long you may find that you're not retaining the information very well. Take regular study breaks. For example, taking five minutes out of every hour to walk briskly, breathing deeply and swinging your arms, can help your mind stay fresh.

As you get to the end of each chapter or section, it's a good idea to do a quick review. Remind yourself of what you learned and work on any difficult parts. When you feel that you've mastered the material, move on to the next part. At the end of your study session, briefly skim through your notes again.

But while review is helpful, cramming last minute is NOT. If at all possible, work ahead so that you won't need to fit all your study into the last day. Cramming overloads your brain with more information than it can process and retain, and your tired mind may struggle to recall even previously learned information when it is overwhelmed with last-minute study. Also, the urgent nature of cramming and the stress placed on your brain contribute to anxiety. You'll be more likely to go to the test feeling unprepared and having trouble thinking clearly.

So don't cram, and don't stay up late before the test, even just to review your notes at a leisurely pace. Your brain needs rest more than it needs to go over the information again. In fact, plan to finish your studies by noon or early afternoon the day before the test. Give your brain the rest of the day to relax or focus on other things, and get a good night's sleep. Then you will be fresh for the test and better able to recall what you've studied.

## STEP 6: TAKE A PRACTICE TEST

Many courses offer sample tests, either online or in the study materials. This is an excellent resource to check whether you have mastered the material, as well as to prepare for the test format and environment.

Check the test format ahead of time: the number of questions, the type (multiple choice, free response, etc.), and the time limit. Then create a plan for working through them. For example, if you have 30 minutes to take a 60-question test, your limit is 30 seconds per question. Spend less time on the questions you know well so that you can take more time on the difficult ones.

If you have time to take several practice tests, take the first one open book, with no time limit. Work through the questions at your own pace and make sure you fully understand them. Gradually work up to taking a test under test conditions: sit at a desk with all study materials put away and set a timer. Pace yourself to make sure you finish the test with time to spare and go back to check your answers if you have time.

After each test, check your answers. On the questions you missed, be sure you understand why you missed them. Did you misread the question (tests can use tricky wording)? Did you forget the information? Or was it something you hadn't learned? Go back and study any shaky areas that the practice tests reveal.

Taking these tests not only helps with your grade, but also aids in combating test anxiety. If you're already used to the test conditions, you're less likely to worry about it, and working through tests until you're scoring well gives you a confidence boost. Go through the practice tests until you feel comfortable, and then you can go into the test knowing that you're ready for it.

# Test Tips

On test day, you should be confident, knowing that you've prepared well and are ready to answer the questions. But aside from preparation, there are several test day strategies you can employ to maximize your performance.

First, as stated before, get a good night's sleep the night before the test (and for several nights before that, if possible). Go into the test with a fresh, alert mind rather than staying up late to study.

Try not to change too much about your normal routine on the day of the test. It's important to eat a nutritious breakfast, but if you normally don't eat breakfast at all, consider eating just a protein bar. If you're a coffee drinker, go ahead and have your normal coffee. Just make sure you time it so that the caffeine doesn't wear off right in the middle of your test. Avoid sugary beverages, and drink enough water to stay hydrated but not so much that you need a restroom break 10 minutes into the test. If your test isn't first thing in the morning, consider going for a walk or doing a light workout before the test to get your blood flowing.

Allow yourself enough time to get ready, and leave for the test with plenty of time to spare so you won't have the anxiety of scrambling to arrive in time. Another reason to be early is to select a good seat. It's helpful to sit away from doors and windows, which can be distracting. Find a good seat, get out your supplies, and settle your mind before the test begins.

When the test begins, start by going over the instructions carefully, even if you already know what to expect. Make sure you avoid any careless mistakes by following the directions.

Then begin working through the questions, pacing yourself as you've practiced. If you're not sure on an answer, don't spend too much time on it, and don't let it shake your confidence. Either skip it and come back later, or eliminate as many wrong answers as possible and guess among the remaining ones. Don't dwell on these questions as you continue—put them out of your mind and focus on what lies ahead.

Be sure to read all of the answer choices, even if you're sure the first one is the right answer. Sometimes you'll find a better one if you keep reading. But don't second-guess yourself if you do immediately know the answer. Your gut instinct is usually right. Don't let test anxiety rob you of the information you know.

If you have time at the end of the test (and if the test format allows), go back and review your answers. Be cautious about changing any, since your first instinct tends to be correct, but make sure you didn't misread any of the questions or accidentally mark the wrong answer choice. Look over any you skipped and make an educated guess.

At the end, leave the test feeling confident. You've done your best, so don't waste time worrying about your performance or wishing you could change anything. Instead, celebrate the successful completion of this test. And finally, use this test to learn how to deal with anxiety even better next time.

> **Review Video: Test Anxiety**
> Visit mometrix.com/academy and enter code: 100340

## Important Qualification

Not all anxiety is created equal. If your test anxiety is causing major issues in your life beyond the classroom or testing center, or if you are experiencing troubling physical symptoms related to your anxiety, it may be a sign of a serious physiological or psychological condition. If this sounds like your situation, we strongly encourage you to seek professional help.

# Additional Bonus Material

Due to our efforts to try to keep this book to a manageable length, we've created a link that will give you access to all of your additional bonus material:

**mometrix.com/bonus948/nurseexec**